Essential Cardiac Electrophysiology

Dedication

To all the students of cardiac electrophysiology
and
To my mentors: Dr. Fred Morady, Dr. Mark Josephson,
Dr. Masood Akhtar, Dr. Warren Jackman, Dr. James Maloney,
Dr. Christopher Wyndham, Dr Eric Prystowsky, Dr George Klein and
Dr Kalyanam Shivkumar
and
To my wife Karuna whose patience and understanding made
this project possible.
and
To my children Moeen, Sakena and Zameer
and my grandchildren Neela and Sameer Yidroose

Essential Cardiac Electrophysiology

The Self-Assessment Approach

Second Edition

Zainul Abedin, MD, FRCP, FHRS

Professor of Clinical Medicine
Paul Foster School of Medicine
Texas Tech University Health Sciences Center;
Adjunct Professor of Electrical Engineering and Computer Science
University of Texas at El Paso
El Paso, TX, USA

WILEY-BLACKWELL

A John Wiley & Sons, Ltd., Publication

This edition first published 2013 © 2013 by Blackwell Publishing Ltd

Blackwell Publishing was acquired by John Wiley & Sons in February 2007. Blackwell's publishing program has been merged with Wiley's global Scientific, Technical and Medical business to form Wiley-Blackwell.

Registered Office
John Wiley & Sons, Ltd, The Atrium, Southern Gate, Chichester, West Sussex, PO19 8SQ, UK

Editorial Offices
9600 Garsington Road, Oxford, OX4 2DQ, UK
The Atrium, Southern Gate, Chichester, West Sussex, PO19 8SQ, UK
111 River Street, Hoboken, NJ 07030-5774, USA

For details of our global editorial offices, for customer services and for information about how to apply for permission to reuse the copyright material in this book please see our website at www.wiley.com/wiley-blackwell

Library of Congress Cataloging-in-Publication Data

Abedin, Zainul, MD.
Essential cardiac electrophysiology : the self-assessment approach / Zainul Abedin. – 2nd ed.
    p. ; cm.
    Includes bibliographical references and index.
    ISBN 978-1-4443-3590-3 (pbk. : alk. paper) – ISBN 978-1-118-52199-1 (obook) –
ISBN 978-1-118-52200-4 (emobi) – ISBN 978-1-118-52201-1 (epdf) –
ISBN 978-1-118-52202-8 (epub)
    I. Title.
[DNLM: 1. Arrhythmias, Cardiac–physiopathology–Handbooks. 2. Arrhythmias,
Cardiac–therapy–Handbooks. 3. Cardiac Electrophysiology–methods–Handbooks.
4. Electrophysiologic Techniques, Cardiac–Handbooks. WG 39]
    612.1'71–dc23
                                    2012043159
A catalogue record for this book is available from the British Library.

Wiley also publishes its books in a variety of electronic formats. Some content that appears in print may not be available in electronic books.

Cover image: courtesy of the author
Cover design by Andy Magee Design Ltd

Set in 9.5/12pt Meridien by SPi Publisher Services, Pondicherry, India
Printed and bound in Malaysia by Vivar Printing Sdn Bhd

1   2013

Contents

Foreword

The second edition of *Essentials of Cardiac Electrophysiology* continues in the same format as the first edition – a concise review in bullet-point fashion of the most important facts dealing with all major topics in clinical cardiac electrophysiology and with selected basic electrophysiology topics that are the most relevant to clinical electrophysiologists. The second edition has been enhanced both by expanding some of the topics previously covered and by the addition of some new topics. For example, additional information useful for those wishing to review cardiac membrane channels has been provided. A notable number of issues directly related to clinical practice have been expanded upon or added, including post-maze arrhythmias, the genetics of atrial fibrillation, new oral anticoagulants, left ventricular non-compaction, the use of magnetic resonance imaging in patients with a device, and management of high defibrillation thresholds.

All in all, this book remains a very useful resource for those seeking a concise review of the most important information on virtually any topic important to clinical cardiac electrophysiologists.

Fred Morady, MD
McKay Professor of Cardiovascular Disease
Professor of Medicine
University of Michigan Health System
Ann Arbor, MI, USA

Preface

I use this quotation with some trepidation because of its use in justifying the Iraq war. But I feel it also describes the state of knowledge in many scientific fields including cardiac electrophysiology.

There has been an exponential increase of information in all facets of cardiac electrophysiology. When the first edition of *Essential Cardiac Electrophysiology* was published there were seven known types of long QT syndromes; by the time this edition went into press the list had expanded to 12 different types of long QT syndromes.

The question is invariably raised as to why we need another book on cardiac electrophysiology when, with the availability of the world wide web and smart handheld devices, the information can be accessed anytime anywhere within a few seconds. The answer to this question lies in the ability of this text to assimilate, synthesize and present only factual and relevant information.

As Albert Einstein has eloquently said, *"Everything should be made as simple as possible, but not one bit simpler."*

Learning is best accomplished by testing, reiteration, and concentration on essential information, accomplished in this book by using a self-assessment approach, illustrations, tables and an enumeration of factual information in bullet format rather than by verbose description.

The first edition has been immensely popular among cardiac electrophysiology and cardiology fellows, residents, and medical students. Keeping the same format, this edition has been expanded by 50% with new information, multiple-choice questions and illustrations.

This has been a long and immensely time-consuming project. The rewards are not financial. These rewards are realized in the form of compliments from students and encouraging remarks from their mentors.

Any project of this magnitude is likely to have errors and or omissions. Any constructive criticism, comments, and suggestions are always welcomed.

Please send comments, critiques and suggestions to, 'essentialep@gmail.com'.

Zainul Abedin

Acknowledgements

I gratefully acknowledge the generous help of Professor Fred Morady, a true scholar and a superb teacher, in reviewing the manuscript and in providing many valuable suggestions.

I am grateful to Ms. Susan Fernandez for secretarial assistance; and to Mr. Thomas Hartman, Ms. Kate Newell, Ms. Cathryn Gates and Ms. Mahabunnisa Mohamed and other members of Wiley-Blackwell editorial, publishing and marketing team.

Abbreviations

4-AP	4-Aminopyridine
AAD	Antiarrhythmic drugs
AAG	Alpha1 acid glycoprotein
ABC	ATP binding cassette protein
Ach	Acetylcholine
Ado	Adenosine
AF	Atrial fibrillation
AIVR	Accelerated idioventricular rhythm
AJT	Automatic junctional tachycardia
AKAP	A kinase anchoring proteins
AP	Action potential
AP	Accessory pathway
APD	Action potential duration
ARP	Atrial refractory period
ARVD/C	Arrhythmogenic right ventricular dysplasia/cardiomyopathy
AT	Atrial tachycardia
AT-II	Angiotensin II
Atp	Adenosine triphosphate
ATP	Anti tachycardia pacing
ATS	Andersen–Tawil Syndrome
AVD	AV dissociation
AVN	Atrioventricular node
AVNRT	AVN re-entry tachycardia
AVRT	AV re-entrant tachycardia
BBB	Bundle branch block
BBRVT	Bundle branch re-entry VT
BRS	Baroreflex sensitivity
Ca	Calcium
CAD	Coronary artery disease
cAMP	Cyclic adenosine monophosphate
CANS	Cardiac autonomic nervous system
CHF	Congestive heart failure
CHB	Complete heart block
CICR	Calcium induced calcium release
CL	Cycle length
Cl$^-$	Chloride
CPVT	Catecholaminergic polymorphic ventricular tachycardia
CS	Coronary sinus
CSF	Cerebrospinal fluid
CSNRT	Corrected sinus node recovery time

CX	Connexion
CYP	Cytochrome P
DAD	Delayed after-depolarization
DCM	Dilated cardiomyopathy
DFT	Defibrillation threshold
EAD	Early after depolarization
EAM	Electroanatomical map
EF	Ejection fraction
EHL	Elimination half life
ER	Eustachian ridge
ERP	Effective refractory period
HB	His bundle
HCM	Hypertrophic cardiomyopathy
HCN	Hyperpolarization activated cyclic nucleotide gated
HERG	Human ether related a-go-go gene protein
HPS	His Purkinje system
HRV	Heart rate variability
HRT	Heart rate turbulence
$I_{Ca\,T}$	Ca current transient or short acting
I_{CaL}	Ca current long acting
ICE	Intracardiac echocardiography
ICD	Implantable cardioverter-defibrillator
I_f	Hyperpolarizing cation current
I_K	Potassium current
I_{K1}	Inward rectifying potassium current
I_{Kach}	Acetylcholine mediated potassium current
$I_{K,ATP}$	ATP dependent potassium current
I_{Kp}	Time independent background plateau current
I_{Kr}	Rapidly activating potassium current
I_{Ks}	Slowly activating potassium current
I_{Kur}	Ultra rapid potassium current
I_{Na}	Sodium current
IP3	Inositol triphosphate
IST	Inappropriate sinus tachycardia
I_{to}	Transient outward current
IVC	Inferior vena cava
K	Potassium
KvLQT1	Voltage-dependent potassium controlling protein
LAFB	Left anterior fascicular block
LCSD	Left cardiac sympathetic denervation
LIPV	Left inferior pulmonary vein
LOC	Loss of consciousness
LQTS	Long QT Syndrome
LSPV	Left superior pulmonary vein
LVH	Left ventricular hypertrophy
LVOT	Left ventricular outflow tract

M	Muscarinic
MHC	Myosin heavy chain
MDP	Maximum diastolic potential
MI	Myocardial infarction
MinK	Minimal potassium current controlling protein
$MnCl_2$	Manganese chloride
MTR	Maximum tracking rate
MVT	Monomorphic VT
Na	Sodium
NAPA	*N*-acetylprocainamide
NAT	*N*-acetyltransferase
NCX	Sodium and calcium exchange
NCC	Noncoronary cusp
NSVT	Nonsustained VT
P	Purinergic
PAC	Premature atrial contractions
PAVB	Paroxysmal AV block
PCA	Pulseless cardiac electrical activity
PCCD	Progressive cardiac conduction disease
PES	Programmed electrical stimulation
PG	P glycoprotein
PJRT	Permanent form of junctional reciprocating tachycardia
PKA	Protein kinase A
PPI	Post pacing interval
PVARP	Postventricular atrial refractory period
PVC	Premature ventricular contractions
QT_c	Corrected QT interval
RB	Right bundle
RCC	Right coronary cusp
RCM	Restrictive cardiomyopathy
RF	Radiofrequency
RNA	Ribonucleic acid
RSPV	Right superior pulmonary vein
RVOT	Right ventricular outflow tract
RyR2	Ryanodine receptor
SACT	Sino atrial conduction time
SAECG	Signal average ECG
SAN	Sinoatrial node
SCD	Sudden cardiac death
SCRC	Sarcoplasmic Ca release channel
SND	Sinus node dysfunction
SMVT	Sustained monomorphic VT
SNRT	Sinus node recovery time
SQTS	Short QT syndrome
SR	Sarcoplasmic reticulum
SSS	Sick sinus syndrome

SUR	Sulfonylurea receptor
SVC	Superior vena cava
SVT	Supraventricular tachycardia
TA	Tricuspid annulus
TCL	Tachycardia cycle length
TDP	Torsades de Pointes
TDR	Transmural dispersion of repolarization
TEE	Transesophageal echocardiography
TIA	Transient ischemic attack
TWA	T wave alternans
ULV	Upper limit of vulnerability
VA	Ventriculoatrial
VF	Ventricular fibrillation
VRP	Ventricular refractory period
VT	Ventricular tachycardia
WCT	Wide complex tachycardia
WPW	Wolff–Parkinson–White syndrome

CHAPTER 1

Ions channels and currents

Self-assessment questions

1.1 Potassium channels and currents

1 In normal Purkinje fibers which one of the following currents is responsible for normal automaticity?
   A I_f hyperpolarization-activated cyclic nucleotide gated current
   B I_{CaL} L-type calcium current
   C I_{Na} rapid inward sodium current
   D I_K delayed rectifier potassium current
   E I_{to} transient outward current

2 Abnormal potassium channel function is unlikely to cause
   A Deafness.
   B Short QT interval.
   C Long QT interval.
   D Catecholaminergic polymorphic ventricular tachycardia.

3 Osborn waves seen in hypothermia are the result of:
   A Uneven distribution of Ito in endocardium and epicardium.
   B Sarcoplasmic calcium overload.
   C Metabolic acidosis.
   D Loss of function of the sodium channel.

4 Which of the following is the result of outward movement of the potassium ions across the cell membrane?
   A Repolarizing current.
   B Depolarizing current.
   C Prolongation of the QT interval.
   D Prominent U waves.

Essential Cardiac Electrophysiology: The Self-Assessment Approach, Second Edition. Zainul Abedin.
© 2013 Blackwell Publishing Ltd. Published 2013 by Blackwell Publishing Ltd.

5 In a diagram of AP shown below, which one of the following currents is active where arrow is pointing?

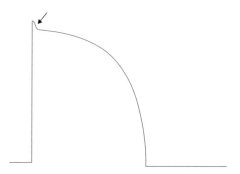

A I_{to}
B I_{K1}
C I_{Na}
D I_{Ca}

6 Which one of the following genes controls the expression of I_{Kr}?
  A *KCNQ1 (KvLQT1)*
  B *KCNH2 (HERG)*
  C *SCN5A*
  D *MinK*

7 Which one of the following actions is likely to activate I_{Katp} current?
  A Rise in intracellular ATP
  B Rise in intracellular calcium
  C Fall of Intracellular ATP
  D Fall of Intracellular calcium

8 How does congestive heart failure affect depolarizing/repolarizing currents?
  A Outward Repolarizing currents are reduced
  B Inward depolarizing currents are reduced
  C Outward repolarizing currents are increased
  D APD is decreased

9 Which one of the following is least likely to occur with prolongation of plateau phase of the AP?
  A Increased strength of contraction
  B Increase in conduction velocity
  C Increased duration of contraction
  D Increased refractoriness

10 Which one of the following is likely to increase the activity of I_{Kr}?
  A Increased extracellular potassium
  B Exposure to Sotalol

    C Decrease extracellular potassium
    D Increase in chloride current

11 When does the reverse use dependent block occur?
    A It occurs with repeated activation of channel
    B It occurs when sodium channel is blocked
    C It occurs at slow heart rate but not at fast heart rate
    D It occurs in the presence of catecholamines

12 Which one of the following is least likely attribute of I_{to}?
    A It is present in ventricular epicardium but not in endocardium
    B It is responsible for spike and dome characteristic
    C It is blocked by Ranolazine
    D It is also present in human atrium

13 Which one of the following is associated with Brugada syndrome?
    A Defect in *SCN5A* gene
    B Loss of I_{Kr}
    C ST segment depression is precordial leads
    D Deafness

14 Which one of the following agents/actions is likely to block I_{Ks}?
    A Aminophylline
    B Indapamide
    C Activation of protein kinase C
    D Erythromycin
    E Increase in intracellular calcium

1.2 Sodium channels and currents

1 Chronic exposure to Na channel blocking antiarrhythmic drugs may result in:
    A Increase in sodium channel messenger RNA, which counteracts the effects of channel blockade.
    B Hyponatremia at cellular level.
    C Decrease in Na/K ATPase.
    D Decrease in sodium channel messenger RNA, resulting in steady state-level.

2 Which of the following statement about Na/K ATPase is incorrect?
    A It is an enzyme responsible for the maintenance of Na^+ and K^+ concentration gradients in the cells.
    B Its operation produces an inwardly directed current as 1 Na^+ ion is removed from the cell in exchange for the influx of 3 K^+.
    C The sodium pump performance determines the level of intracellular Na^+ level and, consequently, cardiac inotropic status.
    D Changes in intracellular Na^+ levels influence the activity of the cardiac Na^+-Ca^{2+} exchanger.

3 SCN5A mutation resulting in loss of function is responsible for which one of the following rhythm disorders?
   A Progressive cardiac conduction disease (PCCD).
   B Long QT syndrome.
   C Catecholaminergic polymorphic ventricular tachycardia.
   D Paroxysmal atrial fibrillation.

4 Which one of the following currents is likely to occur when the Na moves across the cell membrane and into the cell?
   A Inward current
   B Outward current
   C Repolarizing current
   D Hyperpolarizing current

5 A patient receiving a Na channel blocker develops AF with rapid ventricular response. What changes on ECG can be anticipated to occur?
   A Narrowing of the QRS complex during tachycardia
   B Widening of the QRS complex during tachycardia
   C Prolongation of the QT interval
   D Shortening of the QT interval

6 What is likely to happen when a Na channel is blocked?
   A Increase in intracellular Ca and increased contractility
   B Increase in EAD and DAD
   C Decrease in contractility
   D Increase in extracellular Na

7 Which one of the following is not associated with Brugada syndrome?
   A Mutation in *SCN5A* resulting in loss of function
   B Increase in Ito current
   C Inhibition of *I*Ca during the plateau phase
   D Mutation in *SCN5A*, resulting in gain of function

8 What type of channel block, by lidocaine, results in effective suppression of arrhythmias during myocardial ischemia?
   A Inactivated state block
   B Resting state block
   C Open state block
   D Closed state block

9 Which one of the following agents is likely to be effective in treating flecainide induced VT?
   A IV magnesium
   B IV lidocaine
   C IV amiodarone
   D IV digoxin

10 Which one of the following metabolic abnormalities is likely to decrease lidocaine dissociation from the channel sites?

A Acidosis
B Ischemia
C Hyperkalemia
D Hyponatremia

11 What electrophysiologic manifestations can be expected when I_{Nab} (the slow component of the background Na current) is blocked?

A Lengthening of the QT interval
B Positive inotropy
C Occurrence of EAD
D Bradycardia

12 Which one of the following interventions is likely to promote occurrence of TDP in patients with LQT3?

A Beta blocker induced bradycardia
B Permanent pacemaker
C Mexiletine
D Exercise-induced sinus tachycardia

1.3 Calcium channels and currents

1 In which one of the following electrical activities there is no contribution from calcium current I_{CaL}?

A EAD
B Electrical remodeling of the atrium during AF
C DAD
D Depolarization of the SA and AV nodes

2 Which of the following statements is incorrect?

A β-Adrenergic agonists increase I_{CaL} channel activity
B Beta-blockers act as Ca channel blockers
C Parasympathetic stimulation decreases I_{CaL} activity
D T-type Ca channel density is increased by growth hormone, endothelin, and pressure overload

3 Which of the following agents has no effect on T-type Ca channel?

A Amiloride
B Flunarizine
C Mibefradil
D Digoxin

4 Which one of the following statements regarding calcium homeostasis in cardiac myocyte is incorrect?

A Ca^{2+}-ATPase contributes substantially to diastolic Ca^{2+} removal from cardiac myocyte.

    B Ca^{2+} in SR lumen is bound to the low-affinity calcium-binding protein calsequestrin

    C Ca^{2+} signal is generated by Ca^{2+} influx through voltage-dependent L-type calcium channels.

    D Sarcoplasmic reticulum is the major reservoir of the calcium.

5 Which one of the following agents increases sensitization to RyR2?

    A Tetracaine

    B Rapamycin

    C Caffeine

    D Doxorubicin

6 Which one of the following statement about ivabradine is incorrect?

    A It produces bradycardia

    B cAMP overload will nullify its effect

    C It produces visual signs and symptoms

    D It has negative inotropic effect.

1.1 Potassium channels/currents[1,2]

- There are more than eight types of potassium currents.
- Plateau phase of the action potential depends on the balance between inward (depolarizing) and outward (repolarizing) currents.
- Potassium currents (outward movement of the K through the potassium channels) are the main contributors to repolarization
- Activity of potassium channel could be either time-dependent or voltage-dependent (K_V).
- Voltage-gated potassium (K_V) channels consist of a tetrameric assembly of α subunits (Figure 1.1). Each α subunit contains six membrane-spanning segments, S1 to S6, with both amino (N) and carboxyl (C) termini located on the intracellular side of the membrane.
- Segments S1 to S4 confer voltage-sensing properties to these channels, whereas S5 and S6 are critical for forming the channel.
- K_V channels fluctuate between open conducting (activated) state(s) and nonconducting state(s), with the kinetics of the transitions depending critically on membrane voltage and channel structure.
- Nonconducting states can be classified as either closed (deactivated) or inactivated states.
- During the course of an action potential, closed K_V channels activate or open in response to membrane depolarization and subsequently enter the inactivated state in a time-dependent manner. Re-entry into the closed state requires membrane repolarization.
- The voltage- and time-dependent transition between these different conformational functional states is called gating.
- Potassium channels catalyze selective transport of K^+ ions across lipid bilayers while remaining impermeable to other biologic cations.
- AP duration determines amount of calcium influx and tissue refractoriness. It is inversely related to heart rate. Prolongation of AP plateau increases the strength and duration of contraction. It also increases refractoriness.
- In congestive heart failure and in left ventricular hypertrophy repolarizing outward currents are reduced by 50%. This increases APD and results in EAD and arrhythmias. Use of class III drugs in patients with CHF needs reevaluation as intended target (K channels) is down regulated or absent.
- In atrial fibrillation repolarizing outward currents (I_K, I_{to}) are reduced. Reduction of these currents may exacerbate arrhythmic effect of hypokalemia and hypomagnesemia.
- Potassium channel expression is decreased in hypothyroid and hypoadrenal states.

Delayed and inwardly rectifying voltage sensitive potassium channels[2]

- Rectification is a diode like property of unidirectional current flow which could be inward or outwards. It limits outward flow of potassium through I_{Kr} and I_{Ks} during plateau. Delayed rectifier potassium channels have slow onset of action.

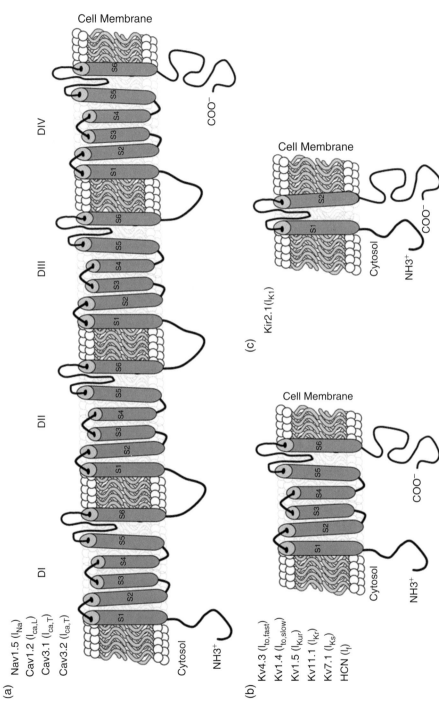

(a)
Nav1.5 (I_{Na})
Cav1.2 ($I_{Ca,L}$)
Cav3.1 ($I_{Ca,T}$)
Cav3.2 ($I_{Ca,T}$)

(b)
Kv4.3 ($I_{to,fast}$)
Kv1.4 ($I_{to,slow}$)
Kv1.5 (I_{Kur})
Kv11.1 (I_{Kr})
Kv7.1 (I_{Ks})
HCN (I_f)

(c)
Kir2.1 (I_{K1})

Figure 1.1 α-Subunits of cardiac ion channels. (a) α-Subunits of Na$^+$ and Ca^{2+} channels consists of four serially linked homologous domains (DI–DIV), each containing six transmembrane segments (S1–S6). (b, c) α-Subunits of channels responsible for I_{to}, I_{Kur}, I_{Kr}, I_{Ks}, I_{K1}, and I_f consist of one single domain with six (B) or two (C) (I_{K1}) transmembrane segments. Four subunits (domains) co-assemble to

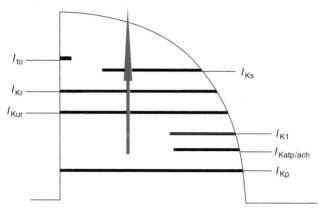

Figure 1.2 Outward currents.

- Voltage gated potassium channels are activated during upstroke of AP.
- Rapidly activating and inactivating voltage sensitive transient outward current I_{to} produces phase 1 of repolarization.
- Inward rectifier I_{K1}, slowly activating delayed rectifier potassium current, which includes fast inactivating rapid component I_{Kr} and slow component I_{Ks}, contributes to plateau and phase 3 of AP.
- K channels carry positive charge which triggers a voltage sensor.
- Potassium channels are closed at resting potential and open after depolarization.
- Two types of voltage-gated channels play major role in repolarization.
  1 Transient outward current (I_{to}) which is characterized by rapid activation and inactivation.
  2 Delayed rectifier I_K which has several components (Figure 1.2)
    I_{Kr} is a rapidly activating current with inward rectification.
    I_{Ks} is a slowly activating current
    I_{Kur} is an ultra rapid current.

Transient outward potassium current (I_{to})
- I_{to} supports early repolarization during phase 1. The transient nature of I_{to} is secondary to its fast activation and inactivation upon depolarization.
- There are two types of I_{to} currents. $I_{to}1$ and $I_{to}2$
- A calcium-activated chloride current ($I_{to}2$) and a classical calcium-independent potassium current ($I_{to}1$) (referred to as I_{to}).
- The calcium-independent I_{to} is of two types: a "rapid" or "fast" $I_{to,f}$ and a slower form, $I_{to,s}$
- $I_{to,s}$ is smaller than $I_{to'f}$
- $I_{to'f}$ recovers rapidly from inactivation, and its α-subunit (Kv4.3) is encoded by *KCND3*. $I_{to,slow}$ recovers slowly from inactivation; its α-subunit (Kv1.4) is encoded by *KCNA4*.

- Kv4.3 and Kv1.4 contain one domain with six transmembrane segments Four subunits co-assemble to form one channel.
- Kv4.3 is strongly expressed in the epicardium and is responsible for shorter AP duration there compared to endocardium, where Kv1.4expression is weak.
- This creates a transmural voltage gradient between epicardium and endocardium.
- $I_{to,f}$ is the primary determinant of the time course of early repolarization (phase 1) of atrial and ventricular action potentials and it varies greatly between regions of the heart.
- Early repolarization modulates L-type calcium current magnitude, thereby regulating excitation-contraction coupling and myocardial contractility.
- $I_{to,f}$ expression is greater in epicardium, right ventricle and the base of the heart, and less in the septum, left ventricular endocardium, and apex of the heart.
- Regional variations in $I_{to,f}$ results in the heterogeneity of action potential, which are responsible for orderly ventricular repolarization.
- Variation in $I_{to,f}$ is responsible for the regional modulation of contractility.
- Electrical heterogeneity associated with the transmural $I_{to,f}$ gradient contributes to synchronization of repolarization and force generation across the ventricular wall.
- The effects of $I_{to,f}$ levels on contractility are related to voltage-dependent modulation of sodium-calcium exchanger which reverses direction during the early repolarization phase.
- The early repolarization period, which is dependent on $I_{to,f}$ levels, controls both the amplitude and the timing of Ca^{2+} release from the SR.
- Reductions in the $I_{to,f}$ and the loss of the notch lead to a slowing of SR Ca^{2+} release.
- The distribution of $I_{to,f}$ in the ventricle synchronizes the timing of force generation between different regions of the ventricle, thereby enhancing mechanical efficiency.
- Generalized downregulation of $I_{to,f}$ occurs in heart failure, slowing the time course of force generation, resulting in reduced myocardial performance.
- Chronic exposure of ventricular myocytes to α-adrenergic agonists (such as phenylephrine) reduces $I_{to,f}$. It also decreased $K_V4.2$, $K_V4.3$, and KChIP2 expression.
- α-adrenergic agonists increase $I_{to,s}$ and $K_V1.4$ expression
- Angiotensin II (AT-II) type 1 (AT-1) receptors stimulation reduces $I_{to,f}$.
- Hypothyroidism prolongs action potential duration reduces $I_{to,f}$ and decreases $K_V4.2$ expression, whereas hyperthyroidism has the reverse effect.
- Aldosterone, induces downregulation of $I_{to,f}$.
- Electrical remodeling in heart disease involves downregulation of $I_{to,f}$ and reductions in $K_V4.2$, $K_V4.3$, and KChIP2, This has been linked to the hypertrophy through the activation of the calcineurin–nuclear factor of activated T cells (NFAT) pathway.
- I_{to} is present in ventricular epicardium but not in endocardium. It is responsible for spike and dome morphology of AP in epicardium.

- In human atrium it recovers rapidly from inactivation thus allowing rapid repolarization at fast heart rate.
- Flecainide, quinidine and ambasilide inhibit I_{to}. Flecainide binds to inactivated $I_{to}1$. It also demonstrates fast unbinding. Quinidine binds to open channel, its slow recovery from block causes rate dependent effect.
- Inhibition of I_{to} prolongs repolarization in diseased human ventricle.
- A gain of function in I_{to} secondary to a mutation in KCNE3 contributes to a Brugada phenotype.

I_{to} mutation and inherited diseases
- *KCNE3* mutation may be responsible for Brugada syndrome. $K_V4.3$, gain of function mutation increases I_{to} fast.
- Increased $I_{to,f}$ induces ST-segment elevation in Brugada syndrome by aggravating transmural voltage gradients.
- *KCNE3* mutation has been identified in familial AF. Mutation increases $I_{to,f}$ and may cause AF by shortening AP duration.

I_{to} expression in acquired cardiac diseases
- I_{to} is reduced in AF, myocardial infarction, and heart failure.
- In myocardial infarction, Ito is down-regulated by the increased activity of calcineurin, a phosphatase that regulates gene transcription by dephosphorylating transcription factors.
- Sustained tachycardia in heart failure reduces I_{to}.
- Ito may be reduced and contribute to QT interval prolongation in diabetes, insulin therapy partially restores Ito, maybe by enhancing $K_V4.3$ expression.

I_{to} and J wave
- J wave (Osborn wave), elevated J point and T wave alternans may be due to transmural gradient between epicardium and endocardium as a result of uneven distribution of I_{to}.
- Prominent J wave are often seen in presence of hypothermia and hypercalcemia.
- The heterogeneity of repolarization generated by $I_{to,f}$ also explains the cardiac T wave memory and Osborne or J wave formation.

Rapidly activating delayed rectifier I_{Kr}
- *KCNH2*, also called the human-ether-a-go-go-related gene (hERG), encodes the α-subunit (Kv11.1) of the channel carrying I_{Kr}.
- I_{Kr} activation upon depolarization is not rapid, but inactivation is fast, resulting in a small outward K^+ current near the end of the AP upstroke.
- During early repolarization, the channel rapidly recovers from inactivation to produce large I_{Kr} amplitudes during AP phases 2 and 3. Channel deactivates (closes) slowly (in contrast to inactivation, deactivation is a voltage-independent process).
- I_{Kr} is responsible for repolarization of most cardiac cells.

- Interaction of Kv11.1 with its β-subunit MiRP1 (encoded by *KCNE2*) induces earlier activation and accelerates deactivation.
- It is blocked by methane sulfonamide, class III agents (D. Sotalol).
- Inward rectification of I_{Kr} results in small outward current.
- It plays an important role in atrial pacemaker cells. It rapidly recovers from inactivation and it peaks at –40 mv.
- *KCNH2* (HERG, Human ether related-a-go-go gene) is responsible for the I_{Kr} current.
- I_{Kr} is increased in the presence of elevated extracellular potassium. Normally increased extracellular potassium will decrease outward potassium current by decreasing chemical gradient but activity of I_{Kr} is increased.
- Increase in serum potassium by 1.4 mEq/L decreases QTc by 24% and decreases QT dispersion.
- Efficacy of I_{Kr} blockers is limited by inverse rate dependency. These drugs are more effective at slower heart rate. High heart rate increases the prevalence of I_{Ks}, which is insensitive to I_{Kr} blockers, thus neutralizes the potassium blocking effects of the I_{Kr} blockers.
- Effect of I_{Ks} but not I_{Kr} is enhanced by β-adrenergic stimulation. Thus effects of pure I_{Kr} blockers will be antagonized by sympathetic stimulation.
- Selective I_{Kr} blockers (D-Sotalol) lose efficiency at high rate and during sympathetic stimulation.
- I_{Kr} and I_{Ks} are present in human atrium and ventricle.
- During phase 3 repolarization, the channels recover from inactivation creating a large repolarizing current, which hastens repolarization and opposes any depolarizing force that would prolong repolarization or create EADs.
- *KCNH2* coassembles with MinK-related peptide 1 (MiRP1) (i.e., *KCNE2*), giving it gating, conductance, regulation, and biphasic inhibition by the methanesulfonilide class III antiarrhythmic drug.

I_{Kr} mutation in inherited diseases
- Loss-of-function mutations in I_{Kr} due to defects in *KCNH2*, (*LQT2*) or MiRP1 (*LQT6*) results in congenital long QT syndromes.
- Gain-of-function mutations in *KCNH2* are associated with short QT syndrome 1 (SQTS1).
- *KCNH2* mutations reduce I_{Kr} *KCNH2 Mutation impairs potassium channel by altering protein Kv11.1.*

I_{Kr} expression in acquired diseases
- In myocardial infarction, Kv11.1 mRNA levels and I_{Kr} are reduced, and AP duration is prolonged
- In diabetes, I_{Kr} reduction contributes to QT interval prolongation. hyperglycemia depresses I_{Kr}, whereas insulin therapy restores I_{Kr} function and shortens QT intervals.
- A high propensity for drug-induced block and acquired long QT syndrome is associated withKCNH2 mutation. I_{Kr} currents are susceptible to drug-induced block particularly in individuals with pre-existing repolarization defects (e.g., patients with LQTS or diabetes)

Slowly activating delayed rectifier I_{Ks}

- Kv7.1, encoded by *KCNQ1*, is the α-subunit of the channel responsible for I_{Ks}. Co-expression of *KCNQ1* with minK (Minimal potassium channel protein) encoding *KCNE1* yields currents that resemble I_{Ks}: a K$^+$ current that activates slowly upon depolarization, displays no inactivation, and deactivates slowly during repolarization.
- I_{Ks} is markedly enhanced by β-adrenergic stimulation through channel phosphorylation by protein kinase A (requiring A-kinase anchoring proteins [AKAPs]) and protein kinase C (requiring minK).
- I_{Ks} contributes to repolarization, especially when β-adrenergic stimulation is present.
- KCNQ1 and KCNE1 are also expressed in the inner ear, where they enable endolymph secretion.
- MinK, a protein, acts as a function altering beta subunit of KCNQ1. Mink modifies KCNQ1 gating and pharmacology.
- Mutation in *KCNE1* and *KCNQ1* causes congenital long QT syndrome (LQTS).
- KCNE1 mutation resulting in MinK suppression leads to inner ear abnormalities and deafness, as seen in Jarvell and Lange–Nielson (JLN) syndrome. Heterozygous mutations in both *KCNQ1* and *KCNE1* cause JLN, which tends to be more lethal than LQT1 or LQT5.
- Reduced activity of I_{Ks} in M cells prolongs APD.
- Bradycardia and class III drugs, which reduce I_{Ks} in M cells, prolong APD and predispose to arrhythmias.
- Slow deactivation of I_{Ks} is important for rate-dependent shortening of AP. As heart rate increases I_{Ks} has less time to deactivate during shortened diastole, it accumulates in open state and contributes to faster repolarization
- Increase in intracellular magnesium decreases and increase in intracellular calcium increases I_{Ks}.
- Indapamide (diuretic), thiopental, propofol (anesthetics) benzodiazepines and chromanol block I_{Ks}.
- Increase cAMP either by β-adrenergic stimulation or by phosphodiesterase inhibitors increases I_{Ks}.
- Activation of protein kinase C increases I_{Ks}.
- Loss-of-function mutations in in *KCNQ1* (LQT1) or KCNE2 (LQT5) results in long QT syndrome. Gain-of-function mutations in *KCNQ1* are associated with short QT syndrome 2 (SQTS2).

I_{Ks} mutation and inherited diseases

- LQTS, type 1 (LQT1), is caused by loss-of-function mutations in *KCNQ1* The resulting IKs reduction is responsible for prolonged AP durations and QT intervals
- Arrhythmia usually occurs during exercise or emotional stress, because mutant I_{Ks} does not increase sufficiently during β-adrenergic stimulation.
- β-adrenergic blocking drugs suppress arrhythmic events in LQT1.
- LQTS type 5 is a result of loss-of-function mutations in *KCNE1* and displays a similar phenotype as LQT1 patients.

- Mutation of *AKAP9*, encoding Yotiao (AKAP9), results in LQTS11. Mutation inhibits the β-adrenergic response of I_{Ks} by disrupting the interaction between Yotiao and Kv7.1. Yotiao mediates phosphorylation of Kv7.1 by protein kinase A upon β-adrenergic stimulation.
- Loss-of-function mutations in both alleles of *KCNQ1* or *KCNE1* cause Jervell and Lange–Nielsen syndrome (JLNS) type 1 or 2, respectively.
- It is characterized by prolonged QT interval, arrhythmia and congenital deafness, the latter due to deficient endolymph secretion.
- *KCNQ1* gain-of-function mutations cause short QT syndrome (type 2).
- *KCNQ1* gain-of-function mutations may cause familial AF by shortening atrial AP duration and facilitating reentry.

I_{Ks} expression in acquired cardiac diseases
- Contradictory reports of *KCNQ1* mutation causing familial AF by increasing I_{Ks} and *KCNE1* polymorphisms increasing AF risk by decreasing I_{Ks} suggest that multiple mechanisms underlie AF.
- Heart failure reduces I_{Ks} in atrial, ventricular, and SA node.

I_{Kur} (ultrarapid) current
- *KCNA5* encodes the α-subunit (Kv1.5) of the channel carrying I_{Kur}.
- Kv1.5 is mainly expressed in the atria, and I_{Kur} is detected only in atrial myocytes. It plays a role in atrial repolarization.
- It activates rapidly upon depolarization but displays very slow inactivation.
- I_{Kur} is sensitive to 4-aminopyridine and is completely blocked by small concentrations.
- It is responsible for atrial repolarization, It is a potassium selective outwardly rectifying current. Short APD of the atria is due to I_{Kur}.
- I_{Kur} is also found in intercalated disks.
- I_{Kur} is absent from human ventricular myocardium.
- It is enhanced by β adrenergic agonists and is inhibited by α-adrenergic agonists.
- Drugs inhibiting I_{Ks} (amiodarone, ambasilide) or I_{Kur} (ambasilide) will be therapeutically superior.
- Presence of I_{Kur} in human atrium makes atrial repolarization relatively insensitive to agents that fail to inhibit this current (d sotalol and flecainide). Quinidine and ambasilide block I_{Kur} in a rate independent fashion.
- I_{Kur} decreases with increasing heart rate.
- Both β- and α-adrenergic stimulation increase I_{Kur} by PKA and PKC effects, respectively.
- Hyperthyroidism can lead to transcriptional upregulation while hypothyroidism leads to decreased expression of $K_V1.5$ channel genes.
- The effects of male sex hormones lead to a reduction in the density of I_{Kur} and $K_V1.5$ expression, which may play a role in gender-specific differences in atrial repolarization.

I_{Kur} mutation and inherited diseases
- *KCNA5* mutations may be responsible for familial AF.
- I_{Kur} loss of function may cause AF through AP prolongation and EAD

Voltage-regulated inward rectifier I_{K1}

- I_{K1} stabilizes the resting membrane potential of atrial and ventricular myocytes during phase 4 and contributes to the terminal portion of phase 3 repolarization.
- I_{K1} channels are closed during AP phases 1 and 2.
- I_{K1} is absent in SAN and AVN myocytes.
- Its α-subunit ($K_{ir}2.1$) is encoded by *KCNJ2* and consists of one domain with two transmembrane segments.
- Blocking of I_{K1} results in depolarization of the resting potential and mild AP prolongation.
- I_{K1} rectification allows it to carry substantial current at negative potentials, which maintains resting potential.
- These channels permit inward potassium flux on membrane hyperpolarization but resist outward potassium flux on depolarization. It prevents potassium ion leak during prolong depolarization.
- I_{K1} is responsible for late phase of repolarization (phase 3) of the cardiac action potential and it sets the resting membrane potential (phase 4).
- Chamber-specific differences in I_{K1} are recognized, with a higher density of I_{K1} in ventricular myocytes but very little I_{K1} current in atrial myocytes.
- Native I_{K1} in human ventricular myocytes is reduced by β-adrenergic receptor stimulation and by the intracellular application of catalytic subunit of PKA.
- Activation of the AT-1 receptors by angiotensin II also appears to downregulate cardiac I_{K1}.
- Kir channels are voltage-regulated despite not having the classic voltage-sensing mechanism – namely, the S1 to S4 segments – of the K_V channels.
- The inward rectifier potassium channel family comprises at least seven subfamilies, $K_{ir}1$ to $K_{ir}7$ (i.e., KCNJ-1 to KCNJ-16).
- Three other inward rectifier (weak) potassium channels are present in the myocardium: 1. TWIK-1 background potassium channels (*KCNK1*), which help to set the resting membrane potential: 2. $I_{K,ACh}$ channels (*KCNJ3*, *KCNJ5*), which regulate heart rate and conduction through the atrioventricular node in response to acetylcholine (ACh); and 3. $I_{K,ATP}$ channels (*KCNJ11*), which respond to changes in metabolic state.
- Loss-of-function mutation in *KCNJ1* is associated with Andersen's syndrome (LQT7), whereas gain-of-function mutations in Kir2.1 (*KCNJ2*) result in short QT syndrome 3 (SQTS3)
- Intracellular magnesium, calcium and polyamines block I_{K1}. Increase in intracellular Ph inactivates I_{K1}. Increase extracellular potassium depolarizes resting membrane.

I_{K1} mutation and inherited diseases[3]

- Loss-of-function mutations in *KCNJ2* are linked to Andersen–Tawil syndrome, characterized by skeletal developmental abnormalities, periodic paralysis, and usually nonsustained ventricular arrhythmia, often associated with prominent U waves and mild QT interval prolongation LQTS type 7.

- *KNCJ2* mutations reduce I_{K1} by encoding defective $K_{ir}2.1$ subunits, which generate nonfunctional channels and/or bind to normal subunits to disrupt their function ("dominant-negative effect").
- I_{K1} reduction may trigger arrhythmia by allowing inward currents, which are no longer counterbalanced by the strong outward I_{K1}, to gradually depolarize the membrane potential during phase 4.
- Membrane depolarization during phase 4 induces arrhythmia by facilitating spontaneous excitability. I_{K1} reduction may trigger arrhythmia by prolonging AP duration and triggering EADs.
- *KCNJ2* gain-of-function mutation, has been linked to short QT syndrome type 3. Increased I_{K1} shorten AP duration and QT interval by accelerating the terminal phase of repolarization.
- *KCNJ2* gain-of-function mutation may cause AF by shortening atrial AP duration

I_{K1} expression in acquired diseases
- In chronic AF, I_{K1} is increased and Kir2.1 mRNA and protein levels are elevated.
- Increased I_{K1} corresponds to more negative resting potentials and, together with reduced $I_{Ca,L}$, accounts for AP shortening in AF.
- In heart failure I_{K1} densities are reduced secondary to increased intracellular Ca^{2+} because Ca^{2+} blocks the outward component of I_{K1}.
- I_{K1} reduction in heart failure or ischemia may facilitate spontaneous excitability and trigger arrhythmia.

ATP-sensitive potassium channel (K_{ATP})
- K_{ATP} channel opens when intracellular ATP level falls and closes when ATP levels rise. ATP produced by glycolytic pathway is preferentially sensed by K_{ATP} channel.
- $I_{K,ATP}$ is a weak inward rectifier but produces a large outward current during depolarization and its activation decreases APD.
- It is responsible for ischemia preconditioning where brief episodes of ischemia protect myocardium from prolonged episodes of ischemia.
- During ischemia intracellular magnesium and sodium levels increase, and extra cellular potassium increases.
- Protons, lactates, oxygen free radicals, and muscarinic receptor stimulation desensitize K_{ATP} channel to the effects of ATP level.
- Sodium and potassium pump and other ATPases degrade ATP.
- Cromakalim, bimakalim, aprikalim, nicorandil, adenosine and protein kinase C open K_{ATP} channel and mimic preconditioning. Sulfonylureas such as glipizide and tolbutamide block K_{ATP} and abolish preconditioning.
- During ischemia there is loss of intracellular potassium and increase in extra cellular potassium resulting in membrane depolarization, slow conduction, and altered refractoriness resulting in reentrant arrhythmias. K_{ATP} counteracts these effects by shortening APD, decreasing workload, promoting inexcitability and increasing potassium conductance during ischemia and hypoxia.

Increased potassium conductance is a result of increased level of intracellular sodium that occurs during ischemia.

- $I_{K,ATP}$ decreases APD and calcium influx. It preserves high-energy phosphates.
- Diazoxide does not activate $I_{K,ATP}$ in sarcolemma but mimics preconditioning. This suggests that there may be other pathways involved in preconditioning.
- $I_{K,ATP}$ causes coronary vasodilatation.

$I_{K,ach}$ (acetylcholine dependent K current)
- Stimulation of muscarinic receptors activates this current. It is mediated by acetylcholine. $I_{K,ach}$ is inwardly rectifying potassium current.
- Parasympathetic stimulation slows heart rate by activating muscarinic receptors which reduces I_f (hyperpolarizing cation current, f stands for funny), in pacemaker cells.
- Effect of potassium channel blockers on atrial repolarization depends on their ability to counteract cholinergic activation of $I_{K,ach}$, either by direct blocked of channel (quinidine) or by muscarinic receptor antagonism (ambasilide, disopyramide).

Two-Pore Potassium Channels (K$_{2P}$)
- K$_{2P}$ channels are composed of four transmembrane domains and two pore-forming P loops arranged in tandem
- Several subfamilies of K$_{2P}$ channels including the TWIK-related acid-sensitive K$^+$ (TASK) channels and TWIK-related K$^+$ (TREK) channels have been identified.
- TASK channels exhibit sensitivity to variations in extracellular pH over a narrow physiological range.
- TREK channels, which comprise TREK-1 *(KCNK2)*, TREK-2 *(KCNK10)*, and TRAAK *(KCNK4)*, display low basal activity, but are stimulated by stretch of the cell membrane, lysophospholipids, and arachidonic acid and are inactivated by hypo osmolarity and phosphorylation by PKA and PKC.
- TREK-1 and TASK-1 in the heart likely to regulate cardiac action potential duration by responding to stretch, polyunsaturated fatty acids, pH, and neurotransmitters.
- TREK-1 may also have a critical role in mediating the vasodilator response of resistance arteries to polyunsaturated fatty acids, thus contributing to their protective effect on the cardiovascular system.
- TASK-1 may have a role in hypoxic vasoconstriction of pulmonary arteries.
- The background current is carried by inward rectifier channels (including I_{K1}, I_{KACh}, and I_{KATP}). Several K$_{2P}$ channels have been proposed to contribute to the cardiac background current.
- TREK-1 activity may play a role in ischemia, when released purinergic agonists such as ADP and ATP lead to arachidonic acid production and activation of TREK-1 by ATP during ischemia.
- As a stretch-activated K$^+$ channel in atrial cells, TREK-1 could be involved in regulating the release of atrial natriuretic peptide, by a stretch-induced increase in intracellular Ca^{2+} concentration.

HCN pacemaker current (I_f)[4]

- The pacemaker current enables spontaneous initiation of cardiac electrical activity.
- It is called the funny current (I_f) because it displays unusual gating properties.
- I_f is a mixed Na^+/K^+ current, which activates slowly upon hyperpolarization and inactivates slowly in a voltage-independent manner (deactivation) upon depolarization.
- I_f conducts an inward current during phases 3 and 4 and may underlie slow membrane depolarization in cells with pacemaker activity (i.e., cells with I_f and little or no I_{K1}).
- I_f activation is accelerated when intracellular cyclic adenosine monophosphate (cAMP) levels are increased.
- I_f mediates heart rate regulation by sympathetic and parasympathetic activity, which control synthesis and degradation of intracellular cAMP, respectively.
- Channels responsible for I_f are named hyperpolarization-activated cyclic nucleotide-gated (HCN) channels.
- Four α-subunit isoforms are described (HCN1–4, encoded by *HCN1–4*), which are preferentially expressed in SAN and AVN myocytes, and Purkinje fibers.
- Their intracellular C-terminus contains cyclic nucleotide-binding domains (CNBDs), which enable direct cAMP binding.
- HCN4 channels carry I_f.

HCN (I_f) mutation and inherited diseases[5]

- Heterozygous *HCN4* mutations were found in individuals with mild to severe sinus bradycardia.
- These mutations decrease HCN channel expression, decelerate I_f activation, or, when located in CNBDs, abolish sensitivity of HCN channels to cAMP.
- *HCN4* mutations cause bradycardia by reducing I_f and the speed of membrane depolarization during phase 4; this results in slower pacemaking rates in SAN myocytes.

HCN expression in acquired diseases[6]

- Increased HCN expression in atrial or ventricular myocytes in pathologic conditions could initiate arrhythmia by triggering spontaneous excitation of non-pacemaker myocytes.
- Increased *HCN2/HCN4* mRNA and protein levels are found in atria of patients with AF and in ventricular tissues of heart failure patients.
- I_f inhibition is believed to lower heart rate without impairing contractility.
- Ivabradine is the only I_f blocker approved for treatment of chronic stable angina and may be useful in the treatment of inappropriate sinus tachycardia

Characteristics of potassium channel block

- Voltage gated potassium channels are activated during upstroke of AP. Rapidly activating and inactivating voltage sensitive transient outward current I_{to} produces phase 1 of repolarization.

- Slowly activating delayed rectifier potassium current, and inward rectifier I_{K1}, which includes fast inactivating rapid component I_{Kr} and slow component I_{Ks}, contributes to plateau and phase 3 of AP.
- Potassium channel blockers prolong APD, a characteristic of Class III action.
- Some potassium channel blockers produce less block at fast heart rates and more blocks at slower heart rates. This phenomenon is called reverse use dependence.
- Potassium channels contribute to repolarization therefore reverse use dependent block will manifest during repolarization at channel level.
- Block of K channel may not consistently affect repolarization because:
    i Many potassium channels are involved in repolarization.
    ii Block of potassium channels (outward currents) maybe counter balanced by inward currents. I_{Ca}, I_{Na}, $I_{Na/Ca}$. Thus no one current dominates repolarization.
    iii Nonspecific effects of potassium channel blockers
    iv Extracellular potassium level may affect K currents.
    v Potassium channel distribution may be variable. Potassium channel expression varies within different layer of myocardium. I_{Kur} is found in atria but not in ventricles
    vi I_{Kr} block could shift repolarization to I_{Ks} at rapid rates. Inability of I_{Ks} to deactivate rapidly and fully will produce less increase in APD.
    vii Many antiarrhythmics are capable of causing potassium channel block and other ion channel block simultaneously.
    viii Drugs that need a long plateau phase to work will be more effective in the ventricle then in the atrium.
- Open channel block occurs when the drug is present during activated or open state.
- Trapping block occurs when the channel closes around the drug without need for drug to unbind. Activation is required to remove the drug from the binding site.
- Drug may bind the channel during inactive state, but cannot bind during resting state.

Effect of pharmacologic agents on the action potential
- Acetylcholine in low concentration prolongs and in high concentration produces abbreviation of epicardial AP. These effects are:
  (a) Reversed by atropine
  (b) Do not occur when I_{to} is blocked
  (c) Accentuated by isoproterenol
  (d) Persist in the presence of propranolol
  (e) Caused by inhibition of I_{Ca} or activation of $I_{K,ach}$.
- Isoproterenol causes more epicardial AP abbreviation than endocardial. It influences I_{to}, I_{Ca}, I_K and I_{Cl}. These currents contribute to phase 1 and phase 3 of AP.
- Organic calcium channel blockers (verapamil) and inorganic calcium channel blocker $MnCl_2$ decreases the I_{Ca} (inward current) and leaves the outward currents unopposed, resulting in decrease of APD and loss of dome in epicardium but not in endocardium.

- I_{to} block may establish electrical homogeneity and abolish arrhythmias due to dispersion of repolarization caused by drugs and ischemia.
- Quinidine inhibits I_{to}.
- Amiloride, a potassium sparing diuretic, prolongs APD and refractoriness.
- Antiarrhythmics, antimicrobials, antihistamines, Psychotropic, GI prokinetic and a host of other pharmacologic agents may alter repolarization.

M cells, potassium currents and APD
- M cells are found in mid myocardium of anterior, lateral wall and outflow tract.
- Electrophysiologically they resemble Purkinje cells.
- M cells show disproportional AP prolongation in response to slow heart rate which may be due to weaker I_{Ks} and stronger late I_{Na}.
- M cells may enforce pump efficiency at slow rates. Long depolarization permits longer efficient contraction.
- Epicardium and endocardium electrically stabilize and abbreviate APD of M cells.
- Loss of either layer by infarction will lead to prolongation of APD. This maybe the mechanism of increased QT interval and QT dispersion seen in non-Q wave MI. These differences could be aggravated by drugs that prolong QT interval or in patients with LQTS.
- M cells play an important role in the inscription of T waves by producing a gradient between epicardium, endocardium and M cells.
- U waves are due to repolarization of His Purkinje cells.
- Amiodarone prolongs APD in epicardium and endocardium and to a lesser extent in M cells which may prevent transmural dispersion of refractoriness.

1.2 Sodium channels and currents[1,7]

- Inward movement of the Na or Ca across the cell membrane through the specific channels produces inward current. Na current depolarizes the cell membrane and is voltage dependent (Figure 1.3).
- The 10 sodium channel subtypes are expressed in cells (Tables 1.1 & 7.3).
- Two sodium channel subtypes are predominant in muscle tissues: NaV1.4 in skeletal muscle and NaV1.5 in the heart.
- NaV1.5 is transiently expressed in developing skeletal muscle but is replaced by NaV1.4 in the adult.
- Most sodium channel subtypes are expressed in neurons.
- The process of channel opening is called activation and the process of closing is called inactivation. During inactivation phase channel enters a nonconducting state while depolarization is maintained.
- Gating process measures current movement rather than ion movement.
- Channels flip between conducting and non-conducting states.
- When all the gates (active or inactive) are open the channel allows the passage of the ions.
- During the early part of repolarization Na channels become inactive. On completion of repolarization the Na channel returns from an inactive to a closed state. During resting potential sodium channels are closed. Na ion conduction

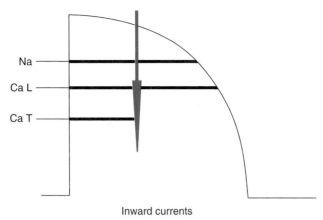

Inward currents

Figure 1.3 Inward currents.

Table 1.1 Membrane current controlling the action potential: pacemaker cells.

Action potential phase	Current	Description	Activation Mechanism	Clone
Phase 4	I_fIKAch	Hyperpolarization-activated current Muscarinic-gated K⁺ current	Membrane hyperpolarization Acetylcholine	HCN2/4 K$_{ir}$ 3.1/3.4
Phase zero	$I_{CaL}I_{Ca-T}$	Calcium current, L type Calcium current, T type	Depolarization Depolarization	Cav 1.2 CaV 3.1/3.2

through the channel occurs when the channel is in the open state and not during the resting or inactive states.
- Movement of sodium occurs through channels and pumps (Figure 1.4).
- Repolarization occurs due to outward K currents. It will be prolonged if the K currents are blocked, as in LQT1 and LQT2, or when inward depolarizing currents persist during repolarization, as in LQT3. In LQT3 (*SCN5A*), a Na channel, remains open during repolarization resulting in continued inward current. This causes prolongation of the QT interval.
- I_{Na} determines cardiac excitability and electrical conduction velocity by enabling phase 0 depolarization in atrial, ventricular, and Purkinje APs,
- The α-subunit of cardiac Na⁺ channels (Nav1.5, encoded by *SCN5A*) encompasses four serially linked homologous domains (DI–DIV), which fold around an ion-conducting pore.
- Each domain contains six transmembrane segments (S1–S6). S4 segment is responsible for voltage-dependent activation (Figure 1.1).
- Voltage dependent opening of Na channel occurs as voltage decreases and conformational change in channel protein occurs (activation).
- There are no β2 subunits of sodium channel in cardiac myocytes. Both β1 and β2 subunits are expressed in the Na channels of the brain neurons.

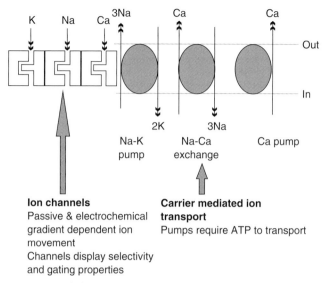

Figure 1.4 Ion pumps and channels.

- Lidocaine inhibits the inactivated state of sodium channels.
- Chronic exposure to Na channel-blocking antiarrhythmic drugs increases sodium channel messenger RNA, which counteracts the effects of channel blockade.

Late Na current (I_{NaL})[8]
- Depolarization of the cell membrane leads to opening of Na^+ channels that gives rise to the action potential (AP).
- Open conformation of the Na^+ channel is unstable, and opening is quickly followed by inactivation.
- Voltage dependence and brevity of Na^+ channel openings restrict Na^+ entry in myocytes to a millisecond, which is sufficient to generate the AP upstroke.
- Inactivated Na^+ channels transition to a resting closed state in response to repolarization of the cell membrane.
- Repolarization of cardiac myocytes (unlike neurons) does not occur until hundreds of milliseconds after Na^+ channel opening, cardiac Na^+ channels spend a long time in inactivated states before closing.
- A failure of Na^+ channels to inactivate leads to continued depolarizing current (sodium channel late current [late I_{Na}]) and Na^+ entry that persists throughout the plateau of the cardiac AP.
- Many Na^+ channel mutations and pathologic conditions either delay or destabilize Na^+ channel inactivation and thereby enhance late I_{Na}.
- The detrimental effects of an enhanced late I_{Na} are
  1 Direct electric effect of an increased inward current during the AP plateau
  2 Indirect effects of increased cellular Na^+ loading
- Both the components are arrhythmogenic.

- AP prolongation and slowing of repolarization, especially at low heart rates, may provide time for reactivation of L-type Ca^{2+} channels and formation of EADs.
- EADs can trigger torsades de pointes (TdP) ventricular tachycardia.
- Late I_{Na} is greater in some cells than in others, and thus late I_{Na}-induced AP prolongation is not uniform and may create an increase transmural dispersion of repolarization.
- The enhancement of late I_{Na} during the AP plateau may potentially lead to a doubling of cellular Na^+ influx, leading to increase intracellular sodium concentration $[Na^+]_i$ in failing and ischemic hearts.
- Increase of $[Na^+]_i$ in turn causes the reversal potential of the sodium–calcium exchanger (NCX) to become more negative. This result is a decreased driving force for Na^+ influx/Ca^{2+} efflux and an increased driving force for Na^+ efflux/Ca^{2+} influx from the cell via NCX.
- Increased Ca^{2+} entry via NCX increases the intracellular calcium concentration $[Ca^{2+}]_i$ and Ca^{2+} uptake in the sarcoplasmic reticulum (SR). This may lead to an increased leak of Ca^{2+} from the SR (ie, Ca^{2+} sparks) during diastole. This leak leads to NCX-induced transient inward currents (I_{TI}) and DADs, which are arrhythmogenic.
- In normal cardiac cells and physiologic settings, Na^+ channel inactivation gating is stable throughout the cardiac AP plateau, and late I_{Na} is small (reported to be 0.2% of peak I_{Na} in the human left ventricle.
- Block of this small physiologic late I_{Na} has not been found to alter electric or contractile function of the heart.
- Block of late I_{Na} shorten AP duration (APD), especially of midmyocardial cells and Purkinje fibers, consistent with findings that the amplitude of late I_{Na} is large in these cells.
- Block of late I_{Na} and reduction of APD in Purkinje fibers and midmyocardial cells is not proarrhythmic; it is associated with reduction of the dispersion of APD, which is antiarrhythmic.
- Many acute causes of an enhanced late I_{Na} have been identified: toxins, angiotensin II, hydrogen peroxide (H_2O_2), nitric oxide, peroxynitrite, hypoxia, ischemic amphiphiles lysophosphatidylcholine and palmitoyl-l-carnitine, glycolytic pathway intermediates thrombin, Ca^{2+} calmodulin, and Na^+ channel phosphorylation.
- The amplitude of late I_{Na} is increased in heart failure; in postinfarction remodeled myocardium in cells expressing mutant forms of scaffolding proteins such as Ankyrin B, Syntrophin, Telethonin and Caveolin 3; and in cells expressing mutant forms of NaV1.5.
- Mutations in the Na^+ channel gene *SCN5A* results in increase in late I_{Na} and causes long QT (LQT) syndrome.
- Ischemia, oxidative stress, and inflamation, reactive oxygen species; intermediary lipid and glycolytic metabolites; acidosis; elevated intracellular Ca^{2+} levels; thrombin; activations of CaMKII, AMPK, PKC, increase late I_{Na}.
- Both late I_{Na} and reverse mode NCX are increased in a failing heart, and late I_{Na} may cause increase of Ca^{2+} loading via NCX.

- K$^+$ outward currents such as background inward rectifier potassium current may be reduced in the failing heart, thus enabling a larger depolarization due to an inward current such as I_{Na} or forward mode sodium–calcium exchange current.
- Depolarization of cells in an ischemic myocardium may lead to increased Na$^+$ window current and further Na$^+$ loading and depolarization.
- A reduction of repolarization reserve because of a decrease of outward K$^+$ current may be associated with an increased proarrhythmic role of late I_{Na}.
- When repolarization reserve is reduced, the effect of an inward current (such as late I_{Na}) to increase APD is amplified.
- Repolarization reserve is reduced in long QT syndromes and by drugs that reduce slow delayed rectifier potassium current (I_Ks) or rapid delayed rectifier potassium current (I_{Kr}) Reduction of late I_{Na} by ranolazine, a drug known to inhibit late I_{Na}, decreases AP prolongation, arrhythmogenesis, and TdP caused by I_{Kr} blockers.
- Reduction of late I_{Na} can reduce the proarrhythmic potential of I_{Kr} blockers and increase repolarization reserve

Late I_{Na} and EADs
- Purkinje fibers seem to be susceptible to EAD formation due to I_{Kr} blockade. Blockers of either Ca^{2+} or Na$^+$ channels can prevent occurrences of EADs.
- High heart rates and cellular Na$^+$ and Ca^{2+} overload are the basis for the formation of DADs.
- Phosphorylations of cardiac ryanodine receptors (RyR2; SR Ca^{2+} release channels) by CaMKII and of SERCA by β-adrenergic receptor-activated protein kinase A are associated with increased spontaneous Ca^{2+} sparks and waves in ventricular myocytes. Overexpression of CaMKIIδc in the heart leads to increased phosphorylation of ryanodine receptors and increased Ca^{2+} spark frequency.
- Conditions associated with excessive Ca^{2+} loading, such as high heart rates; inhibition of Na$^+$,K$^+$-ATPase activity by cardiac glycosides; or enhancement of late I_{Na} (e.g., by ischemia, oxidative stress) result in increased spark frequency and in DADs.
- The increased influx and concentration of intracellular Na$^+$ caused by late I_{Na} reduce Ca^{2+} extrusion via NCX. The resultant Ca^{2+} overload can lead to not only increased diastolic tension but also DADs.
- Reduction by ranolazine of an enhanced late I_{Na} has been shown to decrease the occurrence of DADs.
- Enhanced late I_{Na} is a risk factor for EADs when combined with low heart rates and drug-induced or inherited reductions of I_{Kr} and is a risk factor for DADs when combined with high heart rates, Ca^{2+} loading, adrenergic activity, and CaMKII activation.
- Amiodarone; propranolol; verapamil; the Na$^+$ channel blockers quinidine, mexiletine, lidocaine, and flecainide; and antiepileptic drugs including phenytoin, are known to reduce late I_{Na} but are rarely used because of a lack of selectivity for inhibition of late I_{Na} relative to peak I_{Na} or other currents.

The antiarrhythmic benefits of inhibiting late I_{Na} in the heart

- The antianginal drug ranolazine and the Pierre Fabre compound F15845 are currently the most selective inhibitors of cardiac late I_{Na}.
- Reduction of late I_{Na} increases repolarization reserve and reduces repolarization variability and its proarrhythmic effects.
- Drugs that selectively reduce late I_{Na} may be effective in the treatment of ischemic heart diseases, including chronic angina, heart failure, and atrial and ventricular arrhythmias, and acute ischemia without causing direct effects on heart rate or blood pressure.
- Late I_{Na} is normally a small current in the heart. It is most prominent in Purkinje fibers and M cells and thus contributes to dispersion of repolarization in the normal myocardium.
- Inhibition of the normal small late I_{Na} has yet to be associated with any electric (or mechanical) consequence for cardiac function.
- An enhancement of late I_{Na} occurs as a result of congenital or acquired Na$^+$ channelopathies, including the commonly acquired conditions of myocardial ischemia, heart failure, oxidative stress, and cardiac remodeling (e.g., atrial fibrillation or postmyocardial infarction).
- Enhancement of late I_{Na}, especially in association with reduction of repolarizing K$^+$ current, is proarrhythmic in both atrial and ventricular myocardium and may provide both the triggers and the substrate for arrhythmic activity.
- Enhancement of late I_{Na} may cause diastolic depolarization, reduction of repolarization reserve, APD prolongation and after-depolarizations, triggered activity, increased dispersion of repolarization, reentrant arrhythmic activity, Na$^+$-induced Ca^{2+} overload associated with AP alternans, and diastolic contractile dysfunction.
- Reduction of an enhanced late I_{Na} has been shown to be protective during ischemia and to reduce arrhythmic activity.

I_{Na} mutation and inherited diseases[9,10]

- LQTS type 3 (LQT3), mutations in *SCN5A* delays repolarization, by enhancing INaL. Delayed repolarization triggers EADs, which may initiate torsades de pointes.
- Drugs that block I_{NaL} (e.g., ranolazine, mexiletine) may shorten repolarization in LQT3. LQTS9, 10 and 12 are the result of mutation in *CAV3*, *SCNB4B* and *SNTA1* resulting in increase sodium current.
- Brugada syndrome is linked to mutations in *SCN5A* that reduce I_{Na} by different mechanisms
- Brugada syndrome has also been linked to mutations in genes encoding Na$^+$ channel β-subunits or a protein involved in intracellular Nav1.5 trafficking
- Cardiac conduction disease is manifested by progressive conduction defects at the atrial, atrioventricular, and/or ventricular level and is commonly associated with *SCN5A* mutations that are also linked to Brugada syndrome.
- *SCN5A* mutation causes atrial and/or ventricular arrhythmia and dilated cardiomyopathy.
- Mutations in *SCN5A* have been linked to sick sinus syndrome, which includes sinus bradycardia, sinus arrest, and/or sinoatrial block. *SCN5A* mutations may

impair sinus node function by slowing AP depolarization or prolonging AP duration in SAN cells.

I_{Na} expression in acquired diseases

- In atrial fibrillation (AF) expression levels of several ion channels in atrial myocytes are altered which may promote and maintain AF ("electrical remodeling").
- Nav1.5 expression is reduced leading to I_{Na} reduction.
- AF (either familial or secondary to cardiac diseases [nonfamilial]) is linked to both SCN5A loss-of-function mutations and gain-of-function mutations.
- I_{Na} loss of function may provoke AF by slowing atrial electrical conduction, whereas gain of function may induce AF by enhancing spontaneous excitability of atrial myocytes.
- In heart failure, peak I_{Na} is reduced, while I_{NaL} is increased.
- Decreased SCN5A expression may underlie peak I_{Na} reduction. I_{NaL} increase is attributed to increased phosphorylation of Na^+ channels, when intracellular Ca^{2+} in heart failure rises.
- In myocardial infarction, myocytes in the surviving border zone of the infarcted area exhibit decreased I_{Na} due to reduced Na^+ channel expression and altered gating.
- Na^+ channel blocking drugs increase the risk for sudden death in patients with ischemic heart disease, possibly by facilitating the initiation of reentrant excitation waves.
- I_{NaL} increases during myocardial ischemia, thus I_{NaL} inhibition may be an effective therapy for chronic stable angina.

Na^+,K^+-ATPase

- The Mg^{2+}-activated Na^+,K^+-ATPase constitutes the sodium pump of cardiac sarcolemma, It is an enzyme responsible for the maintenance of Na^+ and K^+ concentration gradients in the cells.
- Its operation is electrogenic, producing an outwardly directed current as 3 Na^+ are removed from the cell in exchange for the influx of 2 K^+.
- This sodium pump helps to maintain the resting potential of cardiac cells, and its short-term inhibition leads to depolarization.
- The sodium pump performance determines the level of intracellular Na^+ level and, consequently, cardiac inotropic status.
- Minor changes in intracellular Na^+ levels exert significant effects on cardiac contractility, because these levels directly influence the activity of the cardiac Na^+-Ca^{2+} exchanger.

Na^+-H^+ exchange

- Na^+-H^+ exchange inhibitors provide cardioprotection during ischemia–reperfusion injury.
- Two classes of NHE1 inhibitors are recognized: amiloride, and its congeners such as ethylisopropylamiloride and 5-N-(methylpropyl)amiloride, and benzoylguanidines and its congeners such as HOE694 and HOE642.

- These inhibitors show high specificity for NHE1 compared with other NHE family members.
- Experimental evidence continues to support cardioprotective, antihypertrophic, and antiproliferative effects for these agents.

Sodium channel block

- There are two types of the Na channel block.
  1 Tonic block results in reduction of peak current with first pulse of the train of pulses. It is seen in drug induced reduction of current during infrequent stimulation.
  2 Phasic block occurs when there is sequential declined in peak current from beat to beat.
- It is also called use dependent or frequency dependent block. It decreases AP upstroke and slows conduction velocity. This type of block increases with repetitive stimulation. If interval between AP is less then four times the recovery constant of the channel, block accumulates.
- During phase 0 Na channels open (open state) for less than 1 millisecond then becomes inactive.
- During phase 2 and 3 (plateau phase) less then one percent of sodium channels remain open (Inactivated State).
- Most depressants of conduction such as elevated extracellular potassium (as may occur in ischemia) produce membrane depolarization and increase fraction of inactivated Na channel. Lidocaine produces inactivated state block therefore it is effective in ischemic zones. The fraction of channels available in open state is reduced during ischemia.
- Quinidine, disopyramide, and propafenone produce open channel block.
- During resting state dissipation of block occurs (drugs dissociates from the site).
- Drugs can produce Na channel block during resting, open or inactivated state. These are called state dependent block. Other type of channel block is voltage dependent.
- Two different sodium channel blocking drugs may act synergistically.
- Class 1A drugs increase APD thus increasing the time sodium channels spend in inactivated state. This will enhance the effectiveness of the drugs that bind to inactivated state (Class 1B drug such as lidocaine).
- Drugs with different binding kinetics may interact. For example drugs with fast kinetic may displace drugs with slower kinetic thus reducing the overall block.
- Lidocaine may reverse the quinidine, propafenone flecainide induced block.
- Ventricular tachycardia due to flecainide, Yew needle toxin, dextropropoxylene can be treated with lidocaine.
- Class 1B drugs have dissociation constant of less then one second thus there is no effect on conduction of normal tissue but will decrease conduction fallowing a closely coupled PVCs and in depressed (ischemic) cells.
- Class 1C drugs have the slowest dissociation of 12 seconds. This results in slowing of conduction and widening of QRS.

- Class 1A drugs have intermediate kinetics more then one second but less then twelve seconds this may result in slowing of conduction and widening of QRS during tachycardia.
- Lidocaine blocks I_{Na} by shifting voltage for inactivation to more negative. It binds to activated and inactivated state of sodium channel.
- Lidocaine, quinidine, and flecainide induce use-dependent block with fast intermediate and slow kinetics respectively.

Drug kinetics and channel state

- Membrane depressants such as increased extracellular potassium, hydrogen, and stretch reduce resting membrane potential. This increases the fraction of inactivated channels and potentiates the effects of the drugs that act on inactivated state. Fewer numbers of channels are available in the open state thus decreasing the effectiveness of the drugs that are open state blockers.
- Decrease in extracellular pH slows the rate of dissociation of lidocaine from sodium channels. Combination of acidosis and membrane depolarization increases the block produced by lidocaine.
- Class 1C drugs are slow to unbind from the channel site and cause slowing of conduction, which may produce incessant tachycardia.
- Marked sinus bradycardia may be pro arrhythmic for drugs with fast half time of recovery form the block because the channels are left unprotected for the major part of APD.

Slow sodium currents (inward)[7]

- Agents that increase slow component of sodium current (diphenylmethyl-piperanzinyl-indole derivatives) are likely to increase inotropy by increasing entry of Na during plateau phase. This leads to increase intracellular calcium through sodium/calcium exchange. Increased intracellular Ca may lead to EAD and PVC.
- Methanesulfonalide-Ibutilide prolongs APD by increasing slow sodium channel current.
- Lidocaine and other class 1B agents block slow component of sodium current and decrease QT in patients with LQT3[6].
- Negative inotropy by sodium channel blockers may be due to blockage of slow sodium channel current.
- Slowing of heart rate produced by class 1B agents is due to block of background sodium current that contributes to the phase 4 of pacemaker AP.
- β-adrenergic stimulation reverses the effects of class I drugs.
- Proarrhythmia from class IC drugs develops during increased heart rate when sympathetic activity is enhanced. β blockers may reverse this phenomenon[7].
- Angiotensin II increases the frequency of reopening of sodium channel and increases Na current.
- Cardiac sodium channels control cardiac excitability by triggering the action potential using pore-forming subunit encoded by *SCN5A*,

- Loss-of-function sodium channelopathies are autosomal-dominant expression resulting from *SCN5A* mutations that conduct less sodium current (I_{Na}).
- Phenotype expression of these mutations includes Brugada syndrome (BrS) and progressive cardiac conduction disease (PCCD).
- Clinical manifestations of PCCD and BrS may overlap in a given patient or same family. Sudden cardiac death (SCD) and syncope, caused by ventricular arrhythmias are the result of reduced cardiac excitability manifested in an electrocardiogram as slowing of conduction.
- *SCN5A* mutations that reduce I_{Na} the most cause the most severe phenotype.
- *SCN5A* mutations may reduce I_{Na} by changing the functional properties (gating) or structural properties by failure to express in the sarcolemma (trafficking) of the sodium channel protein.
- Missense (M) mutations, in which a single amino acid is replaced by an aberrant amino acid, disrupt gating of the channel.
- Truncation (T) mutations, in which the sodium channel protein is truncated because of the presence of a premature stop codon, are not inserted into the sarcolemma, and cause haploinsufficiency.
- T mutations potentially reduce I_{Na} more than M mutations.

1.3 Calcium channels and currents[11,12]

The sarcoplasmic reticulum (SR)
- The sarcoplasmic reticulum (SR) is a cellular organelle present in cardiac myocytes.
- Its function is to amplify the transient Ca^{2+} signals that initiate muscle contraction.
- The primary Ca^{2+} signal is generated by Ca^{2+} influx through voltage-dependent L-type calcium channels during the action potential.
- This Ca^{2+} signal is subsequently amplified by Ca^{2+} release from the SR in a process termed excitation-contraction coupling.
- The mechanism driving the amplification is calcium-induced calcium release (CICR).
- The large fraction of Ca^{2+} in SR lumen is bound to the low-affinity calcium-binding protein calsequestrin.

Calcium channels
- Ten calcium channel genes have been identified.
- Calcium channels are very selective and allow Ca permeability a thousand-fold faster.
- There are four types of calcium channel expressed in the heart:
  1 L type, expressed on surface membrane.
  2 T type expressed on surface membrane.
  3 Sarcoplasmic reticulum (SR) Ca release channel.
  4 Inositol triphosphate (IP3) receptor channels are present on internal membrane.

L type calcium channel (LTCC)

- The L-type (long-lasting) inward Ca^{2+} current (ICa,L) is responsible for the AP plateau. Ca^{2+} influx by I_{CaL} activates Ca^{2+} release channels (ryanodine receptor [RyR2]), located in the SR membrane.
- SR Ca^{2+} release (Ca^{2+} transients) via RyR2 channels couples excitation to contraction in myocytes.
- *CACNA1C* encodes the α-subunit (Cav1.2) of L-type channels.
- Cav1.2 gating is voltage dependent.
- I_{CaL} is blocked by several cations (e.g., Mg^{2+}, Ni^{2+}, Zn^{2+}) and drugs (dihydropyridines, phenylalkylamines, benzothiazepines).
- Its amplitude increases markedly during β-adrenergic stimulation.
- It is a major source of Ca entry in to the cell. It opens when depolarization reaches positive to −40 mv.
- PKA-dependent phosphorylation of LTCC (L=Large) causes several-fold increases in $I_{Ca,L}$.
- It produces inward current that is responsible for depolarization of SA and AV node and contributions to the plateau phase of action potential.
- Increased calcium current prolongs depolarization and increases height of action potential plateau.
- Calcium channel dependent inward current causes EAD.
- I_{CaL} is responsible for excitation, contraction and coupling. Blockade of these channels results in negative inotropic effects.
- In atrial fibrillation (AF) decrease activity of I_{CaL} channel shortens APD and perpetuates arrhythmia (electrical remodeling).

I_{CaL} mutation and inherited diseases

- *CACNA1C* mutations are linked to Timothy syndrome, a rare multisystem disease with QT interval prolongation (LQTS type 8), ventricular tachyarrhythmia, and structural heart disease.
- *CACNA1C* gain-of-function mutations delay repolarization by increasing $I_{Ca,L}$.
- Loss-of-function mutations in *CACNA1C* or *CACNB2* may cause Brugada syndrome.
- RyR2 mutations cause catecholaminergic polymorphic ventricular tachycardia, a disease associated with exercise- and emotion-induced arrhythmia.
- Mutant RyR2 channels permit Ca^{2+} leakage from the SR into the cytoplasm. Ca^{2+} leakage induces extrusion of Ca^{2+} to the extracellular matrix by the Na^+/Ca^{2+} exchanger, which exchanges one Ca^{2+} ion for three Na^+ ions.
- The Na^+/Ca^{2+} exchanger generates an inward Na^+ current, which causes DAD (abnormal depolarization during phase 4 due to activation of Na^+ channels).
- DADs may be responsible for ventricular tachyarrhythmia.

I_{CaL} expression in acquired diseases

- In AF, Cav1.2 mRNA and protein levels are down-regulated, resulting in I_{CaL} reduction, which contributes to AP shortening.

- Sarcoplasmic reticulum Ca^{2+} transients are smaller and slower in heart failure, causing contractile dysfunction.
- In myocardial infarction, I_{CaL} is reduced in the border zone of the infarcted area.
- Acute ischemia inhibits I_{CaL} due to extracellular acidosis and intracellular Ca^{2+} and Mg^{2+} accumulation.

Regulation of pacemaker and Ca currents:

β-Adrenergic receptor stimulation
- It increases L type calcium channel activity.
- This results in increased contractility, heart rate, and conduction velocity.
- Stimulation of receptors activates guanosine triphosphate binding protein Gs which in turn stimulates adenylyl cyclase activity thus increasing the cAMP level.
- Beta-blockers have no direct affect on calcium channels.
- Sympathetic stimulation may also activate alpha1 receptors.

Parasympathetic stimulation
- It decreases L type calcium activity through muscarinic and cholinergic receptors.
- Acetylcholine, through G protein, activates inwardly rectifying $I_{K,ach}$, which makes MDP more negative and decreases slope of diastolic depolarization. This results in slowing of the heart rate.
- Magnesium acts as an L type calcium channel blocker.

T type calcium channel (TTCC)
- I_{CaL} is present in all cardiac myocytes, whereas cardiac I_{CaT} is more prominent in atrial cells and cardiac Purkinje cells.
- I_{CaT} is present in pacemaker and conducting cells, and may have a role in atrial pacemaking and myocyte development.
- I_{CaL} is involved in triggering SR Ca^{2+} release and refilling SR Ca^{2+} stores, rather than pacemaking.
- These are found in cardiac and vascular smooth muscles, including coronary arteries.
  1 Opens at more negative potential.
  2 Inactivates rapidly (Transient T).
  3 Has low conductance (tiny T).
- Occurs in high density in SA and AV node.
- Does not contribute to AP upstroke (which is dominated by sodium channel).
- It is implicated in cell growth.
- T type Ca channel density is increased in the presence of growth hormone, endothelin-1 and pressure overload.
- Failing myocytes also demonstrate increase density of T type Ca channels.
- Drugs and compounds that block T type Ca channels include[5,6]:
  - Amiloride.

- o 3, 4-Dichrobenzamil.
- o Verapamil.
- o Diltiazem.
- o Flunarizine.
- o Tetradrine.
- o Nickel.
- o Cadmium.
- o Mibefradil.
- TTCC is up-regulated by norepinephrine, alpha agonist (phenylephrine), extracellular ATP and LVH.
- It has been implicated in the secretion of neurohormones, such as aldosterone, renin, atrial naturietic factor, and insulin, all of which regulate heart function.
- Mibefradil selectively blocks TTCC.
- Efonidipine, a dihydropyridine derivative, has been found to inhibit both LTCC and TTCC.

Sarcolemmal Ca^{2+}-ATPase
- It serves prominent roles in Ca^{2+} extrusion.
- This enzyme removes intracellular Ca^{2+} in parallel with the Na^+-Ca^{2+} exchange system. Ca^{2+} efflux is essential for myocardial cell function,
- Ca^{2+}-ATPase does not appear to contribute substantially to diastolic Ca^{2+} removal, this role is played primarily by the cardiac Na^+-Ca^{2+} exchanger.

Sarcoplasmic calcium release channels (ryanodine receptors)
- Three mammalian isoforms have been identified: RyR1, RyR2, and RyR3.
- RyR1 is found in skeletal muscle.
- RyR2 is the dominant isoform in cardiac muscle and also is found in smooth muscle RyR3 is expressed in brain, skeletal, cardiac, smooth muscle and in other tissues.
- These are intracellular channels that are regulated by calcium.
- These channels mediate influx of calcium from SR into cytosol.
- It provides calcium for cardiac contraction. SR controls cytoplasmic Ca level by release or uptake during systole and diastole respectively.
- Calcium release from SR is triggered by increase in intracellular calcium, produced by L type Ca channels. It is called calcium-induced calcium release.
- When a cell is calcium overloaded SR releases calcium spontaneously and asynchronously causing DAD, seen in digitalis toxicity.
- Caffeine releases calcium from SR.
- Doxorubicin decreases cardiac contractility by depleting SR calcium.
- Magnesium and ATP potentiates channel flux.
- In ischemia decreased intracellular ATP decreases calcium release and causes ischemic contractile failure.
- Verapamil has no effect on SCRC.
- SR also has potassium, sodium, and hydrogen channels.

SR Ca²⁺ overload

- SR Ca^{2+} overload can generate arrhythmias.
- Mutations of the skeletal muscle RyR_1 have been linked to malignant hyperthermia.
- Mutations of the RyR_2 protein result in Ca^{2+} sensitivity when the SR is overloaded; this results in arrhythmias during β-adrenergic stimulation.
- These arrhythmias manifest as exercise-induced catecholaminergic polymorphic ventricular tachycardias (CPVTs).
- Caffeine causes sensitization of RyR_2 to Ca^{2+}
- Tetracaine and Ruthenium red inhibits the RyR_2
- Scorpion toxins imperatoxin A and imperatoxin I may affect the gating of RyR_2.
- Anticancer drugs (e.g., doxorubicin) cause redox modification of the RyR_2 resulting in decrease contractility and drug induced cardiomyopathy.
- The immunosuppressants FK506 and rapamycin cause cardiotoxic effects by interfering with the stability of calstabin2 binding to the RyR_2.
- The benzothiazepine derivative JTV-519 (K201) can stabilize calstabin2 on the RyR_2 protein and slow down or prevent its dissociation.

Inositol triphosphate (IP3) receptors

- Found in smooth muscles and in specialized conduction tissue.
- Up regulated by angiotensin II and alpha adrenergic stimulation.
- Stimulation of myocytes angiotensin II receptors by angiotensin increases intracellular IP3.
- Arrhythmogenic effect of angiotensin II in congestive heart failure maybe due to elevated IP3.
- IP3 receptors have been implicated in apoptosis.

Sodium and calcium exchange

- Opening of voltage-operated calcium channels, during the plateau phase of APD, increases flux of calcium into cytoplasm resulting in calcium induced calcium release (CICR) from SR.
- During diastole calcium is removed from the cell by sodium/calcium exchange located in the cell membrane.
- Lowering of pH blocks sodium/calcium exchange.
- SR calcium ATPases, sarcolemmal calcium ATPases and sodium/calcium exchange decrease cytoplasmic calcium from elevated systolic level to baseline diastolic level by pumping Ca back into sarcoplasmic reticulum or by extruding Ca from the cell.
- During calcium removal inwardly directed current is observed, which may cause DAD.
- DAD occurs when there is pathologically high calcium load as seen in digitalis toxicity or fallowing reperfusion.
- Na/Ca exchange is able to transport calcium bidirectionally. Reverse mode will increase intracellular calcium, which may trigger SR calcium release.

Effect of antiarrhythmic drugs on calcium channel

- Most Na and K channel blocking agents also affect Ca channels.
- Quinidine, disopyramide, lidocaine, mexiletine, diphenylhydantoin, flecainide, propafenone, moricizine, and azimilide suppress L type calcium currents.
- Amiodarone blocks both L and T type Ca currents.
- Sotalol has no effect on Ca channels.
- Digoxin inhibits sodium/potassium ATPases. This inhibition results in an increase in intracellular Na, which in turn leads to increase in intracellular Ca through Na/Ca exchange.
- Verapamil blocks Ca current and decrease calcium activated chloride current.

HCN (hyperpolarization-activated cyclic nucleotide gated) I_f channels[6,13,14]

- It is activated not on depolarization of the membrane (as are most voltage-gated ion channels) but on membrane hyperpolarization.
- The channel is permeable for K^+ and Na^+ ions, with a three-fold higher selectivity for K^+ than for Na^+.
- At the maximum diastolic potential of sinoatrial node cells (approximately -60 to -75 mV), I_f channels carry an inward current that depolarizes the membrane potential toward the activation range of T-type and then L-type calcium channels.
- Voltage dependence of I_f channel activation is regulated by cyclic adenosine monophosphate (cAMP).
- Direct binding of cAMP to the channel shifts the activation curve to more depolarized voltage, allowing the channel to opens.
- The increase in heart rate in response to β-adrenergic agonists (which increase the intracellular cAMP level) has been attributed to this direct effect of cAMP on the I_f channel.
- Lowering of cAMP level by muscarinic agonists inhibits the channel resulting in a reduced heart rate.
- Four different genes *HCN1* to *HCN4* have been identified
- The channels are composed of six transmembrane segments (S1 to S6), including a positively charged S4 segment constituting the voltage sensor.
- S4 is the ion-conducting pore region.
- The proteins contain a cyclic nucleotide binding
- HCN channels contain structural features of both voltage- and cyclic nucleotide-gated ion channels, and are modulated by both membrane potential and cyclic nucleotides.
- Acidic pH values shift the channel activation curve to more hyperpolarized potentials, inhibiting channel activity
- HCN4 is most commonly expressed isoform in humans.
- Ventricular myocytes from patients with ischemic cardiomyopathy have twice the density of I_f compared to control subjects. This may generate pathologic depolarizing currents responsible for ventricular arrhythmias

I_f blockers as bradycardic drugs

- HCN currents are responsible for the spontaneous slow diastolic depolarization rate (DDR) of the sinus node.
- Drugs that block this current can delay the DDR, thereby prolonging diastole.
- HCN blocker, ivabradine (Procoralan), produces bradycardia using this mechanism.
- It influences only chronotropy but not inotropy.
- Ivabradine, and the related experimental drugs cilobradine and zatebradine, blocks HCN currents in dose- and use-dependent fashion.
- This drug does not discriminate among the four HCN subtypes – all HCN isoforms are equally blocked.
- Ivabradine blocks sinoatrial I_f. It does not reach neuronal HCN channels.
- It blocks retinal HCN1, producing visual signs and symptoms.
- I_f blockers do not arrest the heart but lower the heart rate to a basal level and leave the heart rate–accelerating response to β-adrenergic stimulation intact.

Gap junction

- Intercellular current flows between cardiac cells by way of gap junction channels. This produces an effective heart beat.
- Cardiac cells form a syncytium that allows for the propagation of both electrical and metabolic signals throughout the tissue.
- Rotigaptide acts by enhancing – or preserving – gap junction communication.
- Enhancement of gap junction communication, under conditions of metabolic stress, may have antiarrhythmic effect.

References

1 Smyth JW, Shaw RM. Forward trafficking of ion channels: what the clinician needs to know. *Heart Rhythm.* 2010;7(8):1135–1140.
2 Jespersen T, Grunnet M, Olesen S-P. The KCNQ1 potassium channel: from gene to physiological function. *Physiology (Bethesda).* 2005;20:408–416.
3 Amin AS, Tan HL, Wilde AAM. Cardiac ion channels in health and disease. *Heart Rhythm.* 2010;7(1):117–126.
4 Baruscotti M, Barbuti A, Bucchi A. The cardiac pacemaker current. *J. Mol. Cell. Cardiol.* 2010;48(1):55–64.
5 Nof E, Antzelevitch C, Glikson M. The Contribution of HCN4 to normal sinus node function in humans and animal models. *Pacing Clin Electrophysiol.* 2010;33(1): 100–106.
6 Biel M, Wahl-Schott C, Michalakis S, Zong X. Hyperpolarization-activated cation channels: from genes to function. *Physiol. Rev.* 2009;89(3):847–885.
7 Darbar D. Cardiac sodium channel variants: action players with many faces. *Heart Rhythm.* 2008;5(10):1441–1443.
8 Hilgemann DW, Yaradanakul A, Wang Y, Fuster D. Molecular control of cardiac sodium homeostasis in health and disease. *J. Cardiovasc. Electrophysiol.* 2006;17 Suppl 1:S47–S56.

9 Clancy CE, Kass RS. Defective cardiac ion channels: from mutations to clinical syndromes. *J. Clin. Invest.* 2002;110(8):1075–1077.

10 London B, Michalec M, Mehdi H, et al. Mutation in glycerol-3-phosphate dehydrogenase 1 like gene (GPD1-L) decreases cardiac Na^+ current and causes inherited arrhythmias. *Circulation.* 2007;116(20):2260–2268.

11 Ter Keurs HEDJ, Boyden PA. Calcium and arrhythmogenesis. *Physiol. Rev.* 2007;87(2):457–506.

12 Bers DM. Calcium cycling and signaling in cardiac myocytes. *Annu. Rev. Physiol.* 2008;70:23–49.

13 Milanesi R, Baruscotti M, Gnecchi-Ruscone T, DiFrancesco D. Familial sinus bradycardia associated with a mutation in the cardiac pacemaker channel. *N. Engl. J. Med.* 2006;354(2):151–157.

14 Bucchi A, Tognati A, Milanesi R, Baruscotti M, DiFrancesco D. Properties of ivabradine-induced block of HCN1 and HCN4 pacemaker channels. *J. Physiol. (Lond.).* 2006;572(Pt 2):335–346.

Answers to self-assessment questions

1.1 Potassium channels

1 A
2 D
3 A
4 A
5 A
6 B
7 C
8 A
9 B
10 A
11 C
12 C
13 A
14 B

1.2 Sodium channels

1 A
2 B
3 A
4 A
5 B
6 C
7 D
8 A
9 B
10 A
11 D
12 A

1.3 Calcium channels

1 C
2 B
3 D
4 A
5 C
6 D

CHAPTER 2

Electrophysiologic effects of cardiac autonomic activity

Self-assessment questions

1 Which one of the following is the likely cardiac manifestation of β_3 receptor stimulation?
   A Increase in contractility
   B Decrease in contractility
   C Decrease in heart rate
   D Increase in heart rate

2 Which of the following muscarinic receptor is predominantly found in the heart?
   A M_1
   B M_2
   C M_3
   D M_4

3 What is the likely cardiac effect of muscarinic receptor stimulation by acetylcholine?
   A Coronary vasoconstriction
   B Positive chronotropic response
   C Enhanced inotropic response
   D Negative dromotropic effect

4 Which one of the following is likely to occur with cardiac adenosine receptor stimulation?
   A Negative chronotropic effect
   B Positive dromotropic effect
   C Enhanced contractility
   D Coronary vasoconstriction

5 Which one of the following currents is activated by purinergic agonists?
   A $K_{Ach, Ado.}$
   B I_{Na}
   C I_{CL}
   D $I_{Ca(T)}$

Essential Cardiac Electrophysiology: The Self-Assessment Approach, Second Edition. Zainul Abedin.
© 2013 Blackwell Publishing Ltd. Published 2013 by Blackwell Publishing Ltd.

6 Which of the following effect is due to adenosine?
A Increase in Ca current
B Decrease in atrial action potential duration (APD) and refractory period
C Stimulation of P_2 receptors
D Decrease in $I_{K,ATP}$ current

7 Which of the following electrophysiologic effects is least likely to occur with vagal denervation of the atrium?
A Increases in atrial APD and effective refractory period (ERP).
B Abolishes sinus arrhythmia
C Decreases heart rate variability and baroreflex sensitivity
D Decreases ventricular effective refractory period

8 Which of the following observations may suggest that in the treatment of CHF nonselective β blockers are likely to be superior to selective β blockers?
A β1 receptors are up regulated.
B β2 and β3 receptors are up regulated
C Peripheral vascular resistance is increased
D Glomerular filtration rate is increased

9 Primary neurotransmitter for sympathetic preganglionic fibers is
A Epinephrine
B Norepinephrine
C Acetylcholine
D cAMP

10 Which of the following agents is unlikely to reduce the cardiac memory?
A Angiotensin II receptor blockade.
B Nifedipine infusion.
C Angiotensin – converting enzyme blockade.
D Adenosine receptor blockade.

11 Which of the following drugs is most likely to shorten the human atrial action potential duration?
A Carvedilol
B Dofetilide
C Adenosine
D Dronedarone

2.1 Adrenergic receptors[1-3]

- The human adrenergic receptor family consists of nine subtypes originating from different genes: α1A, α1B, α1D, α2A, α2B, α2C, β1, β2, and β3.
- Autonomic innervation of the heart involves both extrinsic and intrinsic cardiac autonomic nervous systems (CANS). The former includes the ganglia in the brain or along the spinal cord and their axons (e.g., the vagosympathetic trunk) en route to the heart; the latter consists of the autonomic ganglia and axons located on the heart itself or along the great vessels within the pericardium.
- The extrinsic and intrinsic CANS can operate interdependently and independently as well.
- α receptors have a greater affinity for norepinephrine, whereas the β receptors have a greater affinity for epinephrine.
- Most postganglionic sympathetic neurons release norepinephrine onto visceral targets.
- All postganglionic parasympathetic neurons release acetylcholine and stimulate muscarinic receptors on visceral targets.
- In both the sympathetic and parasympathetic divisions, synaptic transmission between preganglionic and postganglionic neurons (termed ganglionic transmission because the synapse is located in a ganglion) is mediated by acetylcholine (ACh) acting on nicotinic receptors (Table 2.1).

β-Adrenergic receptors[4-6]

- β_1 is a predominant adrenergic receptor in the myocardium. 75% of total β receptor population is β_1.
- β_1 stimulation causes positive inotropic, chronotropic and lusitropic (relaxation) response. cAMP dependent activation of protein kinase A (PKA) phosphorylates and activates β adrenergic receptor.

Table 2.1 Properties of the sympathetic and parasympathetic system.

	Location of neuron cell bodies	Primary neurotransmitter	Primary postsynaptic receptor	Myelination
Parasympathetic preganglionic	Brainstem and sacral spinal cord (S2–S4)	Acetylcholine	Nicotinic	Yes
Parasympathetic postganglionic	Terminal ganglia in or near target organ	Acetylcholine	Muscarinic	No
Sympathetic preganglionic	Intermediolateral cell column in the spinal cord (T1–L3)	Acetylcholine	Nicotinic	Yes
Sympathetic postganglionic	Prevertebral and paravertebral ganglia	Norepinephrine	Adrenergic	No

Table 2.2 Characteristics of the subtypes of adrenergic receptors.

Receptor	Agonist	Antagonist	Tissue	Responses
α_1	Epi>NE>>Iso phenylephrine	Prazosin	Heart,	↑contractility, arrhythmias.
			Intestinal SM	Relaxation.
			Urinary & vascular SM	Contraction.
			Liver.	Glycogenolysis gluconeogenesis
α_2	Epi>NE>>Iso, clonidine	Yohimbine	Pancreatic β cell	↓Insulin
			Platelets	Aggregation
			Nerve terminal	↓NE
			Vascular SM	Contraction
β_1	Iso>Epi=NE, dobutamine	Metoprolol	Heart	↑Inotropy, chronotropy & AV conduction.
			Juxtaglomerular	↑Renin
β_2	Iso>Epi>>NE Terbutaline	Propranolol	Heart	↑Inotropy Automaticity Arrhythmias
			Vascular GI GU bronchial SM.	Relaxation.
			Skeletal muscle	Glycogenolysis K uptake.
			Liver	Glycogenolysis
β_3	Iso=NE>Epi		Adipose tissue	Lipolysis.
			Heart	↓contractility

AV=atrioventricular. Epi=epinephrine. GI=gastrointestinal. GU=genitourinary. Iso=isoproterenol. NE=norepinephrine. SM=smooth muscle. ↑=increased release. ↓=decreased release.

- Even in the presence of continuing β stimulation cAMP response wanes. This phenomenon is called receptor desensitization. Persistent agonist stimulation decreases total number of receptors (receptor down regulation).
- In ageing heart β_1 receptor is down regulated and β_2 becomes dominant.
- In congestive heart failure (CHF) sustained adrenergic stimulation leads to desensitization and down regulation of β_1 receptors. β_2 receptor expression is preserved. α1 receptor subtypes remains constant or may even be up-regulated. Under these conditions β_2 and α1 stimulation results in atrial and ventricular arrhythmias.
- This supports the observation that non selective beta blockers reduce cardiac mortality in post myocardial infarction (MI) and CHF patients.
- In general, the type-2 adrenergic receptors (α2 and β2) are found at the prejunctional site in the central and peripheral sympathetic nervous system, where activation of α2 receptors inhibits, and activation of β2 receptors enhances norepinephrine release (Table 2.2).

- Presynaptic α2A and α2C receptor subtypes are important in decreasing sympathetic activity in the central nervous system as well as in decreasing the norepinephrine release in cardiac sympathetic nerve terminals.
- β_2 receptor is up-regulated in denervated, transplanted heart.
- Stimulation of the β_2 receptors of the sinoatrial (SA) node results in sinus tachycardia.
- β_2 receptor stimulation elevates intracellular pH, which increases responsiveness to calcium.
- β adrenergic stimulation increases I_K.
- In cardiomyocytes, endothelial or smooth muscle cells, the type-2 adrenergic receptors are also present postsynaptically together with α1, β1, and β3 receptors.
- Acute changes in myocardial function are exclusively governed by the β receptors.
- α1-receptor contribution is negligible in humans under normal conditions.
- Although all three types of α1 receptors are expressed in the heart, the α1A is the dominant subtype.
- No direct α2 receptor mediated effects are discernible on the myocardium.
- α1 adrenergic receptor stimulation induces growth.

β_3 receptors

- The β3 receptor is an important regulator of adipose tissue and gastrointestinal tract. It is also present in human heart and is implicated as an inhibitor of cardiac contractile function. In normal heart β3-adrenoceptors protects myocardium from the deleterious effects of excess catecholamines that may occur in hyperadrenergic states including heart failure.
- The negative inotropic effects of β3-adrenoceptors are mediated through activation of constitutively expressed endothelial nitric oxide synthase. This action opposes the positive inotropic effects of catecholamines on β1- and β2-receptors, which are mediated via cyclic adenosine monophosphate (cAMP).
- β3-adrenoceptor stimulation decreases $I_{Ca,L}$ type calcium current in ventricular myocytes.
- Whereas β3 receptor activation may protect against cardiac myocyte damage due to catecholamine excess during the early stage of heart failure, β3-adrenoceptor up-regulation may contribute to decrease contractility in the later phases of disease.
- β3-adrenoceptors are desensitization-resistant and their action may exceed that of impaired, down-regulated or desensitized β1- and β2-adrenoceptors. This may result in depression of contractility and exacerbation of heart failure.
- This supports the observation that nonselective beta-blockers reduce cardiac mortality in patients with recent MI and CHF.

2.2 Cholinergic receptors[7,8]

- Cholinergic receptors are nicotinic or muscarinic depending on their ability to interact with nicotine or muscarine.

- Cholinergic receptors are activated by acetylcholine from parasympathetic nerve terminals.
- Effects of acetylcholine that are mimicked by muscarine and blocked by atropine are called muscarinic effects. Other effects of acetylcholine that are mimicked by nicotine and are not antagonized by atropine but are blocked by tubocurarine are called as nicotinic effects.
- Cardiac effects of acetylcholine are mediated by muscarinic cholinergic receptors.
- Five types of (M1–M5) muscarinic receptors have been identified.
- M1 and M3 receptors cause mobilization of intracellular Ca by activating phospholipase C. M2 and M4 receptors inhibit adenylyl cyclase and enhance K conductance through K channels.
- M1 receptor is found in autonomic ganglia and CNS.
- M2 is a dominant muscarinic receptor of cardiac myocytes.
- M3 is predominant receptor in smooth muscle cells, where its stimulation causes contraction, and in secretory glands.
- Inhibitory effects of acetylcholine on calcium current and contractility are due to M2 receptors and can be blocked by M2 antagonist.
- Acetylcholine (ACh) is hydrolyzed by acetylcholinesterase. Cardiac effects of ACh are characterized by vasodilatation, negative chronotropic effect, negative dromotropic effect (decrease in conduction in SA and atrioventricular (AV) nodes) and negative inotropic effect.
- Commonly used synthetic choline derivatives are methacholine, carbachol and bethanechol.
- Muscarine, pilocarpine and arecoline are naturally occurring alkaloid with pharmacological properties similar to acetylcholine.
- Atropine and scopolamine are naturally occurring alkaloids that act as muscarinic receptor antagonist.

2.3 Purinergic receptors[9]

- Autonomic nonadrenergic and noncholinergic nerves were suggested to contain ATP.
- Nerves utilizing ATP as their principal transmitter were named "purinergic" based on the actions of purine nucleotides and nucleosides in a wide variety of tissues, P1- and P2-receptor classification was proposed (Figure 2.1).
- There are two types of purinergic receptors, P1 and P2.
- P1 is activated by adenosine.
- P2 is activated by extracellular ATP.
- Two types of P2 receptors have been identified. P2X are ion channels, while P2Y are G protein coupled receptor.
- P1 purinoceptors are much more sensitive to adenosine and AMP than to ADP and ATP. The reverse is true for P2 purinoceptors.
- P2 receptors are unaffected by methylxanthines such as caffeine and theophylline that selectively and completely inhibits the P1 purinoceptors.
- Subclasses of P1 adenosine receptors were introduced when their stimulation was shown to inhibit (A1 subtype) or activate (A2 subtype) adenylyl cyclase activity.

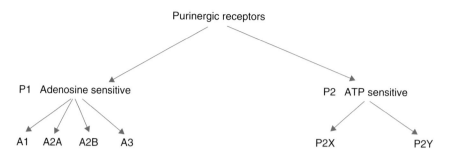

▼ Negative chronotropic, dromotropic,
  inotropic and anti β adrenergic effects.

▼ Inhibited by methylxanthines.

▼ In vascular endothelium and smooth
  muscles of coronary arteries cause
  adenosine induced coronary
  vasodilatation.

Figure 2.1 Purinergic receptors.

Adenosine

- There are four subtypes of adenosine (P1 purinergic) receptors; A_1, A_2A, A_2B and A_3. All four are expressed in the heart.
- A_1 and A_2 receptors are antagonized by xanthines.
- Electrophysiologic actions of adenosine on heart are mediated by A_1 receptors. Blockade of this receptor abolishes negative chronotropic, dromotropic, inotropic and anti β adrenergic effects of adenosine.
- A_1 receptors inhibit adenylyl cyclase and activate K current and phospholipase C.
- A_2 receptors activate adenylyl cyclase.
- A_2A receptors are present in vascular endothelium and smooth muscles of coronary arteries and cause adenosine induced coronary vasodilatation.
- Effects of extracellular ATP, before its degradation to adenosine, are mediated by P_2 purinergic receptors.
- Stimulation of muscarinic and adenosine receptors cause activation of inhibitory guanine (G) proteins. This leads to production of cAMP mediated activation of I_{CaL}, I_K and I_{CL}.
- Density of A_1 adenosine and M_2 muscarinic cholinergic receptor is greater in the atrium.

Acetylcholine and adenosine sensitive potassium currents

- Cholinergic and purinergic agonist activate inwardly rectifying potassium currents $I_{K,ach, ado}$.
- *Inwardly rectifying* means it is easier for the current to flow inward than outward through $I_{Kach,Ado}$ channels. Inward rectification is attributed to voltage dependent block of potassium channels by intracellular Mg and polyamines (spermine and spermidine).

Table 2.3 Effect of acetylcholine, adenosine and extra cellular ATP on cardiac currents.

	Acetylcholine	Adenosine	ATP
Receptor	M_2	A_1	P_2
$I_{Kach,Ado}$	↑	↑	↑
I_K	No effect	No effect	↑
$I_{K,ATP}$	↑	↑	↑
I_{CaL}	↓	↓	↑ in atria ↓ in V
I_{Na}	No effect	No effect	Variable
I_f	↓	↓	No effect
I_{CL}	No effect	↓ if stimulated	↑

↑ = Increase. ↓ = Decrease. V = Ventricle.

- These currents are also activated by extra cellular ATP, arachidonic acid (prostacyclin), somatostatin, and sphingosine-1-phosphate.
- Lipoxygenase potentiates and cyclo-oxygenase inhibits $I_{K,ach,Ado}$.
- Hyperpolarizing current (I_f) is an inward current, and is responsible for diastolic depolarization of the SA node. This is a time-dependent, nonspecific cation current.
- Acetylcholine and adenosine inhibit I_f due to inhibition of adenylate cyclase.
- Adenosine has no effect on ventricular AP of myocytes.
- In the SA and AV node adenosine and acetylcholine cause hyperpolarization and reduce the rate of diastolic depolarization. These actions result in slowing of heart rate (negative chronotropy) and delay in AV node conduction (negative dromotropy).
- Adenosine's effects occur at atrial-His and nodal region, but has no effect on nodal-His bundle region (NH) region of the AV node.
- Acetylcholine and adenosine decrease atrial APD and contractile force (in the absence of β adrenergic stimulation) due to activation of $I_{K,ach,Ado}$ and inhibition of I_{CaL}.
- Adenosine and acetylcholine attenuate β-adrenergic stimulated I_{CaL} in ventricular and atrial myocytes and inhibit transient inward current and delayed after-depolarization (DAD). Adenosine may be effective in catecholamine sensitive ventricular tachycardia (VT) by abolishing cAMP-dependent triggered activity.
- Acetylcholine and adenosine decrease atrial action potential duration (APD) and effective refractory period (ERP) and facilitate induction of AF.
- During AV nodal ischemia local production of adenosine may be responsible for bradycardia seen in patients with inferior wall MI.
- Extra cellular ATP causes DAD, and early after-depolarization (EAD) by stimulating P_2 receptors and inducing I_{CaL} (Table 2.3).

2.4 Cardiac autonomic innervations

- Vagal postganglionic neurons to the sinus node are located in left pulmonary vein left atrial junction, and neurons to AV node are found in the inferior vena cava/left atrium (IVC/LA) fat pad.
- Superior vena cava (SVC)/aorta fat pad innervates both atria.
- Vagal denervation of atria prevents induction of acute atrial fibrillation (AF), abolishes sinus arrhythmias, decreases heart rate variability and eliminates baroreflex sensitivity without affecting vagal innervation to the ventricle.
- Efferent vagal fibers to ventricle do not travel through three epicardial fat pads.
- Changes in sinus node function may not reflect changes at ventricular level.
- Sympathetic efferent fibers are epicardial located along the coronary arteries parasympathetic efferent fibers are subendocardial in the ventricle.
- Block of nitric oxide synthase attenuates cholinergic action and increases calcium current. L arginine reverses these effects.
- L arginine also reduces the effects of sympathetic stimulation such as shortening of ERP and induction of ventricular arrhythmias.
- Vagal stimulation facilitates AF.
- Decrease in atrial refractory period maybe due to activation of sodium/hydrogen exchanger induced by atrial ischemia during AF.
- After MI there is regional sympathetic denervation which results in post denervation supersensitivity to circulating catecholamines and predisposes to ventricular arrhythmias.
- Beneficial effects of beta-blockers in reducing incidence of sudden cardiac death in post MI patients are due to reduction in heart rate and other anti sympathetic activities.
- Initial sympathetic stimulation and subsequent withdrawal resulting in hypotension and bradycardia may be responsible for neurocardiogenic syncope.
- Pure I_{Kr} blockers may not reduce sudden death (SWORD and DIAMOND trials) because sympathetic stimulation may activate I_{Ks} and I_K.
- I_{Ks} blockers prolong APD and refractoriness but this effect is lost with sympathetic stimulation.
- Alpha blocking agents have no antifibrillatory effects.
- In post-MI patients left cardiac sympathetic denervation confers the same survival benefit as beta-blockers (3% mortality). Providing an alternative to patients who cannot take beta-blockers.
- Vagal stimulation decrease heart rate and ischemia induced lethal arrhythmias. These effects are reversed by atropine.
- Muscarinic agonists such as morphine, methacholine and oxotremorine reduce ischemic ventricular arrhythmias.
- Exercise training increases parasympathetic tone, increases heart rate variability, baroreflex sensitivity and decreases density of β-adrenergic receptor. In HRV low frequency component reflects sympathetic and high frequency component reflects vagal activity.

Baseline   V pacing   15 days later

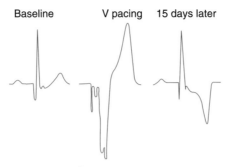

Figure 2.2 Cardiac memory T wave changes.

Cardiac memory[10,11]

- Cardiac memory (Figure 2.2) is characterized by a T-wave change that is neither primary (i.e., activation-dependent and following the vector of the QRS complex that preceded it) nor secondary (i.e., completely independent of the QRS complex and intrinsic to repolarization alone).
- It is a result of abnormal prior ventricular activation (due to pacing, preexcitation etc.) producing T-wave morphology that is maintained during subsequent sinus rhythm.
- It may be a manifestation of altered myocardial stretch.
- T wave "remembered" the abnormal QRS vector; hence the name cardiac memory.
- It has been noted in association with intermittent left bundle branch block, ventricular extrasystoles, right ventricular pacing, post-tachycardia syndrome, and ventricular pre-excitation.
- Cardiac memory is a form of electrocardiographic remodeling that occurs from altered cardiac stretch resulting in increased cardiac angiotensin II synthesis/release.
- Short-term memory results from angiotensin II-induced trafficking of an angiotensin1 receptor. This results in reduction of I_{to}.
- Long-term memory is initiated by angiotensin II binding to its receptor leading to reduction of the transcription factor cAMP response element binding protein (CREB).
- CREB phosphorylation and degradation, results in reduced KChIP2 transcription and expression and decreased I_{to}.
- $I_{Ca,L}$ and I_{Kr}. Connexin43 are also altered in memory.
- Short-term memory lasts for minutes to hours and long-term memory persists from weeks to months.
- Memory is not associated with altered coronary flow, ischemia, or structural remodeling.
- Altered ventricular stretch but not altered ventricular activation initiates memory.
- Altered stretch causes rapid synthesis/release of angiotensin II that engages stretch-initiated signal transduction pathways.

- Angiotensin II receptor blockade, angiotensin-converting enzyme inhibition, or tissue protease inhibition reduces the accumulation of short-term cardiac memory.
- The tissue protease involvement suggests the angiotensin II is locally synthesized rather than circulating.
- Calcium is an important cofactor in memory initiation.
- Nifedipine infusion prevents induction of short-term memory and chronic administration of amlodipine reduces the magnitude of long-term memory.
- AP notch is determined by the transient outward potassium current, I_{to}.
- I_{to} density is higher in epicardial than endocardial myocytes.
- Induction of short-term memory can be prevented by infusing 4-aminopyridine to block I_{to}. This may reduce the gradient between the epicardium and endocardium I_{to}.
- I_{to} might be critically involved in cardiac memory.
- I_{to} and angiotensin II initiates short-term memory via one mechanism (ion channel trafficking) and long-term memory via a second mechanism (gene transcription).
- Angiotensin II-induced trafficking of the channel carrying I_{to} is responsible for pacing induced stretch that lead to the T-wave change of short-term cardiac memory.
- Long-term memory is associated with increased APD in left ventricular epicardium , epicardial AP shows loss of the notch (determined by I_{to}) and endocardium, but not midmyocardium. This may be due to altered transmyocardial repolarization gradient.
- Neonates have no I_{to}, no action potential notch, and no pacing-induced cardiac memory. At approximately 6 weeks of age, I_{to}, the notch, and inducible memory evolve, and with advancing age and a larger I_{to}, memory is ever more inducible.

References

1 Metra M, Nodari S, Dei Cas L. Beta-blockade in heart failure: selective versus nonselective agents. *Am J Cardiovasc Drugs.* 2001;1(1):3–14.
2 Reiter MJ. Cardiovascular drug class specificity: beta-blockers. *Prog Cardiovasc Dis.* 2004;47(1):11–33.
3 Kvetnansky R, Sabban EL, Palkovits M. Catecholaminergic systems in stress: structural and molecular genetic approaches. *Physiol. Rev.* 2009;89(2):535–606.
4 Taylor MRG, Bristow MR. The emerging pharmacogenomics of the beta-adrenergic receptors. *Congest Heart Fail.* 2004;10(6):281–288.
5 Brodde OE, Bruck H, Leineweber K, Seyfarth T. Presence, distribution and physiological function of adrenergic and muscarinic receptor subtypes in the human heart. *Basic Res. Cardiol.* 2001;96(6):528–538.
6 Dinicolantonio JJ, Hackam DG. Carvedilol: a third-generation β-blocker should be a first-choice β-blocker. *Expert Rev Cardiovasc Ther.* 2012;10(1):13–25.
7 Harvey RD, Belevych AE. Muscarinic regulation of cardiac ion channels. *Br. J. Pharmacol.* 2003;139(6):1074–1084.
8 Olshansky B, Sabbah HN, Hauptman PJ, Colucci WS. Parasympathetic nervous system and heart failure: pathophysiology and potential implications for therapy. *Circulation.* 2008;118(8):863–871.

9 Vassort G. Adenosine 5′-triphosphate: a P2-purinergic agonist in the myocardium. *Physiol. Rev.* 2001;81(2):767–806.

10 Rosen MR. Why T waves change: a reminiscence and essay. *Heart Rhythm.* 2009;6(11 Suppl):S56–61.

11 Ozgen N, Rosen MR. Cardiac memory: a work in progress. *Heart Rhythm.* 2009;6(4):564–570.

Answers to self-assessment questions

1 B
2 B
3 D
4 A
5 A
6 B
7 D
8 B
9 C
10 D
11 C

CHAPTER 3
Mechanisms of arrhythmias

Self-assessment questions

1 Osborn wave is least likely to be seen when
  A Transmural voltage gradient is present.
  B In the presence of hypothermia.
  C Hypercalcemia is present.
  D Following intracranial bleed.

2 Which of the following statements about delayed after-depolarization (DAD) is *incorrect*?
  A It is caused by inward currents produced by Ca overload.
  B Long AP durations favor DAD.
  C Occurs during phase 2 of APD.
  D Lidocaine may decrease the tendency for DAD.

3 Which of the following statement about early after-depolarization (EAD) is correct?
  A Occurs after the completion of the action potential (AP).
  B Occurs during tachycardia.
  C It is caused by reactivation of the I_{CaL} during plateau phase.
  D It is caused by Na channel blockers.

4 Arrhythmias due to re-entry occur when there is:
  A Prolongation of the phase 2 of AP.
  B Spontaneous depolarization during phase 4.
  C Sarcoplasmic reticulum Ca overload.
  D An area of slow conduction and unidirectional block present.

5 Which one of the following is not a characteristic of supernormal conduction?
  A The impulse conducts better than expected.
  B The impulse conducts when block was expected.
  C It is faster than normal.
  D It occurs during the recovery phase of APD.

Essential Cardiac Electrophysiology: The Self-Assessment Approach, Second Edition. Zainul Abedin.
© 2013 Blackwell Publishing Ltd. Published 2013 by Blackwell Publishing Ltd.

3.1 Conduction and block

Electrophysiology of action potential[1]

- Normal action potential duration (APD) is 180 ms.
- Maximum negative membrane potential is defined as a resting potential.
- I_K repolarizes the membrane to the resting potential.
- When the membrane potential reaches threshold level it results in the onset of the action potential (AP). When threshold stimulus excites the cell, I_{Na} depolarizes membrane at 382 V/s. This produces Phase 0 of AP. Phase 1 of AP is a result of early repolarization produced by I_{to}. Plateau phase is the phase 2 of AP.
- Phase 0 correlates with the onset of the QRS complex (Figure 3.1).
- I_{CaL} (inward current) supports AP plateau against repolarizing (outward current) I_k. I_{CaL} triggers calcium release from sarcoplasmic reticulum (SR) through calcium-induced calcium release (CICR).
- $I_{Na/Ca}$ pump, during repolarization, extrudes calcium, taking in three sodium ions for each calcium ion that is removed. This causes significant inward current, which slows repolarization and prolongs APD.
- I_{Kr} increases during early phase of AP. I_{Kr} is potassium selective.
- I_{Ks} attains a large magnitude during plateau phase. It is a major repolarizing current.
- End of the plateau phase heralds the beginning of phase 3 of AP. During this phase depolarizing Ca and Na currents decline and K currents enhance repolarization. End of phase 3 occurs when the resting potential is reached.

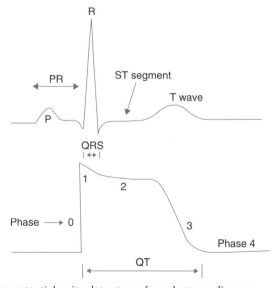

Figure 3.1 Action potential as it relates to surface electrocardiogram.

- Phase 3 correlates with the T waves on the surface electrocardiogram.
- Cells capable of producing spontaneous depolarization initiate phase 4 of AP.

Depolarizing and repolarizing currents[2]

- Inward movement of positive ion depolarizes cell by increasing the positive charge on the inner surface of the cell membrane as compared to the outer surface of the membrane. Outward movement of positive ions repolarizes the cell membrane by making the inner surface more negative than the outer surface.
- Potassium currents are outward currents.
- During plateau phase of action potential current flow activity is reduced, separating phase 2 from the phase 3 of AP.
- The length of the plateau phase of the AP determines the strength and duration of cardiac contraction and produces cardio protective window during which reexcitation by sodium and calcium channel cannot occur.
- A small net current is needed to maintain plateau and small change in current markedly influences the time course of plateau.
- Repolarization begins when net current flow turns outward either by increase in outward or by decrease in inward currents.
- Sinoatrial node cells have little inward rectifier current (I_{K1}) and large quantities of the "funny current" I_f, sometimes called "pacemaker current."
- Most currents are highly selective for a specific ionic species (e.g., Na⁺, K⁺, or Ca²⁺ for each respective channel type), I_f is relatively nonselective, with mixed permeability to both Na⁺ and K⁺[3].
- Each ion channel produces a current with a characteristic "reversal potential" that depends on the channel's permeability and ionic concentrations on either side of the membrane.
- A channel that is highly permeable to K⁺ and not to other ions, such as I_{K1}, allows only K⁺ to cross the cell membrane.
- K⁺ is much more concentrated inside than outside the cell, K⁺ ions will leave the cell through I_{K1} channels, and the loss of positively charged K⁺ will create a negative intracellular voltage charge.
- This negative intracellular charge attracts K⁺ and keeps it from leaving the cell, opposing the chemical force causing K⁺ to leave the cell. At a certain voltage level, the electrical force holding K⁺ inside the cell will be equal and opposite to the chemical force driving K⁺ out. The voltage at which this occurs is called the K⁺ "equilibrium potential" and under normal conditions is approximately −80 to −90 mV.
- The "reversal potential" is the voltage at which the electrical and chemical forces across a channel are balanced and no ionic movement occurs (no current passes across the channel). For channels that are highly selective to K⁺, the reversal potential is very close to the K⁺ equilibrium potential.
- For channels largely permeable to Na⁺ (e.g., those underlying phase 0 action potential upstroke), the reversal potential will be dominated by Na⁺, which is much more concentrated outside than inside the cell, creating a very positive equilibrium potential of approximately +60 mV.

- I_f channels, with mixed permeability to Na$^+$ and K$^+$, have a reversal potential between the equilibrium potentials of Na$^+$ and K$^+$, approximately -25 mV.
- I_f induces automaticity because it activates in a time-dependent way after cells repolarize during phase 3.
- Following repolarization, I_f begins to activate; as it does, it causes the intracellular potential to depolarize in the direction of the I_f equilibrium potential of approximately -25 mV. If I_f is sufficiently strong, the cell depolarizes to its threshold potential and generates spontaneous activity.
- The rate of spontaneous cellular activity depends on the amount of I_f but also on the amount of background K$^+$ current, I_{K1}.
- When I_{K1} is very strong (as in working ventricular muscle), a very large amount of I_f is needed to depolarize the cell because the large I_{K1} holds the cell very close to the K$^+$ equilibrium potential. That is why normal ventricular muscle shows little spontaneous automaticity.
- To induce spontaneous automaticity in ventricular muscle, either I_f can be enhanced or I_{K1} reduced, creating a balance in favor of spontaneous phase 4 depolarization.

Supernormal conduction
- During the recovery phase of APD supernormal conduction may exist when a subthreshold stimulus may evoke a response. Same stimulus may fail to produce response before or after supernormal conduction period.
- An impulse arriving during supernormal excitability conducts better than expected or conducts when block was expected. It is not faster than normal.
- Supernormal conduction depends on super normal excitability and exists only in Purkinje fibers not in the His bundle or myocardium. It may be noted in the presence of complete atrioventricular (AV) block.
- Supernormal conduction could be recorded in diseased cardiac tissue.
- Examples of improved AV conduction not due to supernormal conduction may be due to gap phenomenon, peeling of refractory period and dual AV nodal physiology.
- Period of supernormal excitability correlates with the end of T wave and the beginning of diastole.
- Supernormal conduction may manifest as unexpected normalization of bundle branch block at a shorter RR interval.
- PR interval remains unchanged or is shorter thereby excluding equal delay in both bundles as a cause of normalization of the QRS.
- In the presence of acceleration dependent aberration during atrial fibrillation (AF) or sinus rhythm with premature atrial contractions (PAC), supernormal conduction may manifest as normalization of QRS.
- An atrial impulse may propagate during supernormal period and result in displacement of subsidiary pacemaker due to concealed conduction.
- Duration of the preceding cycle length determines the location of supernormal conduction. Longer cycle length shifts the supernormal period distally.

- During AV block a sinus impulse may conduct or electronic pacemaker may capture during the period of supernormal excitability.

Concealed conduction

- It is characterized by unexpected behavior of subsequent impulse in response to incomplete conduction of a preceding electrical impulse. Its diagnosis is made by deductive analysis and exclusion of the other conduction abnormalities such as block of conduction.
- A concealed impulse may become intermittently manifest in the other parts of the same tracing.
- ECG reflects conduction and electrophysiologic properties of the myocardium.
- Propagation of an impulse through specialized conduction tissue is not recorded on surface electrocardiogram but can be inferred.
- Concealment is commonly encountered at the level of the AV node or bundle branches.

Exit Block[3]

- Exit block is commonly seen in sinoatrial, junctional and ventricular pacemakers.
- A repetitive pattern or group beating of type I or II periodicity is suggestive of exit block.
- Type I exit block presents with gradual shortening of the PP or RR interval with eventual failure to record a P or R wave. The resulting pause, which is less than the sum of two basic cycle lengths is typical of Wenckebach periodicity.
- Atypical Wenckebach delay may resemble sinus arrhythmia.
- Type II exit block is characterized by a pause that is multiple of basic cycle length.
- In a parasystole, failure of the impulse to manifest may be due to an exit block or physiologic refractoriness.

Gap junction[4]

- Gap junctions are responsible for intercellular transfer of current. Connexin 43 (CX43) is a major gap junction protein found in human atrium and ventricles.
- More than 50% reduction in CX43 produces slowing of conduction velocity.
- Gap junctions are located at or near the ends of working atrial and ventricular myocytes where intercalated discs connect adjacent cells.
- Longitudinal conduction velocity in myocardium is 0.7 m/s and transverse velocity of 0.2 m/s; the result is a substrate for anisotropic conduction.
- In crista terminalis ratio of longitudinal to transverse conduction is 10:1.
- Slow conduction in sinoatrial (SA) and AV nodes is due to small and sparsely distributed gap junctions.
- Gap junctions in Purkinje tissue facilitate rapid conduction.

- CX40 is a major conductor of intercellular currents in atrium. CX43 is a major conductor of intercellular current in ventricle.

Continuous and discontinuous conduction
- The difference between the electrical potential of excited and nonexcited tissue produces a flow of current.
- As the current flows through the cell membrane it shifts membrane potential to threshold potential by activating sodium and calcium currents.
- During normal propagation, sodium (inward) current provides charge for membrane depolarization except in AV and SA nodes.
- Delay in propagation may occur in gap junctions. Calcium inward current is essential for allowing the current to pass through the cell junction.
- Atrial trabeculation may contribute to conduction discontinuities.
- In the ventricle, connective tissue, hypertrophy, or the scar from myocardial infarction may add to discontinuities.
- Impedance of scar is lower then that of normal myocardium.
- Capillaries may contribute to anisotropic conduction.

Gap phenomenon
- The gap phenomenon in AV conduction is when AV block at longer coupling intervals is followed paradoxically by restored AV conduction at shorter coupling intervals. The proximal site is atrioventricular node and the distal site is His-Purkinje system.
- It can also occur at different sites in the conduction system.
- It occurs when the initial site of block is in the distal conduction system. As the coupling interval is further decreased, a critical delay occurs in the proximal conducting site, which gives the distal site time to recover excitability.
- Gap phenomenon occurs when the effective refractory period of the distal site is longer than the functional refractory period of the proximal site.

Electrical heterogeneity
- AP of ventricular epicardium and M cells shows prominent notch due to I_{to} mediated phase 1.
- Absence of notch in endocardium correlates with weaker I_{to}.
- Spike and dome morphology of AP is absent in the neonate. Its gradual appearance correlates with the appearance of I_{to}.
- I_{to2} is a calcium-activated chloride current.
- The magnitude of I_{to} and spike and dome in right ventricular epicardium is more prominent then in the left ventricular epicardium.

I_{to} and J wave
- Transmural voltage gradient between epicardium and endocardium due to I_{to} results in J wave (Osborn wave).
- Prominent J waves may occur in the presence of hypothermia and hypercalcemia.
- Occurrence of elevated J point may be due to transmural gradient and dispersion of early repolarization.

3.2 Automaticity[5,6]

- Automaticity occurs due to spontaneous diastolic depolarization as a result of inward Na currents or due to decay of outward K currents during phase 4 of AP.
- Normal automaticity occurs during physiologic conditions utilizing the currents that are normally involved in impulse generation. It is present in the SA node, some atrial tissue such as crista terminalis and Bachmann's bundle, the AV node and His Purkinje fibers.
- Ionic currents which are normally not involved in generating pacemaker current may produce these currents in the presence of disease state and cause abnormal automaticity and induce arrhythmias.
- Rate of impulse formation in the pacemaker cell depends on resting potential, slope of diastolic depolarization and threshold (take off) potential.
- Norepinephrine accelerates spontaneous depolarization of the SA node by stimulating β_1 receptors. Acetylcholine slows spontaneous depolarization via muscarinic receptors.
- Increase in adenylyl cyclase and cAMP and I_f current activity accelerates and decrease in the activity slows the sinus rate.
- Acetylcholine slows the sinus rate by opening $I_{K,ach}$, resulting in a more negative max diastolic potential.
- Ventricular myocytes also have pacemaker current (I_f). β stimulation increases pacemaker current in Purkinje fibers. Acetylcholine reverses the effects of β stimulation by reducing cAMP generated by β stimulation; it has no direct effect on pacemaker current.
- Pacemaker cell depolarization is inhibited when it is driven faster than its intrinsic rate (overdrive suppression). This is mediated by sodium/potassium exchange pump and possible inactivation of I_{CaL} current.
- Atrial and ventricular myocytes do not exhibit spontaneous diastolic depolarization.
- When membrane potential is depolarized to less then −60 mV spontaneous depolarization may occur (abnormal automaticity). This is mediated by slow inward calcium current.
- Decrease in membrane potential maybe due to ischemia.
- Extracellular Na and Ca may affect abnormal automaticity.
- Overdrive suppression is less likely to affect abnormal automaticity.

Pacemaker channels[2]
- Pacemaker channels are dominant in SA nodes and subsidiary pacemakers.
- Subsidiary pacemakers are located in AV nodes and Hi Purkinje fibers.
- Cells from SA node demonstrate steeper diastolic depolarization and therefore reach threshold earlier than subsidiary pacemakers, resulting in overdrive suppression of subsidiary cells.
- Diastolic depolarization is caused by activating inward currents or by deactivating outward currents. At least one of these currents is time dependent.
- Delayed rectifier (I_K I_{Kr} I_{Ks}) and I_f are present in the SA node.

- I_f is a hyperpolarizing current. Its conductance is increased by extracellular hyperkalemia.
- L and T type calcium currents are also present in pacemaker cells.
- Inward rectifying I_{K1} is present in Purkinje cells but not in the SA node. This current increases with elevated extracellular potassium, and may contribute to suppression of pacemaker activity in HPS during hyperkalemia.
- Decay of I_K appears to facilitate pacemaker current.

Autonomic regulation of pacemaker currents
- β agonists stimulates G protein through the β receptors located on the cell membrane. This increases the level of cAMP and promotes phosphorylation of I_{CaL}, I_f, I_K and $I_{Na/K}$ pump through protein kinase A, promoting an increase in heart rate as a result of increased in MDP (maximum diastolic potential) and increase in the slope of diastolic depolarization.
- Parasympathetic agonist acetylcholine activates muscarinic receptors.
- Acetylcholine, through G protein, activates inwardly rectifying $I_{K,ach}$, which makes MDP more negative and decreases slope of diastolic depolarization. This results in slowing of the heart rate.

Triggered activity[7]
- Triggered activity is initiated by after-depolarization. There are 2 types of after-depolarizations, early and delayed (EAD and DAD).
- EAD occurs before and DAD occurs after the completion of AP repolarization.

Delayed after depolarization (DAD)[8]
- DAD occurs after repolarization of AP. It is caused by inward currents produced by increase intracellular Ca load.
- Increase level of catecholamines and cAMP enhance Ca uptake and cause DAD in atrial and ventricular myocytes.
- Catecholamines increase sarcolemmal calcium by stimulating sodium/calcium exchange.
- Most common cause of DAD is digoxin. It inhibits sodium/potassium pump and leads to increased in intracellular calcium.
- Increase in extracellular ATP levels potentiates the DAD effect of catecholamines.
- Withdrawal of cholinergic stimulation increases calcium in atrial myocytes and may cause DAD.
- Longer APD favors DAD. Longer cycle length allows for more calcium entry into cells. Amplitude of the DAD depends on cycle length.
- Quinidine may increase DAD by prolonging APD. Lidocaine shortens APD, thereby decreasing DAD.

Sodium and calcium exchange and DAD
- Opening of voltage operated calcium channels, during plateau phase of APD, increases flux of calcium into cytoplasm, causing CICR from SR.

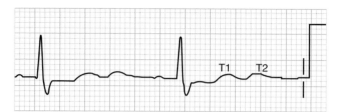

Figure 3.2 Bifid T wave.

- During diastole calcium is removed from the cell by sodium/calcium exchange pump, located in cell membrane.
- Lowering of pH blocks sodium/calcium exchange.
- SR calcium ATPase, sarcolemmal calcium ATPase and sodium/calcium exchange decrease cytoplasmic calcium from elevated systolic level to baseline diastolic level by pumping Ca back into SR or by extruding Ca from the cell.
- During calcium removal inwardly directed current $I_{Na/Ca}$ is observed, which may cause DAD.
- DAD occurs when there is pathologically high calcium load either due to digitalis toxicity or following reperfusion.
- Na/Ca exchange is able to transport calcium bidirectionally. Reverse mode will increase intracellular calcium, which may trigger SR calcium release.
- DAD is induced by spontaneous release of calcium from overloaded SR that in turn activates Na/Ca exchanger to extrude Ca from the cell. This generates, because of 3:1 ratio of Na/Ca exchange, large inward current that causes depolarization and DAD. I_{CaL} does not participate in DAD.
- It is likely that the arrhythmias documented during digitalis toxicity and those that occur during catecholaminergic polymorphic ventricular tachycardia share the same mechanism, and are probably triggered by DAD.
- DADs coincide with U waves.
- If the T wave is bifid the first component is labeled as T1 and second component as T2 (Figure 3.2).
- U wave occurs after the T wave has reached the baseline.
- Increased transmural dispersion of repolarization plays a role in degeneration of polymorphic ventricular tachycardia (VT) to ventricular fibrillation in CPVT.
- The ECG surrogate of transmural dispersion of repolarization is T peak to T end interval TPE. U waves is not included into this measurement, T2 should be distinguished from U wave.
- U waves are not often seen in leads I, aVR, and aVL, so measurement of the QT interval in these leads is unlikely to include U wave.
- High-amplitude T2 waves are the ECG correlates of early after-depolarizations.

Early after-depolarizations (EAD)[8–10]

Phase2 EAD
- EAD occurs when large inward current during plateau phase occurs resulting in prolongation of plateau. This provides time for reactivation of I_{CaL}. It is

this second phase of reactivation of inward I_{CaL} that produces EAD by depolarizing cell membrane.

- EAD does not require spontaneous release of calcium from SR and does not require inward activation of $I_{Na/Ca}$.
- I_{CaL} is a primary depolarizing factor responsible for EAD.
- A delicate balance between depolarizing and repolarizing currents controls the plateau phase of the AP. An increase in inward current and/or decrease in outward current may induce EADs. Examples include persistent inward I_{Na} in LQT3 and reduced I_{Kr} and I_{Ks} in LQT2 and LQT1, respectively[4].
- Once the plateau is prolonged reactivation of I_{CaL} induces EAD. This mechanism applies to phase 2 (plateau) EAD.
- EADs occur in Purkinje fibers and M cells of the myocardium.
- Other conditions that can cause EAD are bradycardia (which reduces outward current caused by delayed rectifier I_K), hypokalemia, and increased calcium current by sympathetic stimulation in the presence of ischemia or injury.
- Pharmacological agents such as potassium channel blockers (quinidine, sotalol), in the presence of hypokalemia and bradycardia prolong repolarization and induce EAD.
- I_{Kr} blockers such as erythromycin, and piperidine derivatives that block histamine H_1 receptors such as astemizole and terfenadine, and cisapride increase APD and cause EAD.
- Magnesium, Flunarizine and Ryanodine can abolish EAD by decreasing intracellular calcium load.
- EAD caused by inward sodium current are abolished by sodium channel blocker mexiletine.

Phase3 EAD
- These occur during fast repolarization and share the mechanism of DAD (spontaneous Ca release from SR and activation of the $I_{Na/Ca}$). They are called EAD because they occur before the completion of AP repolarization (Figure 3.3).
- EAD may occur during plateau phase and are caused by L type Ca current. EAD that occur during phase 3 of APD are due to Na/Ca exchange current.

His Purkinje electrical activity
- Conduction through the His bundle (conduction velocity 1–3 m/s) and bundle branches occurs during the isoelectric interval between the end of the P wave and the beginning of the QRS complex.
- Conduction through His Purkinje cells is little affected by vagal stimulation, epinephrine, or removal of stellate ganglia.
- Purkinje cells stain lightly, presumably due to the reduced, but still significant, myofibrillar content and enhanced glycogen. Electron microscopic studies show that Purkinje cells lack t-tubules.
- Connexin40 (CX40) protein is a Purkinje connexin isoform.
- A Purkinje fiber does not show automaticity when it is being overdriven by excitatory waves from the rapidly firing sinus node. This phenomenon, called overdrive suppression, results from enhanced electrogenic Na/K pump activity.

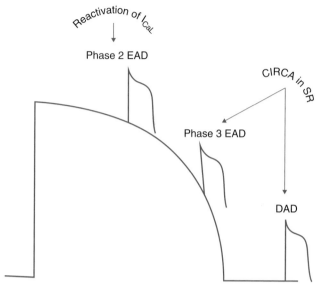

Figure 3.3 Mechanisms of EAD and DAD.

- I_f current in the Purkinje myocytes play a role in generating phase 4 depolarization and contributes to normal automaticity.
- I_f activation occurs in Purkinje cells at physiologic potentials (-80 to -130 mV), whereas in ventricular cells I_f activation occurs at more negative potentials (-120 to -170 mV).
- HCN4 and HCN2 proteins in Purkinje fibers characterize I_f current.
- Ryanodine and Thapsigargin suppress the Ca^{2+} wave and the accompanying membrane depolarization. This is an example of reverse excitation–contraction coupling, where intracellular Ca^{2+} produces a change in ionic conductances and resultant change in membrane voltage.
- Spontaneous Ca^{2+} release and ensuing Ca^{2+} waves modulate normal Purkinje cell pacemaker function.
- The mechanism of propagation is not electrical, but chemical. Ca^{2+} influx binds to Ca^{2+} release ryanodine receptor (RyR) channel. This leads to opening of the RyR channel and release of a greater amount of Ca^{2+} from the SR. This Ca^{2+} diffuses to adjacent RyR to cause further Ca^{2+} release from SR stores. Hence, released Ca^{2+} continues to propagate along a cell. This is called Ca^{2+}-induced Ca^{2+} release.
- A portion of the Ca^{2+} is pumped out of the cell via the Na/Ca exchanger, and the resulting current depolarizes the membrane. This current, Iti (transient inward current) causes DADs. It is dependent on Na/Ca exchange and Ca^{2+}-dependent chloride currents.
- Reactivation of the Ca^{2+} current and/or the late Na^+ current has been shown to produce the inward currents contributing to EADs observed during APs with prolonged repolarization. Such EADs occur in the relatively depolarized myocyte or Purkinje cell.

Torsades de Pointes (TDP)

- TDP is a polymorphic ventricular tachycardia associated with LQTS.
- Quinidine and hypokalemia produce EAD and triggered activity resulting in TDP. Initial event in TDP is EAD induced triggered activity.
- TDP often follows short–long–short cycle length.

Excitability and conduction

- Excitability is dependent on availability of sodium channels thus reduced Na channel activity will reduce excitability and conduction velocity.
- Reduced membrane excitability and reduced gap junction coupling slows conduction which may predispose to reentrant arrhythmias.
- Reduced gap junction coupling also slows conduction velocity which may allow I_{CaL} to induce inward depolarizing currents.
- I_{CaL} plays a dominant role in maintaining conduction in the setting of reduced coupling. While I_{Na} controls excitability, I_{CaL} influences conduction during reduced coupling.

Summary

- DADs occur during calcium over load due to Ca release from SR. This activates $I_{Na/Ca}$.
- EAD is generated by recovery and reactivation of I_{CaL}.
- Phase 3 EAD share mechanism of DAD.
- Slow conduction could be due to decrease membrane excitability or reduced gap junction coupling.
- Decrease in I_{Na} causes slow conduction, due to decreased excitability.
- Slow conduction due to decrease gap junction coupling requires contribution of IcaL.

3.3 Re-entry

- Size of re-entry circuit depends on tissue excitability.
- It suppresses normal pacemaker by overdrive suppression.
- Decreased conduction velocity, increase in refractory period and/or decrease in circuit length will make re-entry less likely.
- Decreasing wave length will increase the tendency to cause re-entry arrhythmias.
- Restitution is described as recovery of excitability after refractory period.
- Multiple re-entries may result in fibrillation.
- Re-entry wave dies when it reaches the border of medium.
- Spiral of re-entry wave may drift or it could be fixed (pin) around the obstacle.
- Re-entry can be anatomical (classic) or functional.
- If a stimulus enters a vulnerable window of an anatomical reentry circuit, it terminates the re-entry impulse.
- Functional re-entry is not terminated by entry of the stimulus inside the vulnerable window.
- Pacing induces a drift in re-entry circuit.

- Decrease in tissue excitability, by slowing conduction, eliminates re-entry.
- When electrical shock is applied to heart, the tissue near cathode (negative electrode) is depolarized (positive charge on the membrane) and tissue near anode (positive electrode) is hyperpolarized (negative charge on the membrane), terminating the arrhythmia.
- For initiation and maintenance of re-entry, anatomic or functional, unidirectional conduction block and the presence of excitable tissue ahead of the propagating wave front (excitable gap) are essential. Slowing of conduction or shortening of refractory period, or both, facilitate the establishment of an excitable gap.
- Half of all cell-to-cell connections are side to side and other half are end to end.
- Gap junction membrane provides resistance to current flow and produces slower conduction transversely than longitudinally, resulting in anisotropic conduction through the myocardium. Reduction in myocardial CX43 results in slowing of conduction velocity.
- During myocardial ischemia slowing of the conduction occurs due to changes in ion channel function and increase resistance at gap junctions. After 60 minutes of ischemia irreversible damage occurs to the gap junction membrane and CX43. This results in slowing and nonuniform conduction.
- Crista terminalis and pectinate muscle produce anisotropic conduction and act as facilitator of reentry. Conduction along the longitudinal axis of the crista and pectinate muscle is faster than along the horizontal axis.
- Crista and the Eustachian ridge act as anatomic barriers (isthmus) during re-entrant activation.
- Discordant activation of atrial epicardium and endocardium at faster rate promotes reentry.
- Crista, pectinate muscles, Backman bundle propagate sinus impulses rapidly.
- Ectopic beats may alter normal conduction and produce changes in refractoriness which promotes reentry.

Phase-2 re-entries (P2R)[2]

- Presence or absence of a spike-and-dome configuration of the AP depends on the balance of membrane currents that are active during the rapid early repolarization phase (phase 1), mainly the transient outward current (I_{to}), the sodium current (I_{Na}), and the current that dominates the beginning of the dome phase, i.e., the L-type calcium current (I_{CaL}).
- P2R refers to a particular type of ectopic discharge in which re-excitation is generated at the interface between cells showing a spike-and-dome action potential morphology and cells lacking such a dome and whose APD is abnormally abbreviated.
- Under such heterogeneous conditions electrotonically mediated re-excitation can be triggered during the dome phase (phase 2) and spread, either retrogradely or anterogradely.
- The P2R wave does not sustain fibrillation, but it can interact with other waves to precipitate VF/VT, as seen in the setting of Brugada syndrome and ischemia.
- Prominent outward current due to I_{to} results in shortening of the APD.

- This may occur during ischemia and may result in a decrease of the plateau phase of AP. These changes may occur nonuniformly throughout the myocardium and cause dispersion of repolarization and phase-2 re-entry.
- When I_{to}, an outward current, is dominant it results in APD shortening and loss of plateau of AP in some epicardial sites producing dispersion of repolarization. This results in local reexcitation and premature beats. This mechanism is termed as phase 2 re-entry.
- Phase 2 re-entry may occur in the presence of potassium channel opener pinacidil, sodium channel blockers flecainide, increased extracellular calcium and ischemia.
- I_{to} blockers restore homogeneity and abolish re-entrant activity.
- I_{to} is present in ventricular epicardium but not in endocardium. I_{to} is responsible for spike and dome morphology of AP in epicardium.
- Reduced activity of I_{Ks} in M cells prolongs APD. Bradycardia and class III drugs prolong APD in M cells and predispose to arrhythmias.
- Repolarization is sensitive to changes in heart rate.

3.4 Pharmacological differences in epicardium and endocardium

- Acetylcholine may alter the epicardial repolarization pattern by blocking I_{Ca} or activating I_{Kach}. It has no effect on I_{to}.
- Isoproterenol causes epicardial AP abbreviation more then it does in endocardium.
- Organic calcium channel blockers (verapamil) and the inorganic calcium channel blocker $MnCl_2$ can cause loss of AP plateau phase in epicardium but only slight abbreviation of AP in endocardium.
- Sodium current block decreases APD in epicardium.
- Block or decrease in calcium current leaves outward currents unopposed which may result in shortening of APD.
- I_{to} block may establish electrical homogeneity and abolish arrhythmias due to dispersion of repolarization caused by drugs and ischemia. Quinidine inhibits I_{to}.
- Amiloride, a potassium sparing diuretic, prolongs APD and refractoriness.
- M cells, found in mid myocardium of anterior and lateral wall and outflow tract of the ventricles, exhibit marked AP prolongation in response to bradycardia and on exposure to class III agents. This may be due to weaker I_{Ks} activity and stronger late I_{Na} activity.
- At slower rates M cells may contribute to pump efficiency because prolonged depolarization permits longer and more efficient contraction.
- Epicardium and endocardium electrically stabilize and abbreviate APD of M cells.
- Loss of either layer by infarction will lead to prolongation of APD. This maybe the mechanism by which QT prolongation and dispersion occurs in non-Q wave myocardial infarction (MI). These differences could be aggravated by drugs that prolong QT interval or in patients with LQTS.

- M cells play important role in the inscription of T waves by producing a gradient between epicardium, endocardium and M cells.
- U waves are due to repolarization of His Purkinje cells.

3.5 Post myocardial infarction arrhythmias

- Post MI hypertrophy of non-infarcted myocytes occurs by 3 weeks due to volume overload.
- Beta-blockers and angiotensin-converting enzyme (ACE) inhibitors may decrease post MI left ventricular hypertrophy.
- APD increases in left ventricular hypertrophy.
- In left ventricular hypertrophy, following ionic current changes occur that favor prolongation of APD and generation EAD:
  1 Decrease I_{to}.
  2 Decrease I_K.
  3 Delayed inactivation of I_{Ca}.
- DAD is easily induced in hypertrophied myocytes in the presence of increased calcium load and β adrenergic agonists.
- Increase intracellular Ca load occurs through Na/Ca exchange mechanism.
- Hyperpolarization activated current (I_f) and T type calcium currents also become active in hypertrophied myocytes.
- Non-homogeneous prolongation of the APD in left ventricular hypertrophy (LVH) results in dispersion of refractoriness and reentrant arrhythmias.
- *Acute* arrhythmias occur within few minutes of onset of ischemia.
- *Delayed* arrhythmias occur 5 to 48 hours after onset of MI. These arrhythmias may be due to abnormal automaticity of Purkinje fibers and may result in accelerated idioventricular rhythm.
- *Late* arrhythmias occur within few days to few weeks after MI; surviving cells within the zone of infarction demonstrate shortening of APD and diminished AP upstroke. Reentrant tachycardia can be easily induced.
- Post MI ventricular tachycardia originates in subendocardial region.
- Infarct size, surviving cells in MI zone, nonhomogeneous sympathetic denervation of myocardium distal to infarct are all arrhythmogenic.
- After successful reperfusion incidence of spontaneous ventricular tachycardia appears to be less then 1%; however inducible arrhythmias occur more frequently which suggests that the substrate for VT is present but triggers such as PVCs, ischemia and increase sympathetic activity may be absent.
- VT often occurs at the border between infracted and normal myocardium close to endocardium.
- Occurrence of the arrhythmias is facilitated by the presence of the *substrate* for arrhythmia such as scar or other conduction slowing abnormalities, electrical *triggers* such as PVCs, *electrical modulating factors* such as altered conduction, transmural dispersion of refractoriness and *physiologic modulating factors* such as ischemia, electrolyte abnormalities, hypoxia and proarrhythmic drugs.
- VF is due to multiple random reentries. Electrical shock results in elimination of these re-entries and renders large portion of myocardium unexcitable

resulting in a successful defibrillation. When 65% or more of myocardium is depolarized VF terminates.

- There is correlation between the shock strength that does not induce VF when applied on T wave during sinus rhythm and the shock energy that successfully defibrillates during VF.

Ionic basis for prolongation of APD in LVH

- Increased activity or slow inactivation of I_{CaL} does not contribute to prolongation of the APD.
- In hypertrophied myocytes there is decrease in density without the change in kinetics of I_{to}. Loss of I_{to} contributes to prolongation of APD.
- Na/Ca exchange generates inward current. This current is increased in LVH and may contribute to prolongation of APD.
- Hyperpolarization activated (I_f) current normally activates at −120 mV; however in hypertrophied myocytes it may activate at less negative potential and cause spontaneous diastolic depolarization.
- In post MI hypertrophy there is decrease in Connexin-43 (more so in endocardium then in epicardium) which results in inhomogeneous conduction.
- In the presence of LQT1 sympathetic stimulation prolongs QT interval and causes Torsades de Pointes. Sympathetic stimulation abbreviates APD in epicardium and endocardium but not in M cell resulting in transmural dispersion.
- Different responses of the three cell types to adrenergic stimulation are related to level of augmentation of I_{Ks}, which is strong in epicardium and endocardium and weak in M cells.
- Augmented I_{Ks} in epicardium and endocardium, but not in M cells, abbreviates APD and causes dispersion of repolarization and broad base T waves.
- D-Sotalol, an I_{Kr} blocker prolongs QT interval and mimics LQT2. It causes greater prolongation of APD in M cells and slows phase-3 repolarization in all cell layers of the myocardium, resulting in prolongation of QT interval and low amplitude T waves.
- Hypokalemia in the presence of I_{Kr} block, results in marked slowing of repolarization and low amplitude and notched T waves.
- Onset of the T wave corresponds to the onset of epicardial AP plateau. Final repolarization of epicardium causes peak of the second component of the T wave. Final repolarization of M cells defines the end of the T wave.
- ATX II augments late I_{Na} by slowing inactivation of I_{Na} and mimics LQT3. This delays onset of the T wave and causes marked prolongation of APD in M cells. M cells have a large late sodium current.

References

1 Wang Y, Rudy Y. Action potential propagation in inhomogeneous cardiac tissue: safety factor considerations and ionic mechanism. *Am. J. Physiol. Heart Circ. Physiol.* 2000;278(4):H1019–1029.
2 Mangoni ME, Nargeot J. Genesis and regulation of the heart automaticity. *Physiol. Rev.* 2008;88(3):919–982.

3 Ufberg JW, Clark JS. Bradydysrhythmias and atrioventricular conduction blocks. *Emerg. Med. Clin. North Am.* 2006;24(1):1–9, v.

4 Rohr S. Role of gap junctions in the propagation of the cardiac action potential. *Cardiovasc. Res.* 2004;62(2):309–322.

5 Dobrzynski H, Boyett MR, Anderson RH. New insights into pacemaker activity: promoting understanding of sick sinus syndrome. *Circulation.* 2007;115(14):1921–1932.

6 Zipes DP. Mechanisms of clinical arrhythmias. *J. Cardiovasc. Electrophysiol.* 2003; 14(8):902–912.

7 Qi X, Yeh Y-H, Chartier D, et al. The calcium/calmodulin/kinase system and arrhythmogenic afterdepolarizations in bradycardia-related acquired long-QT syndrome. *Circ Arrhythm Electrophysiol.* 2009;2(3):295–304.

8 Huffaker R, Lamp ST, Weiss JN, Kogan B. Intracellular calcium cycling, early after depolarizations, and reentry in simulated long QT syndrome. *Heart Rhythm.* 2004; 1(4):441–448.

9 Gilmour RF Jr. Early afterdepolarization-induced triggered activity: Initiation and reinitiation of reentrant arrhythmias. *Heart Rhythm.* 2004;1(4):449–450.

10 el-Sherif N. Early afterdepolarizations and arrhythmogenesis. Experimental and clinical aspects. *Arch Mal Coeur Vaiss.* 1991;84(2):227–234.

Answers to self-assessment questions

1 D
2 C
3 C
4 D
5 C

CHAPTER 4

Sinus node dysfunction and AV blocks

Self-assessment questions

1 Which of the following currents does not contribute to the AP of the SAN?
  A I_{CaL}
  B I_{Na}
  C I_f
  D I_{to}

2 What are the characteristics of type I SA exit block?
  A There is progressive lengthening of the PP interval preceding the pause.
  B Duration of the pause is less than the sum of the two preceding sinus beats.
  C It is caused by non-conducted PACs.
  D It may progress to complete AV block.

3 A 65-year-old man presents with an AV block in which the PR interval of all captured complexes are constant in spite of varying RP intervals. These characteristics are suggestive of which type of AV block?
  A Type I second degree AV block.
  B Fascicular block.
  C Type II second degree AV block.
  D Functional block.

4 Which one of the following statements is incorrect regarding paroxysmal AV block?
  A It occurs below the His bundle.
  B It is initiated by concealed conduction of the P waves.
  C Resumption of the normal conduction is due to peeling of the refractory period.
  D Permanent pacing is not indicated.

Essential Cardiac Electrophysiology: The Self-Assessment Approach, Second Edition. Zainul Abedin.
© 2013 Blackwell Publishing Ltd. Published 2013 by Blackwell Publishing Ltd.

5 A 65-year-old female presents with acute anterior MI. RBBB, left anterior fascicular block and intermittent complete AV block. What are the likely characteristics of this AV block?

A Permanent pacemaker is indicated.

B Mortality is less than 5%.

C Complete AV block is preceded by progressive changes in AV conduction.

D Site of the AV block is in AV node.

6 A 25-year-old male was admitted to a hospital following an episode of syncope. He was diagnosed to have myotonic dystrophy 5 years ago. Echocardiogram revealed left ventricular hypertrophy. Most likely cause of his syncope is:

A Ventricular tachycardia.

B Preexcitation.

C Seizure disorder.

D Complete AV block.

7 A 72-year-old male had an episode of syncope. Perfusion studies and the echocardiogram are normal. ECG rhythm strip, recorded during a syncopal episode is shown below.

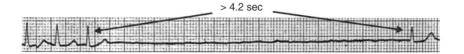

Which of the following is the most appropriate choice of therapy?

A Dual chamber permanent pacemaker implant.

B Biventricular pacemaker implant.

C VVI pacemaker implant.

D Oral theophylline administration.

8 The ECG shown below was recorded in an 81-year-old patient who presented with episodes of dizziness. What is the likely diagnosis?

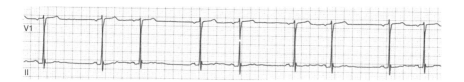

A Type 1 sino atrial exit block.

B Type 1 second degree AVN block.

C Type II Sino atrial exit block.

D Non conducted PACs.

9 Blockade of HCN4 channel is likely to produce
   A Sinus tachycardia.
   B Hypotension.
   C Sinus bradycardia.
   D Premature ventricular complexes.

10 Which one of the following is least likely to be present in a patient with inappropriate sinus tachycardia?
   A Resting heart rate of more than 100 bpm.
   B Increased circulating immunoglobulin G (IgG) autoantibodies to β-adrenergic receptor.
   C P wave morphology similar to sinus P wave.
   D Sweating, tremors and TSH level of 0.02.

11 A patient presents with 2:1 AV block. Which one of the following electrocardiographic characteristics likely to favor the diagnosis of type II second-degree AV block?
   A PR interval <0.16 seconds.
   B A normal QRS morphology.
   C Nonconducted PAC and concealed conduction.
   D Presence of Atrial fusion beats.

12 A 55-year-old female patient presents with syncope. Following electrocardiographic tracing was recorded while she was being monitored in telemetry. Which one of the following is the most appropriate explanation of these electrocardiographic finding

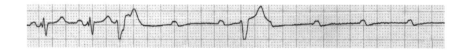

   A Tachycardia dependent phase 3 AV block.
   B Pause dependent phase 4 AV block.
   C Vagal AV block.
   D Concealed conduction.

13 A 68-year-old woman presents for a routine evaluation. She has no complaints other than arthritis in her back. She is active and participates in yoga classes three times per week. Her medications include levothyroxine for hypothyroidism and hydrochlorothiazide for hypertension. On physical examination, her pulse is 46/min. On further questioning, she notes that during a yoga class, she experienced palpitations. She undergoes 24-hour electrocardiographic monitoring, which demonstrates a heart rate between 39 and 82/min, with an average of 45/min, and occasional pauses of up to 2.9 seconds. Her laboratory data include a normal thyroid-stimulating hormone level.

Which is the best management option for this patient?

A Pacemaker implantation.

B Exercise stress test.

C Electrophysiologic study.

D Reassurance and observation.

14 A 50-year-old man was admitted to the hospital following a broken ankle. While the patient was asleep sinus bradycardia at a rate of 30 bpm, nonsustained ventricular tachycardia, and episodes of nonsustained atrial tachycardia were recorded. Patient is not aware of any arrhythmias.

What will be your recommendations?

A Prescribe metoprolol.

B Start warfarin.

C Implant permanent pacemaker.

D Order a sleep study.

15 In human sinus node cells, the pacemaker current, I_f, is generated by which of the following?

A L type calcium channel.

B Sodium channel HCN5A.

C T type calcium channel.

D Hyperpolarization activated cyclic nucleotide gated channel (HCN4).

4.1 Sinoatrial node[1]

- Upstroke velocity of the action potential (AP) in the sinoatrial node (SAN) cells is 4–9 V/s. The maximum diastolic potential (MDP) is –40 to –70 mV. AP amplitude is 70–80 mV. The action potential duration (APD) is 100–120 ms.
- I_f current is activated at less then –50 to –60 mV. It is an inward current, carried by Na and K ions (decay of I_K).
- I_f current is found in spider cells. It is a safety current.
- I_{CaL} is responsible for upstroke of AP. It is activated in the last third of diastolic depolarization. Block of I_{CaL} stops spontaneous depolarization.
- I_{CaT} is present in SAN cells, has more a negative threshold and more rapid rate of inactivation.
- I_{Na} does not contribute to AP in SAN, more positive MDP of the pacemaker cells inactivates this current; however in the presence of hyperpolarizing agents such as acetylcholine it may contribute to increased upstroke.
- $I_{Nab'}$ is a background inward current selective for sodium and potassium. Like I_f current it contributes to spontaneous depolarization.
- I_K is also present in pacemaker cells and influences APD by the rate of its inactivation. Blockade of this current may cause loss of spontaneous activity in pacemaker cells.
- $I_{K,ach}$ is present in pacemaker cells. It is a strong outward current and is responsible for hyperpolarization of the membrane.
- I_{to} and I_{K1} are not present in pacemaker cells. Absence of I_{K1} in pacemaker cells is responsible for diastolic depolarization.
- $I_{Na/K'}$ a sodium/potassium pump current, produces significant outward current during diastolic depolarization. It can be blocked by ouabain.
- Sodium calcium, exchanger $I_{Na/Ca'}$ contributes to diastolic depolarization and produces increase inward current in later third of diastolic depolarization. Elimination of these currents stops spontaneous activity.
- Adrenergic stimulation increases I_{CaL} and I_f.
- Cholinergic stimulation decrease I_{CaL} and I_f by shifting activation to more negative potential.
- I_{CaL} block slows the rate of propagation velocity in pacemaker cells but not in the atrium.
- Cholinergic stimulation activates $I_{K,ach}$ and hyperpolarizes SA cells by producing outward current. This outward current can result in sinus arrest and make cells unexcitable to normal levels of the currents.
- Adrenergic and cholinergic activity is modulated by β_1 and M_1 receptors respectively. These receptors activate and increase level of the cAMP.
- SA node has large number of the β_1 receptors, which play a role in chronotropic response.
- Increase in atrial pressure increases the heart rate by stimulating mechanically sensitive ion channels. This phenomenon is called *Bainbridge effect*.
- The sinoatrial node remodels with age, increasing the risk for bradycardia and atrial fibrillation (AF). The underlying substrate may involve a reduction in

the density of L-type Ca current in the sinoatrial node and in CaV1.2 protein.

Sinus tachycardia and SA re-entry tachycardia

- The sinus node is located in epicardial groove of sulcus terminalis and its activity may extend along crista terminalis. The sinus node artery runs through the center of the node.
- With increasing heart rate the site of impulse formation moves superiorly and with decreasing rate it shifts inferiorly.
- The resting potential of sinus pacemaker cells is −55 mv.
- Parasympathetic stimulation decreases sinus rate while sympathetic stimulation increases it.
- Common causes of sinus tachycardia include fever, anemia, hypotension, hyperthyroidism and drugs such as atropine, catecholamines, caffeine, nicotine, aminophylline and amphetamines.
- A high resting heart rate (>100 bpm) confers higher risk of cardiac mortality than a low resting heart rate (≤60 bpm).
- The increased risk is comparable to the risk that arises from moderately severe left ventricular dysfunction.
- An elevated resting heart rate has same predictive value for mortality as hypertension, diabetes or a prior myocardial infarction.
- *CASQ2* mutations causes sinus bradycardia.

Inappropriate sinus tachycardia[2]

- Persistent sinus tachycardia in the absence of any identifiable cause is called inappropriate sinus tachycardia (IST). Possible mechanisms include:
  1 Autonomic dysfunction increased sympathetic and/or decreased parasympathetic tone.
  2 Abnormal sinus node automaticity.
  3 Atrial tachycardia arising in close proximity of the sinus node.
  4 Increased circulating immunoglobulin G (IgG) autoantibodies to β-adrenergic receptor may induce a persistent increase in cAMP production.
  5 The tachycardic effect of β-receptor autoantibodies is inhibited by propranolol.
- Unpredictable sudden onset suggests presence of atrial tachycardia.
- Diagnostic features of inappropriate sinus tachycardia include:
  ○ Resting heart rate is more than 100 bpm.
  ○ P wave morphology similar to sinus P wave.
  ○ Persistent tachycardia in the absence of any physiologic cause.
- Symptoms include palpitation, near syncope and exercise intolerance.
- It is common in females. It is not associated with mitral valve prolapse.
- Diagnostic evaluation includes EKG, 24-hour Holter monitor, stress test and assessment of intrinsic heart rate using autonomic blockade by IV administration of 0.2 mg/kg of propranolol and 0.4 mg/kg of atropine.
- Intrinsic heart rate = 118.1 − (0.57 × age).

- Electrophysiologic study may be helpful in excluding atrial tachycardia or sinus node reentry tachycardia.
- Reentrant tachycardias are induced by extra stimulus.
- Most right atrial tachycardias arise from crista terminalis. With adrenergic stimulation the rate of atrial tachycardia increases without any shift of the focus. Onset is often abrupt.
- In IST, rate and focus shift gradually with adrenergic stimulation.

Treatment of IST[2-4]
- Ivabradine, a HCN4 blocker, specifically inhibits the pacemaker current (I_f) in the sinoatrial node and lower heart rate. The does is 5–10 mg daily.
- Other treatment options include beta-blockers and/or calcium channel blockers.
- Amiodarone, propafenone and flecainide decrease SN automaticity and may be useful in severe cases.
- Successful radiofrequency ablation of IST or sinus node modification remains difficult. Although short-term success rates may be favorable (range 76–100%), long-term outcomes are disappointing.
- The endpoint of successful sinus node ablation remains unclear. Heart rate below 80 to 90 bpm, with or without isoproterenol infusion (usually 1–2 µg/min), at the conclusion of the procedure are considered as reasonable end points.
- Most of the cardiac and extracardiac symptoms persist despite documented slower heart rates suggesting that sinus tachycardia and symptoms of palpitations are likely secondary manifestations of autonomic dysregulation.
- Three dimensional mapping or intracardiac echocardiography in localizing the crista, may improve the outcome of the ablation.
- Surgical or radiofrequency ablation of the SA node and insertion of permanent pacemaker may be considered. Fatigue, awareness of the paced rhythm and other symptoms may persist in spite of rate reduction.
- To avoid diaphragmatic paralysis high output pacing should be performed with ablation catheter along the crista terminalis before delivering RF current.
- The clinical features of inappropriate sinus tachycardia significantly overlap with postural orthostatic tachycardia syndrome (POTS).
- A multidisciplinary approach involving neurologist, cardiovascular rehabilitation and psychiatrist may be necessary in managing patients with inappropriate sinus tachycardia[4].

Sinus node dysfunction (SND)[1]
- Sick sinus syndrome (SSS) refers to a spectrum of cardiac arrhythmias that includes sinus arrest, sinoatrial block, sinus bradycardia, or alternating paroxysmal atrial tachyarrhythmias with bradycardia (tachy-brady syndrome).
- When the SAN fails to initiate the heartbeat, other subsidiary sites take over and become the dominant pacemaker.
- In the SAN cells, the mechanism of spontaneous diastolic depolarization has been attributed to hyperpolarization-activated pacemaker current (I_f).
- Ca^{2+} release from the sarcoplasmic reticulum (SR) contributes to depolarization.

Box 4.1 Extrinsic causes of SND

Hypothyroidism.
SAN or atrial ischemia.
Postatrial surgery.
Medications: Antiarrhythmics: Class I agents, amiodarone
　　　　　Beta-blockers.
　　　　　Ca channel blockers
　　　　　H2 receptor blockers: ranitidine, cimetidine
　　　　　Psychotropic drugs: lithium, tricyclic antidepressants,
　　　　　phenothiazines.
Neurologic diseases: Myotonic dystrophy, Emery–Dreifuss syndrome,
　　　　　tuberous sclerosis
Infiltrative disorders: Amyloidosis, hemochromatosis, systemic lupus,
　　　　　sarcoidosis, lymphoma
Myocarditis
Familial
Carotid sinus hypersensitivity
Increased vagal tone
Jaundice
Hypothermia
Elevated intracranial pressure

Causes of SND
- Intrinsic (primary) SND may result from fibrosis, ageing related loss of pacemaker cells.
- Extrinsic (secondary) causes of SND are listed in Box 4.1.

Pathophysiology
- The sinus node is located near the superior anterolateral portion of right atrium near the superior vena cava junction and the superior end of crista terminalis.
- Cells in the SAN demonstrate diastolic depolarization and its AP is calcium channel-dependent. Phase 0 demonstrates slow upstroke velocity.
- SAN cells do not have connexin-43 gap junctions.
- Impulses may originate along crista. With sympathetic stimulation the source of impulse formation shifts more superiorly and with vagal stimulation it shifts more inferiorly.
- The primary pacemaker area is located in the center of the node. Sympathetic and parasympathetic nerves innervate it.
- AP of the pacemaker cells is characterized by phase 4 depolarization, relatively positive maximum diastolic potential and slow upstroke velocity.
- Phase 4 depolarization is the result of four different ionic currents.
  1 Decay of I_K delayed rectifier
  2 Increase I_f inward current

3 Inward calcium current.

4 Background current.

- Sympathetic stimulation enhances phase 4 depolarization by increasing I_f and I_{Ca}.
- Parasympathetic stimulation decreases phase 4 depolarization.
- Drugs causing negative chronotropic response aggravate SND.
- Sensitivity to parasympathetic transmitters increases with age.
- Increase in AP duration of atrial myocardium may cause bradycardia this may be mechanism of bradycardia in long QT syndrome.
- Bradycardia-related dispersion of refractoriness may result in tachyarrhythmia.

Clinical manifestations

- SAN intrinsic rate decreases as number of cells decline with increasing age.
- Long pauses may occur due to exit block from SAN after PAC or termination of the tachycardia. This may result in syncope or near syncope. Bradycardia may cause fatigue and/or dyspnea.
- Atrial asystole may predispose to thromboembolic complications.
- SND may present as abnormality of impulse formation such as bradycardia or sinus arrest or as abnormality of impulse conduction such as exit block or loss of physiologic responsiveness such as chronotropic incompetence.
- Sinus node dysfunction could be intrinsic due to structural disease of the sinus node or it could be due to extrinsic influences (Box 4.1).
- Bradycardia, SA exit block, sinus arrest, chronotropic incompetence, atrial fibrillation or arrhythmias are the common manifestations of SND.
- SND may appear intermittently.
- Extrinsic factors causing sinus bradycardia include carotid sinus syndrome, vasovagal syncope and increase vagal tone.
- Bradycardia may cause fatigue, or dyspnea. Palpitations or embolism may occur due to AF.
- Carotid sinus pressure or tilt test may uncover abnormalities.
- Carotid sinus hypersensitivity, sternocleidomastoid denervation syndrome and neurocardiogenic syncope may coexist with SND.

Electrocardiographic characteristics of SND

- Persistent sinus bradycardia, in the absence of drugs, is common.
- Sinus pause of 3 seconds or more may occur (Figure 4.1). Duration of the pause is not multiple of basic heart rate. Fallowing the pause heart rate may accelerate (not seen in exit block).
- Nonconducted PAC may mimic sinus pauses.
- SA exit block is a common manifestation of SND. In type 1 SA exit block there is progressive shortening of the PP interval preceding the pause. The pause is less than the sum of two preceding sinus cycle lengths.
- In type 2 SA block the pause is equal to multiple of sinus cycle length (Figure 4.2).
- In SND there may be concomitant suppression of subsidiary pacemaker.

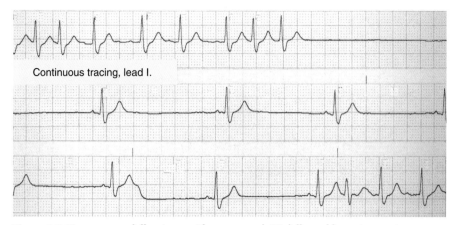

Continuous tracing, lead I.

Figure 4.1 Sinus pauses following rapid paroxysmal AF, followed by extreme sinus bradycardia. Typical of "Brady Tachy" syndrome.

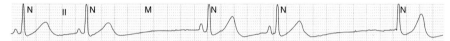

Figure 4.2 SA exit block.

Diagnosis
- Exercise test may uncover chronotropic incompetence.
- Administration of adenosine bolus, if results in slowing of sinus cycle length, by more than 2 standard deviations, is indicative of SND.
- Sinus node recovery time (SNRT) is an interval from the last paced beat to first sinus impulse. It is considered abnormal if it exceeds 1400 ms.
- Corrected SNRT is derived by subtracting base line sinus cycle length from SNRT. A CSNRT of greater than 530 ms is considered abnormal.
- CSNRT, if divided by 2, yields sinoatrial conduction time (SACT). Normal SACT ranges from 70 to 120 ms.
- Atropine by decreasing vagal tone and enhancing retrograde conduction into the SN may worsen SNRT.
- Low intrinsic heart rate after autonomic blockade is suggestive of SND.
- After complete autonomic blockade the intrinsic heart rate can be calculated by $118.1 - (0.57 \times age)$.
- During electrophysiologic study a normal corrected sinus node recovery time does not exclude the possibility of SND.

Prognosis and treatment
- Prognosis is good; however occurrence of stroke in the presence of AF, congestive heart failure and atrioventricular (AV) block may alter the outcome.
- Atrial based pacing for symptomatic bradycardia lowers the incidence of AF, thromboembolic events and congestive heart failure.
- Atrial based pacing should be considered for symptomatic patients. Incidence of AV block is 1% per year.

- Drugs responsible for bradycardia should be discontinued.
- DDD pacing should be considered for patient with His Purkinje disease and neurocardiogenic syncope.
- Pacing may allow use of antiarrhythmic drugs.
- Anticoagulation should be considered in the presence of atrial flutter/fibrillation.
- Anticholinergics, sympathomimetic or methylated xanthines can be used for patients with mildly symptomatic bradycardia.
- Discontinuation of offending agents, treatment of hypothyroidism, and use of vagolytic agents or theophylline may be helpful in short term.
- VVI pacemaker implant is the treatment of choice for patients who present with pause related syncope but otherwise have normal AV node conduction.

4.2 Atrioventricular node (AVN) anatomy and electrophysiology[5,6]

- The AVN is located in triangle of Koch, bound by tendon of Todaro, orifice of the CS and septal leaflet of the tricuspid valve.
- There are anterior and posterior inputs to the AVN from the atrium.
- There are two types of cells in the AVN: rod and ovoid-shaped cells.
- Spontaneous activity correlates with I_f current, which is far greater in ovoid cells.
- I_{Na} and I_{to} are present in rod cells.
- AVN conduction delay is inversely related to the prematurity of the impulse that it receives from the atrium.
- Occurrence of longer S2–H2 interval with shorter S1–S2 is due to slow recovery of excitability of N cells.
- Slow AVN pathway (posterior input) is located posteriorly and inferiorly between orifice of the CS and septal leaflet of the tricuspid valve.
- Fast pathway is located anteriorly and superiorly in the interatrial septum. It has shorter distance to travel to AVN but demonstrates longer ERP.
- Sudden change in AH interval with minimal change in input interval may be due to shift of conduction from anterior (fast) to posterior (slow) pathway.
- After successful elimination of the AVNRT, discontinuous conduction may still be present.
- In AF slow pathway elimination may not alter heart rate if impulse can reach the AVN via another route.
- Subthreshold stimuli delivered in the triangle of Koch causes postganglionic release of acetylcholine, resulting in hyperpolarization of N cells and slowing AVN conduction.
- The function of the AVN can be summarized as follows:
  1 Synchronization of the atrial and ventricular contractions with appropriate delay.
  2 Protection of the ventricles from excessive rates in case of an atrial tachyarrhythmia.
  3 As a back-up pacemaker in case of sinus node dysfunction.
- Conduction from the atria to the ventricles or the reverse occurs via a number of atrionodal connections.

- The fast pathway is located outside the triangle of Koch, superior to the tendon of Todaro, and is connected with the AVN by transitional cells inserting into the common AV bundle distal to most of the compact AVN.
- The slow pathway is located within the triangle of Koch, between the tricuspid annulus and the ostium of the coronary sinus, and is connected with the compact AVN by the rightward posterior extension of the AVN.
- There is evidence for an additional slow pathway that does not run between the tricuspid annulus and the ostium of the coronary sinus but is connected with the compact AVN by its leftward posterior extension.
- In AF, a complete AV block can be created by ablating all atrionodal inputs while AV-junctional rhythm is still manifest.
- Blocking of I_f current slowed the spontaneous rate of pacemakers in the AV nodal region three times more than it slowed the rate of pacemakers in the sinoatrial node.
- HCN4 is the major isoform of I_f. Regions of the inferior right atrium and the tricuspid and mitral valves left atrial appendage and left atrial wall have automatic properties perhaps related to expression of I_f.

Left bundle branch block (LBBB)

- Normal ventricular activation proceeds rapidly via Purkinje fibers, resulting in synchronous activation of both ventricles.
- In LBBB, right ventricular activation precedes left ventricular activation. Left ventricular activation may proceed via slow right to left transseptal activation or via slow left bundle branch conduction.
- Intraventricular conduction delay adds to abnormal left ventricular activation, resulting in interventricular and intraventricular dyssynchrony and impairment of cardiac function.
- LBBB adversely affects patients who present with myocardial infarction because:
  1 Diagnosis of myocardial infarction in the presence of LBBB can be difficult, potentially leading to delayed diagnosis and a delay or lack of appropriate therapy.
  2 Combination of myocardial infarction and LBBB tend to have higher in-hospital mortality.
  3 Presence of new LBBB is associated with heart failure perhaps due to ventricular dyssynchrony.
  4 LBBB is a predictor of nonfatal myocardial infarction.

Right bundle branch block (RBBB)

Mechanisms of intermittent RBBB

First- and second-degree RBBB
- Analogous to traditional first- and second-degree AV block there could be an ECG pattern of "complete" or 1:1 right BBB during sinus rhythm, on the basis of first-degree right bundle branch delay (rather than block).

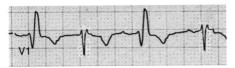

Figure 4.3 2:1 block at right bundle.

- This may manifest by repetitive delayed (but not blocked) anterograde conduction into the right bundle branch. During sinus rhythm, conduction delay may allow ventricular activation to be completed solely via the left bundle branch. However, delayed conduction (first-degree block) and refractoriness in the right bundle branch may prevent transseptal retrograde penetration of depolarization of the right bundle branch system.
- As in first-degree AV "block" where an increase in the atrial rate may induce second-degree AV block, a similar mechanism could account for the transition from first- to second-degree 2:1 RBBB driven by an increase in rate (phase 3, 2:1 RBBB). During 2:1 RBBB, every alternate impulse may block (rather than delayed) in the right bundle branch. The block in the right bundle branch may provide sufficient time for refractoriness to recover so that the next beat could be conducted normally along the right bundle branch (Figure 4.3).

Linking
- The term linking is used specifically to describe the mechanism for perpetuation of functional anterograde BBB, namely, repetitive transseptal retrograde concealed penetration by impulses propagating along the contralateral bundle.
- Linking is known to occur during functional 1:1 BBB (sustained for at least several consecutive beats) in orthodromic AV reentrant and AV nodal reentrant tachycardia.

Electrical alternans or aberrancy
- Rate-related aberrancy of every other beat (based on cycle length alternans) may manifest as intermittent bundle branch block.

Bradycardia-dependent BBB
- Phase 4 bradycardia-dependent block may be responsible for BBB of alternate beats.

Alternating bundle branch block
- Whereas alternating bundle branch block at slow heart rates without an intervening normal QRS is pathologic and requires a pacemaker, alternating bundle branch block during rapid heart rates interrupted by a single normal QRS is not uncommon and is physiologic.

HCN4 chanellopathy and sinus bradycardia[3]
- The hyperpolarization-activated nucleotide-gated channel HCN4 plays a major role in diastolic depolarization of SAN cells. Mutant HCN4 channels have been found to be associated with inherited sinus bradycardia.

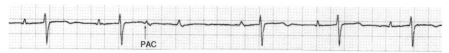

Figure 4.4 PAC resulting in concealed conduction and blocked sinus beat.

- Despite its critical location, this mutation carries a favorable prognosis without the need for pacemaker implantation during long-term follow-up.
- Deletion in *RYR2*, which leads to extended clinical phenotypes (e.g., SAN and AVN dysfunction, AF, atrial standstill, and dilated cardiomyopathy).
- The density of the major current determining the sinoatrial nodal action potential, the L-type calcium current, decreases with age.
- Omega-3 polyunsaturated fatty acids (ω-3 PUFAs) found in fish oils lower resting heart rate.
- HCN blockers such as ivabradine are able to slow heart rate without other cardiovascular side effects.

Concealed conduction
- It is characterized by unexpected behavior of subsequent impulse in response to incomplete conduction of a preceding electrical impulse. Its diagnosis is made by deductive analysis and exclusion of the other conduction abnormalities such as block of conduction (Figure 4.4).
- A concealed impulse may become intermittently manifest in the other parts of the same tracing.
- ECG reflects conduction and electrophysiologic properties of the myocardium.
- Propagation of an impulse through specialized conduction tissue is not recorded on surface electrocardiogram but can be inferred.
- Concealment is commonly encountered at the level of AVN or bundle branches.

Exit block
- Exit block is commonly seen in sinoatrial, junctional and ventricular pacemakers.
- A repetitive pattern or group beating of type I or II periodicity is suggestive of exit block.
- Type I exit block presents with gradual shortening of the PP or RR interval with eventual failure to record a P or R wave. The resulting pause, which is less than the sum of two basic cycle lengths is typical of Wenckebach periodicity.
- Atypical Wenckebach delay may resemble sinus arrhythmia.
- Type II exit block is characterized by a pause that is multiple of basic cycle length.
- In a parasystole, failure of the impulse to manifest may be due to an exit block or physiologic refractoriness.
- If a tachycardia presents with two different cycle lengths in which short CL is longer then basic CL and long CL is less than sum of two basic CL and sum of short and long CL equal three basic CL, then 3:2 type I exit block is present.

Box 4.2 Causes of variable PR interval

1 Intermittent conduction over slow pathway
2 Intermittent conduction over accessory pathway
3 Type I (Wenckebach) AV block
4 Concealed conduction from premature beats in to AV junction
5 Intermittent junction rhythm and AV dissociation
6 High adrenergic/vagal tone
7 Paced rhythm with dynamic AV delay

AV block and AV dissociation[7]

- Brady arrhythmias may be responsible for sudden cardiac death in up to 20% of patients.
- This may be due to asystole resulting from AV block without escape rhythm or due to torsades de pointes in the setting of repolarization abnormalities.
- AV dissociation can be due to AV block or due to physiologic refractoriness resulting in failure of transmission of atrial impulse to the ventricle.
- AV block is due to failure of conduction of the atrial impulse to the ventricle in the absence of physiologic refractoriness. It is generally due to interruption of the normal conduction pathway or due to pathologic refractoriness.
- AV block can be at the level of the AV node (above the His bundle) or intra-Hisian or it can be distal to the His bundle (infra-Hisian).
- Prognosis depends on the site of AV block. Block distal to the His bundle implies poor prognosis.

Prolonged PR interval (first degree AV block)

- It occurs when PR interval exceeds 200 ms.
- This may represent conduction delay in atrium, AV node or His Purkinje system.
- All P waves are conducted to the ventricle with prolonged but constant interval. Causes of variable PR interval are enumerated in Box 4.2.
- If the QRS duration is normal the delay is invariably in the AVN; 90% of these cases will demonstrate prolonged AH interval.
- If the QRS duration is prolonged then the delay could be in the AVN (60%) or in the His Purkinje system.
- Very long PR intervals favor delay in the AVN.
- Prognosis of patients with prolonged PR interval is good and no therapy is indicated.
- In patients with prolonged PR interval and bifascicular block, the rate of progression to complete heart block (CHB) is low and in asymptomatic patients pacing is not indicated even if patient requires general anesthesia.
- If the HV interval exceeds 100 ms, prophylactic pacing is indicated.
- Prolongation of the PR interval is associated with increased risks of AF, pacemaker implantation.

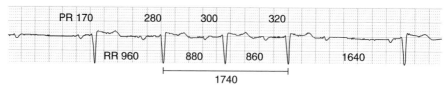

Figure 4.5 Type 1 AV block. (Intervals are in ms.)

Second degree AV blocks[7,8]

These are of two types.

- Type I AV block[11] (Mobitz I or Wenckebach) is characterized by the following (Figure 4.5):
  1 Progressive prolongation of the PR interval at decreasing increments.
  2 Progressive shortening of RR interval.
  3 Pause encompassing the blocked P wave. The duration of the pause is less than the sum of two PP intervals.
- Typical type I AV block is seen in 50% of cases others are atypical and characterized by varying sequence of PR and RR intervals. For example PR and RR intervals that terminates the cycle may be longest and PR interval may be constant or decrease.
- Long Wenckebach cycles tend to be atypical.
- Concealed conduction may be the mechanism for prolongation of PR RR in atypical sequence.
- Type I AV block, in asymptomatic subjects with normal heart, has excellent prognosis and requires no treatment.
- Type I AV block with normal QRS complex is likely to be AV nodal, however if the QRS duration is prolonged, block may be in the AVN, His bundle or infra-Hisian.
- Symptomatic patients with syncope, near syncope, worsening of CHF or angina due to bradycardia produced by type I AV block may require pacing.
- Patients with three sequentially blocked P are likely to have bilevel block within the AV node: 2:1 block proximally, with Wenckebach conduction distally. This pattern of bilevel block could be responsible for two sequentially blocked P waves.
- Bilevel AV block, is also known as alternating Wenckebach (aW) periods. Every other beat of atrial tachycardia is completely blocked. The conducted beats undergo AV Wenckebach conduction with progressive PR prolongation and reducing RR interval until one fails to conduct to the ventricle. Thus there is 2:1 AV block at one level and 5:2 AV Wenckebach at another level.

Type II AV block is characterized by the following:
  1 Constant PP and RR intervals.
  2 Constant PR interval before the blocked P wave.
  3 Pause encompassing the P wave is twice as long as preceding PP interval (Figure 4.6).
- It often accompanies bundle branch block.
- Site of block is invariably in the His or is infra-Hisian (Figure 4.7).
- Second degree AV block with narrow QRS complex is likely to be Type I AV block with minimal increments in PR interval, and may be mistaken for type II block.

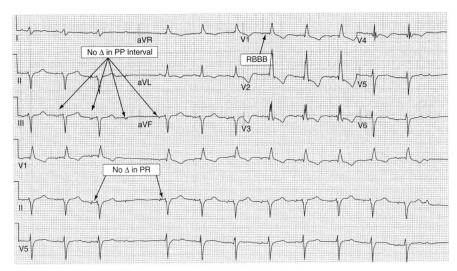

Figure 4.6 Type II AV block.

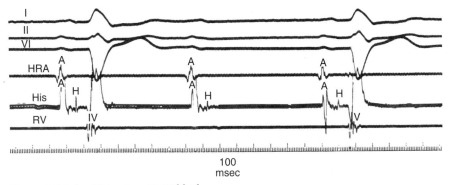

Figure 4.7 Infra-Hisian type II AV block.

- 2:1 AV block with very long PR interval and narrow QRS suggests AV nodal block.
- Constant PR interval of all captured complexes, in spite of varying RP interval, suggests type II AV block. If the PR interval varies inversely with RP interval it is likely to be due to type I AV block.
- Functional infra-Hisian block may occur in the presence of long short HH cycle lengths preceding the block. Rapid atrial pacing will not reproduce this type of block. Pacing is not indicated for functional infra-Hisian AV block.
- Type II AV block often progresses to complete AV block and requires pacing even in an asymptomatic patient.
- Type II AV block accompanied by alternating BBB would require permanent pacemaker.
- In 2:1 AV block, the site of block cannot be reliably determined by the surface ECG, but the PR interval of the conducted P wave and QRS width may give clues about the site of the block.

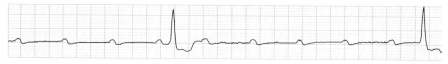

Figure 4.8 Complete AV block.

  1 A PR interval >300 ms suggests block in the AV node, whereas a PR interval <160 ms suggests block in the His Purkinje system or His bundle.

  2 A normal QRS morphology suggests that the site of block is in the AV node or His bundle.

- Second-degree intra-Hisian block, is defined as intermittent conduction between the proximal and distal segment of His bundle.
- An intra-Hisian site of block should be suspected if in the presence of a narrow QRS, block fails to improve with isoproterenol or atropine, and there is paradoxical improvement in conduction with carotid pressure.
- Unusual electrocardiographic findings that suggest pseudo-AV block secondary to nonpropagated His bundle extrasystoles are:
  1 Sudden appearance of unexplained PR prolongations;
  2 Appearance of both type I and type II block in the same patient;
  3 Occurrence of type II block in a patient with normal QRS duration complexes;
  4 Apparent blocked premature atrial contractions; and
  5 Atrial fusion beats.
- Presence of His bundle extrasystoles may be a reflection of diseased His bundle, in those situations the prognosis would be similar to infra-Hisian block.
- If the AV conduction is normal, the therapy should be directed at suppressing automaticity.

Complete AV block[9–11]
- It could present as:
  1 Acquired heart block.
  2 Congenital heart block.
  3 Vagally mediated AV block.
  4 Paroxysmal AV block.
- It can be classified depending on the site of block:
  1 AV nodal block.
  2 Infranodal block.
- It is characterized by failure of all the P waves to conduct to the ventricle.
- Escape rhythm can be junctional with a rate of 40–60 bpm and narrow QRS complex or 20–40 bpm with wide QRS if it arises from the ventricle (Figure 4.8).
- Drug induced AV block may persist after discontinuing the offending agent[5].
- Other causes of AV block are listed in Table 4.1.

Congenital AV blocks

Kearns–Sayre syndrome (KSS)
- It is a rare mitochondrial cytopathy.
- The phenotypic expression includes:

Table 4.1 Causes of complete AV block.

CAD	MI, ischemia.
Congenital	Fibroelastosis, transposition of vessels, septal defects, collagen diseases in mother[6]. *KCNQ1* mutation, Kearns–Sayre syndrome (KSS)
Connective tissue diseases[6]	Ankylosing spondylitis, Reiter disease, polychondritis, scleroderma, rheumatoid arthritis.
Degenerative diseases	Lenegre disease, Lev disease, sclerosis of conduction system.
Drugs[5]	Beta-blockers, Ca channel blockers, quinidine, procainamide, amiodarone.
Infection	Rheumatic fever, myocarditis, Lyme disease, Chagas disease, diphtheria
Infiltrative disorders	Amyloidosis, sarcoidosis, tumors, Hodgkin disease, myeloma, glycogen storage cardiomyopathy, a genetic disorder caused by *PRKAG2* gene mutation
Metabolic	Hypoxia, electrolyte disorders
Neurologic disorders	Becker muscular dystrophy, myotonic dystrophy
Traumatic	Surgical trauma, cardiac contusion, alcohol/surgical septal ablation

CAD = coronary artery disease; MI = myocardial infarction.

1 Progressive external ophthalmoplegia.
2 Atypical pigmentary degeneration of the retina.
3 Complete heart block.
4 Sensorineural deafness.
5 Impaired intellectual function.
6 Short stature.
7 Endocrine and renal abnormalities.
- It is a mitochondrial disorder accompanied by deletions of mitochondrial DNA in skeletal muscle.
- Cardiac histopathological studies show fatty infiltration and fibrosis of the bundle branches and SAN and AVN.
- Cardiac involvement includes conduction defects such as fascicular blocks and first-degree AV block followed by complete heart block.
- Conduction defects appear later in the disease after signs of other organ systems involvement are apparent.
- Conduction defect is progressive from fascicular blocks to complete AV block by second or third decade of life.
- Long QT interval due to *KCNQ1* mutation and torsades de pointes may occur.

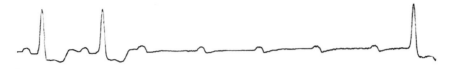

Figure 4.9 Paroxysmal AV block.

- Clinical presentation may include syncope and sudden death from complete heart block or torsades de pointes.

Glycogen storage cardiomyopathy
- Glycogen storage cardiomyopathy, a genetic disorder caused by *PRKAG2* gene mutation.
- These patients present with atrioventricular connections and preexcitation.
- Mechanism of death is AF with fast heart rate causing ventricular fibrillation.
- Patients with the *PRKAG2* mutation are known to be at high risk for dying from fast AF at an early age (20–30 years) and from complete AV block at a later age.
- The clinical picture of glycogen storage cardiomyopathy includes left ventricular hypertrophy, sinus bradycardia, AV conduction disturbances, and atrial tachyarrhythmias.

AV blocks due to gene mutation
- Wild-type human *KCNQ1* mutation may present with AV block phenotypes.
- AF patients with the *KCNQ1* mutation may demonstrate bradycardia or slow ventricular response.
- Pacing is recommended for congenital AV block if:
  1 The patient is symptomatic
  2 QRS is wide
  3 Rate is less then 50 bpm
  4 The block is infra-Hisian

Paroxysmal AV block[12,13]
- Paroxysmal atrioventricular block (PAVB) is defined as the sudden and unexpected repetitive block of transmission of the atrial impulse to the ventricles accompanied by delayed emergence of an adequate escape rhythm (Figure 4.9).
- It is an important cause of syncope.
- It presents as sudden change from apparently normal 1:1 AV conduction to complete heart block.
- Heart disease and conduction abnormality in resting electrocardiograms (ECGs) may not be evident.
- Normal cells are characterized by a more negative resting potential, larger action potential amplitude, and fast depolarizing sodium current.
- Refractoriness depends on a normal voltage–time course of the sodium current, and the end of repolarization usually signals full recovery of excitability.

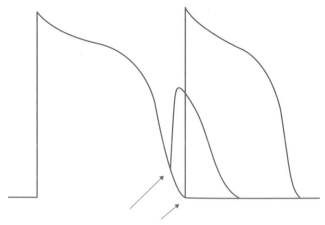

Figure 4.10 Voltage-dependent block (phase 3 block).

- Depolarization during phase 3 may result in conduction block. This is the mechanism of phase 3 AVB, which is correctly referred to as voltage-dependent block (Figure 4.10).
- Recovery of excitability depends on the balance between inward depolarizing currents (i.e., I_{Na} and I_{Ca}) and outward repolarizing potassium currents (I_{K1}, I_{Kr}, and I_{Ks}).
- Diseased cells have less negative resting potential, smaller action potential amplitude of shorter duration, and a much slower depolarizing current carried by a sodium current with depressed kinetics.
- In these cells repolarizing currents during the early phase of diastole become dominant as sodium current tend to be weak.
- These outward currents oppose depolarization, and thus recovery of excitability extends beyond the end of repolarization.
- This is referred to as "postrepolarization refractoriness" and implies that, contrary to a normal cell, a premature stimulus has to fall later in diastole before it can result in a propagating action potential.
- The depolarized action potential has slower conduction properties and is susceptible to conduction block.
- At a more depolarized resting potential, the sodium current cannot be activated, but a slow depolarizing current through the calcium channel can be induced by a strong stimulus.
- This action potential is referred to as the "slow response" and is also characterized by slow conduction properties and postrepolarization refractoriness.

Classification of paroxysmal AV block[13]

1 Tachycardia dependent paroxysmal AV block (TD-PAVB).
2 Pause or bradycardia-dependent paroxysmal AV block (PD-PAVB) (also described as phase 4 block).

Tachycardia-dependent paroxysmal AV block (TD-PAVB)

- It occurs in association with Mobitz type II block.
- Mechanisms include the following:
  1 Concealed conduction of non-conducted P waves in to AV junction.
  2 Deceleration dependent depolarization of lower AV junction.
- Resumption of normal AV conduction fallowing paroxysmal block has been attributed to:
  1 Wedensky facilitation, where properly timed retrograde impulse allows sub-threshold antegrade impulse to conduct.
  2 Peeling of refractory period (shortening of the refractory period with increasing frequency of stimulation).
- TD-PAVB develops in conjunction with increased rate of the atrial input to the AV conduction. The increase in atrial rate could be spontaneous, gradual or sudden or it could be in response to pharmacological agents.
- There may be changes in the AV conduction system secondary to alteration in coronary perfusion, autonomic tone, or circulating catecholamine.
- TD-PAVB is a result of concealed conduction into His Purkinje system.
- Rate-dependent concealed conduction in to the diseased His Purkinje system is responsible for the repetitive conduction block.

Pause dependent paroxysmal AV block (PD-PAVB)

- Sudden, pause dependent phase 4 AV block occurs in diseased conduction system.
- Evidence of distal conduction disease at baseline is often present, RBBB being the most common finding.
- It is produced by blocked or conducted PAC or PVC resulting in a pause.
- It occurs below the His.
- Concealed His extrasystole may mimic AV block.
- AV block may occur when the atrial rate is slow, this may be due to phase 4 block, also referred to as bradycardia-dependent block.
- Phase 4 bradycardia-dependent block or aberrancy results when a supra-ventricular or ventricular impulse reaches a diseased His Purkinje system during phase 4 of the action potential at a time when sodium channels are inactive.
- Consequently, subsequent impulses can no longer depolarize the diseased tissue, leading to asystole (Figure 4.11).
- Phase 4 block usually occurs in the His Purkinje system; therefore the likely site of block is infranodal. Normal AV conduction may resume at faster atrial rate.
- Although phase-4 or bradycardia-dependent paroxysmal AV block is usually induced by critical slowing of the sinus rate, it can occur after a premature beat of atrial, junctional, or ventricular origin. During the postextrasystolic pause, the postextrasystolic beat fails to conduct because of phase 4 block (Figure 4.12).
- Phase 4 AV block is associated with an injured distal conduction system. Possible mechanisms postulated include
  1 Prolonged recovery induced hypopolarization.
  2 Spontaneous diastolic depolarization.
  3 Shift in threshold potential, and decrease in membrane responsiveness (hyperpolarization) without phase 4 depolarization.

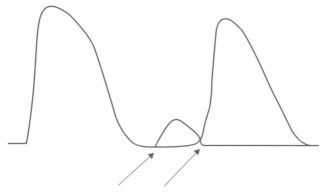

Figure 4.11 Postrepolarization refractoriness and phase 4 block.

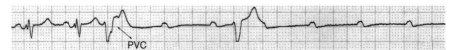

Figure 4.12 PD- PAVB.

- Phase 4 hyperpolarization takes the membrane away from the threshold potential. It therefore impairs conduction and leads to block.
- Bradycardia-dependent BBB may be a result of exit block associated with slow diastolic depolarization in conducting fibers proximal to an area of impaired conductivity.
- Paroxysmal AVB is a disorder of the His Purkinje system, and is secondary to local phase 4 block in the His bundle or in the bundle branches after a critical change in the H-H interval.
- During a long pause (prolonged diastolic period), the fibers of the diseased His Purkinje system spontaneously depolarize (membrane potential becomes less negative) and become less responsive to subsequent impulses due to sodium channel inactivation.
- On a surface ECG, an increased H-H interval may manifest as a lengthened P-P interval, although prolonged P-P is not mandatory and may not be observed before paroxysmal AVB.
- Prolongation of the H-H interval may result from spontaneous sinus rate slowing (prolonged P-P), and post-extrasystolic pauses in association with atrial, ventricular, His extrasystoles.

Differentiation between vagal AV block and paroxysmal AV block[13]

- Differentiation between the often benign and reversible causes of vagal AVB from paroxysmal AVB is essential because there is no benefit from prophylactic pacemaker implantation in vagal AVB (Table 4.2).

Table 4.2 Comparison of vagal versus paroxysmal AVB.

	Vagal AVB	Paroxysmal AVB
Level of block	AV nodal	Infranodal
Initiated by APB, VPB, HES	No	Yes
Tachycardia before initiation	No	May be seen
Resumption of conduction	Sinus acceleration (P-P shortening) or withdrawal of vagal input	Appropriately timed escape beat, or premature beats (sinus or ectopic APB, VPB, HES)
P-P lengthening	Present	May occur
PR prolongation	Present	Not present
CSM	Prolong PR before block	PP lengthening without change in preceding PR

APB = atrial premature beat; AV = atrioventricular; AVB = atrioventricular block; CSM = carotid sinus massage; HES = His extrasystole; VPB = ventricular premature beat.

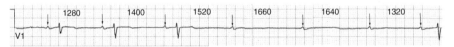

Figure 4.13 Vagal AV block.

- Clinical features suggestive of paroxysmal AVB include:
  1 Paroxysmal AVB is often initiated by atrial, His, or ventricular premature extrasystole that initiates the pause.
  2 Tachycardia can initiate paroxysmal AVB via suppression of AV conduction.
  3 Sinus acceleration (i.e., shortening of P-P interval) has been observed during ventricular asystole without affecting the block.
  4 Slowing of a heart rate before initiation of AVB and/or sudden development of AVB alone does not occur.
  5 Unidirectional anterograde block with preservation of retrograde conduction, as is seen in infra-nodal block but not in AV nodal block. This mechanism allows VPB to reset and resume 1:1 AV conduction in paroxysmal AVB.
- Features suggestive of parasympathetic or vagal AV block include (Figure 4.13)
  1 Gradual slowing of the sinus rate (P-P lengthening) and AV conduction (prolonging PR), which are occasionally followed by sinus arrest (complete SA block) or complete AV block. Sudden block may also occur with heightened vagal tone.
  2 Resumption of AV conduction on sinus acceleration (shortening of P-P interval)
  3 Significant PR prolongation or Wenckebach before initiation of AVB,
  4 Prolonging P-P interval during ventricular asystole,
  5 Significant PR prolongation on resumption of AV conduction,

Table 4.3 Characteristics of AV block in the setting of acute MI.

	Inferior MI	Anterior MI
Characteristic	Preceded by type I AV block	Preceded by type II AV block
Onset	Occurs in first 2–3 days	Occurs in the first week
Duration	May last for 3–14 days	Could be permanent
Site	Nodal	Infra nodal
Pathology	AV nodal ischemia	Necrosis of conduction tissue
QRS duration	Narrow	Wide. Bundle branch block
Treatment	Temporary pacing	Permanent pacing
Mortality	10–20%	60–80%

6 Clinical history highly suggestive of heightened vagal tone (i.e., during micturition, phlebotomy, etc.).
7 No retrograde activation of the His bundle with a ventricular or His extrasystole to reset and abolish AVB.
- Ajmaline or procainamide induced infranodal block or HV lengthening has been used in diagnosing infra-Hisian AVB.
- Positive ajmaline or procainamide response suggest infranodal conduction disorder, and is not specific for identifying patients at risk of developing paroxysmal phase 4 AVB over other types of acquired AVB.
- Paroxysmal AVB may be reproduced in an electrophysiology laboratory via critically timed atrial or ventricular extrastimulus, or rapid ventricular pacing.
- Normal HV interval does not exclude the risk of developing paroxysmal AVB.
- Paroxysmal AVB is a marker of HPS disease with unpredictable escape mechanism, implantation of permanent pacemaker is recommended.

AV block in patients with acute myocardial infarction (MI)[7,8]
- It is common with inferior MI.
- It is probably due to increase vagal tone that accompanies early after an acute inferior MI. It presents as prolong PR or Type I AV block or advanced AV block.
- It responds to atropine.
- AV block occurring late after an acute MI is secondary to ischemia of AV node resulting in increase levels of adenosine in the AVN area. These effects can be blocked by theophylline.
- Characteristics of AV block in the setting of inferior and anterior MI differ and are listed in Table 4.3.
- In the Cardiac Arrhythmias and Risk Stratification After Acute Myocardial Infarction (CARISMA) study 10% of the patients with LVEF ≤ 40% after acute myocardial infarction had high-degree AV block. It was associated with a very high risk of cardiac death[12].

AV dissociation

- During AV dissociation atrial and ventricular activity is independent.
- The mechanisms of AV dissociation could be physiologic or pathologic.
  1 Physiologic refractoriness with interference. (Impulse may conduct if occurs during non refractory window of cycle length)
     - Rate of primary pacemaker (sinus) is slower then subsidiary (junctional) pacemaker resulting in non-conduction of some of the impulses due to physiologic refractoriness.
     - Inappropriate acceleration of subsidiary pacemaker. Accelerated junctional rhythm or ventricular tachycardia.
     - Due to physiologic refractoriness and physiologic AV conduction delay when primary pacemaker accelerates (sinus or atrial tachycardia).
  2 Pathologic failure of conduction of sinus impulses resulting in more P waves then QRS complexes as in complete AV block. (Impulse does not conduct even if it occurs during non-refractory period of the cycle length.)

References

1 James TN. Structure and function of the sinus node, AV node and His bundle of the human heart: part I-structure. *Prog Cardiovasc Dis.* 2002;45(3):235–267.
2 Shen WK. How to manage patients with inappropriate sinus tachycardia. *Heart Rhythm.* 2005;2(9):1015–1019.
3 Thollon C, Bedut S, Villeneuve N, et al. Use-dependent inhibition of hHCN4 by ivabradine and relationship with reduction in pacemaker activity. *Br. J. Pharmacol.* 2007;150(1):37–46.
4 Shen W-K. Modification and ablation for inappropriate sinus tachycardia: current status. *Card Electrophysiol Rev.* 2002;6(4):349–355.
5 Rosenblueth A. Mechanism of the Wenckebach–Luciani cycles. *Am. J. Physiol.* 1958; 194(3):491–494.
6 Bakker ML, Moorman AFM, Christoffels VM. The atrioventricular node: origin, development, and genetic program. *Trends Cardiovasc. Med.* 2010;20(5):164–171.
7 Abidov A, Kaluski E, Hod H, et al. Influence of conduction disturbances on clinical outcome in patients with acute myocardial infarction receiving thrombolysis (results from the ARGAMI-2 study). *Am. J. Cardiol.* 2004;93(1):76–80.
8 Brady WJ Jr, Harrigan RA. Diagnosis and management of bradycardia and atrioventricular block associated with acute coronary ischemia. *Emerg. Med. Clin. North Am.* 2001;19(2):371–384, xi-xii.
9 Hucker WJ, Nikolski VP, Efimov IR. Autonomic control and innervation of the atrioventricular junctional pacemaker. *Heart Rhythm.* 2007;4(10):1326–1335.
10 Zeltser D, Justo D, Halkin A, et al. Drug-induced atrioventricular block: prognosis after discontinuation of the culprit drug. *J. Am. Coll. Cardiol.* 2004;44(1):105–108.
11 Qu Y, Xiao GQ, Chen L, Boutjdir M. Autoantibodies from mothers of children with congenital heart block downregulate cardiac L-type Ca channels. *J. Mol. Cell. Cardiol.* 2001;33(6):1153–1163.
12 Silvetti MS, Grutter G, Di Ciommo V, Drago F. Paroxysmal atrioventricular block in young patients. *Pediatr Cardiol.* 2004;25(5):506–512.
13 El-Sherif N, Jalife J. Paroxysmal atrioventricular block: are phase 3 and phase 4 block mechanisms or misnomers? *Heart Rhythm.* 2009;6(10):1514–1521.

Answers to self-assessment questions

1 D
2 B
3 C
4 D
5 A
6 D
7 C
8 A
9 C
10 D
11 A
12 B
13 D
14 D
15 D

CHAPTER 5
Supraventricular tachycardia

Self-assessment questions

5.1 Atrial flutter

1 A 54-year-old male presents with progressively increasing dyspnea. ECG is shown below. Serum potassium was 3.2 mEq/L. Perfusion studies are normal. Echocardiogram revealed biatrial enlargement, enlarged and diffusely hypokinetic left ventricle and ejection fraction of 26%. Eight months ago on a routine examination blood pressure of 120/70 and heart rate of 70 bpm was recorded. Six months ago spot check in a drug store revealed a blood pressure of 110/70 and heart rate of 150 bpm. Patient was asymptomatic.

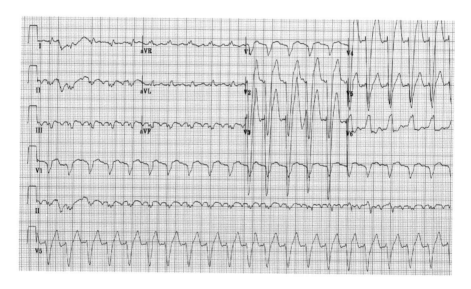

What will you recommend?
A IV lidocaine.
B Bi V defibrillator implant.

Essential Cardiac Electrophysiology: The Self-Assessment Approach, Second Edition. Zainul Abedin.
© 2013 Blackwell Publishing Ltd. Published 2013 by Blackwell Publishing Ltd.

C Radiofrequency ablation

D Ca channel blockers.

2 A 36-year-old sales representative was found to have an atrial flutter. Physical examination and echocardiogram were normal. Serum potassium was 3.9 mEq/L.

Next day he reported to hospital outpatient area for chemical cardioversion. He received 1 mg of ibutilide intravenously and converted to sinus rhythm within 10 minutes. Two hours later he insisted on leaving the hospital. While in a meeting he had an episode of syncope. Subsequent evaluation revealed sinus rhythm and blood pressure was normal.

What is the most likely cause of his syncope?

A Recurrence of atrial flutter with rapid ventricular response

B Neurocardiogenic syncope

C Polymorphic Ventricular tachycardia

D Embolic stroke from left atrial clot

3 A 45-year-old male who has persistent atrial flutter, undergoes radiofrequency ablation. During second application of the energy flutter is terminated. What will you consider as a satisfactory end point for this procedure?

A Termination of atrial flutter is a satisfactory end point

B Bidirectional block across isthmus should be demonstrated

C Rapid atrial pacing should be performed in an attempt to induce flutter

D Additional RF lesions should be delivered near CS ostium

4 A 77-year-old female had paroxysmal atrial fibrillation. Echocardiogram and perfusion studies were normal. She was treated with propafenone 150 mg TID. Five weeks later she came to the clinic complaining of palpitations. ECG revealed persistent atrial flutter.

What will be your recommendation?

A Continue propafenone and consider ablation for atrial flutter

B Discontinue propafenone

C Consider ablation for atrial fibrillation

D Consider rate control using Ca channel blockers and β blockers.

5 A 75-year-old woman is admitted to the hospital for the painful swelling of the left knee. Patient has chronic obstructive pulmonary disease. She has been treated for congestive heart failure (left ventricular ejection fraction of 30%). She takes digoxin 0.125 mg daily. Two years ago cardiac catheterization performed elsewhere had revealed normal coronary arteries and global left ventricular dysfunction. An electrocardiogram done at that time had revealed sinus rhythm with a conduction defect.

She has been aware of palpitations.

The laboratory data:

Blood urea nitrogen	43 mg/dL
Serum creatinine	3.0 mg/dL
Serum Sodium	133 mEq/L
Serum potassium	4.3 mEq/L
Serum magnesium	2.0 mEq/L

An electrocardiogram was performed.

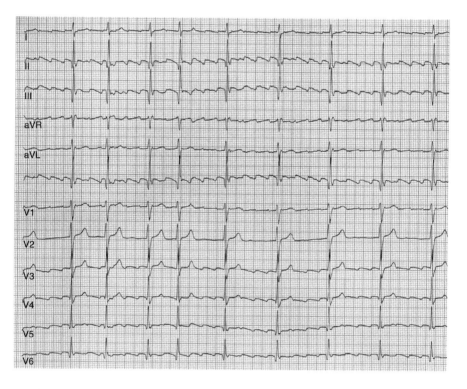

Which of the following is most appropriate?

A Initiate sotalol 120 mg PO BID.

B Initiate flecainide 100 mg PO BID.

C Consider radiofrequency ablation.

D Increase the dose of digoxin to 0.25 mg PO daily.

6 A 75-year-old man is referred to you because of the abnormal electrocardiogram (shown below) obtained during preoperative clearance for an elective cholecystectomy. There is no history of coronary artery disease or peripheral vascular disease. He reports recent decrease in exercise tolerance. Electrocardiogram and echocardiogram obtained 6 months ago were normal.

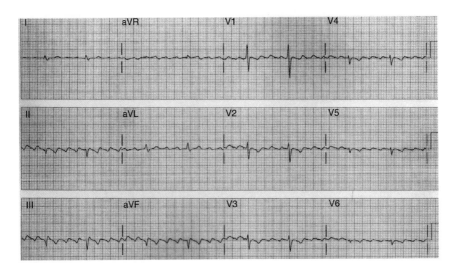

What will be your recommendation?
A Chemical cardioversion using ibutilide
B Aspirin for two weeks followed by elective direct current cardioversion.
C Warfarin for three weeks, followed by elective direct current cardioversion.
D Transesophageal echocardiography followed by elective direct current cardioversion and aspirin.
E Radiofrequency catheter ablation.

7 A 60-year-old man was admitted to the hospital because of palpitations and lightheadedness. He had similar episode 2 years ago. There is no history of coronary artery disease or hypertension. Electrocardiogram (shown below) showed atrial flutter.

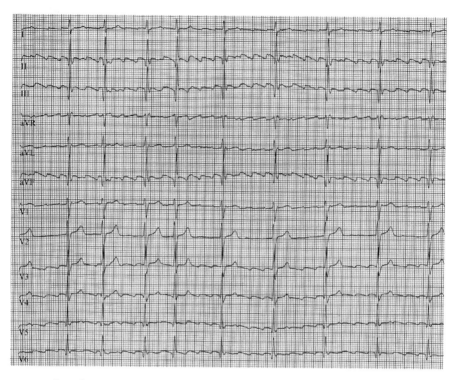

Next day after receiving the third dose of flecainide he developed a rapid heart rate. Electrocardiogram was recorded.

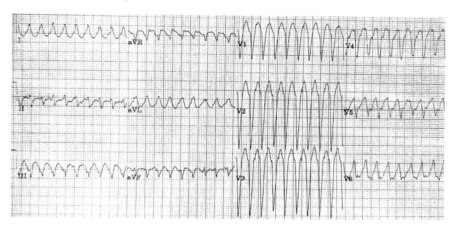

Which of the following is the most likely diagnosis?

A Antidromic reentrant tachycardia.

B Ventricular tachycardia.

C Atrial flutter with 1:1 conduction.

D AV node reentry tachycardia utilizing bystander fascicular-ventricular connection.

5.2 Atrial tachycardias

1 A 56-year-old nurse presents with recurrent episodes of tachycardia. The ECG is shown.

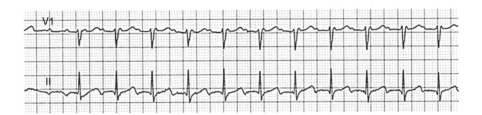

What is the most likely diagnosis?
A Sinus tachycardia
B Atrial tachycardia
C AVRT
D Atypical AVNRT

2 Ablation at which of the following sites is likely to cure the tachycardia?
A Accessory pathway
B AV nodal slow pathway
C Atrial tachycardia focus
D AV junction

3 A 25-year-old man is referred to you because of sustained tachycardia. During electrophysiologic study, the following tracing was obtained.

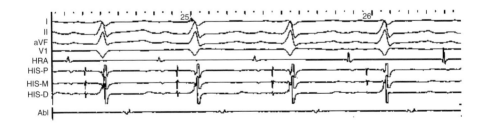

The ablation catheter is located in mid segment of crista terminalis
Which of the following is the most likely diagnosis?
A Atrial tachycardia
B Atypical AV re-entrant tachycardia using a slowly conducting pathway as the retrograde limb
C Atypical (fast-slow) AV nodal reentrant tachycardia
D Sinus node re-entrant tachycardia

5.3 Atrial fibrillation

1 A 35-year-old female with mitral valve disease presents with history of several episodes of atrial fibrillation that lasted for 2–4 hours and spontaneously terminates. This could be classified as:
   A Persistent AF
   B Chronic AF
   C Paroxysmal AF
   D Lone AF

2 The most common symptom of the AF is:
   A TIA/stroke
   B Fatigue and tiredness
   C Syncope
   D Chest pain

3 Which of the following is not a risk factor for thromboembolic complication in a patient with AF and therefore not an indication for anticoagulation with warfarin?
   A The patient is 57 years old
   B Hypertension
   C LVF
   D Diabetes

4 A 48-year-old patient presents with AF that has lasted for more than 48 hours. TEE is negative for intracardiac clots. What will be your recommendation following a successful cardioversion?
   A Begin warfarin and continue indefinitely
   B Begin aspirin
   C Begin warfarin for 3 weeks
   D Patient does not need anticoagulation or antiplatelet therapy

5 Attempted cardioversion for AF is unsuccessful in a 60-year-old patient. His EF is 25%. Should he undergo repeat cardioversion after administration of IV ibutilide?
   A True
   B False

6 A 50-year-old female patient presents with paroxysmal AF. She was recently diagnosed to have chronic active hepatitis and abnormal liver function test. To maintain sinus rhythm which of the following drugs could be safely prescribed?
   A Sotalol
   B Mexiletine
   C Amiodarone
   D Procainamide

7 A 76-year-old woman has had persistent atrial fibrillation for 3 years. She also has hypertension and asthma. Current medications are warfarin; digoxin, 0.25 mg daily; atenolol, 25 mg twice daily; diltiazem, 30 mg every 8 hours; and inhaled bronchodilators. During 24-hour ambulatory ECG monitoring, the average ventricular response was 130 beats per minute (bpm.) with occasional episodes of 150 bpm. Echocardiogram shows a 6 cm left atrium and a dilated left ventricle. Estimated left ventricular ejection fraction is 35%.
Which of the following is the best treatment plan?
A Increase the dose of atenolol
B Increase the dose of diltiazem
C Initiate amiodarone and consider elective cardioversion 4 weeks later
D Radiofrequency catheter ablation of the AV junction, and insertion of ventricular pacemaker.

8 A 58-year-old woman, who has long-standing hypertension, reports approximately one episode of paroxysmal atrial fibrillation (AF) monthly. She has no history of diabetes mellitus, congestive heart failure, or stroke. Episodes of AF persist as long as 12 hours and are characterized by palpitations, dizziness, and fatigue. Three episodes have resulted in hospital admission; however, records show that her heart rate was 86 to 90 bpm. A trial of amiodarone was discontinued because of changes in liver function. Current medications are sustained-release metoprolol, 100 mg daily, and aspirin, 81 mg daily.

Serum thyroid-stimulating hormone level is normal. Electrocardiogram in sinus rhythm shows normal intervals, left atrial abnormality, and left ventricular hypertrophy.

Baseline echocardiogram shows left ventricular ejection fraction of 65%. Left atrial dimension is 4.2 cm. Wall thickness of the interventricular septum and the posterior wall is 1.4 cm. Exercise echocardiogram reveals no ischemia.
Which of the following should be recommended?
A Addition of diltiazem
B Addition of flecainide
C Addition of disopyramide
D Catheter-based pulmonary vein isolation
E Radiofrequency catheter ablation of the atrioventricular junction and pacemaker implantation.

5.4 Automatic junctional tachycardia

1 To differentiate AJT from AVNRT which of the following maneuvers could be helpful?
A PAC delivered near slow pathway when septal A has occurred
B Adenosine infusion
C Parahisian pacing
D Assessment of prematurity index

2 Which of the following therapeutic options is least likely to help in the treatment of AJT?
  A AV node ablation and insertion of permanent pacemaker
  B Amiodarone
  C Digoxin
  D Propafenone

5.5 AV node re-entry tachycardias

1 Dual AV node physiology is defined as:
  A 50 milliseconds increase in H1H2 for 10 milliseconds decrease in A1A2 interval
  B 50 milliseconds increase in A2H2 for 10 milliseconds decrease in A1A2 interval
  C 50 milliseconds increase in H2V2 for 10 milliseconds decrease in A1A2 interval
  D Occurrence of atrial echo beats in response to any A1A2

2 Which of the following properties is the result of distal insertion of fast pathway into AV junction?
  A Increased decremental conduction
  B Increased response to AV node blocking agents
  C Greater response to Na channel blocking agents
  D Preexcitation on surface electrocardiogram

3 After slow pathway ablation, the presence of A2H2 jump without induction of tachycardia is indicative of unsuccessful ablation.
  A True
  B False

4 In which of the following conditions is the HA interval during tachycardia likely to be shorter than the HA interval during RV pacing?
  A AVNRT
  B AVRT
  C Bundle branch re-entry VT
  D Atrial tachycardia

5 Which of the following conditions are likely to present with variable HA interval?
  A AVNRT
  B AVRT
  C Atrial tachycardia
  D Atriofascicular tachycardia

6 A 25-year-old female had recurrent episodes of palpitation. During electro-physiologic study wide complex tachycardia was induced. Tachycardia could be entrained by right atrial pacing; however, on repeated occasions, on termination of atrial pacing tachycardia resumed without the change in the VA interval as shown in the following tracing.

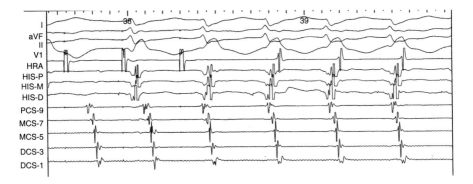

What is the most likely mechanism of this tachycardia?

A AVNRT

B AVRT

C Atrial tachycardia

D LVVT (fascicular tachycardia)

7 A 50-year-old female had recurrent episodes of tachycardia. During electrophysiologic study the following observations were made.

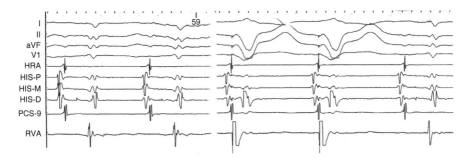

Ablation at which of the following sites is mostly likely to cure the tachycardia?

A Subeustachian isthmus

B Accessory pathway

C AV nodal slow pathway

D Atrial tachycardia focus

8 A 26-year-old woman, who is in the last trimester of pregnancy, complains of palpitations. First episode that occurred 4 months ago, lasted for several minutes and terminated spontaneously; It was not associated with dizziness, chest pain, or syncope. Second episode was recorded while in primary care physician's office.

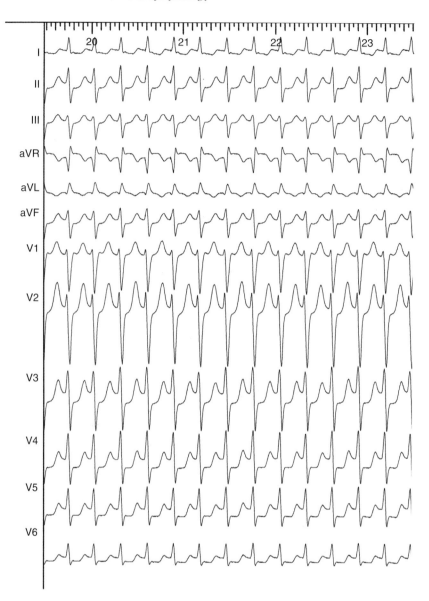

Tachycardia terminates spontaneously. Baseline ECG and echocardiogram are normal.

Which of the following is most appropriate at this time?

A Deliver the fetus as soon as possible

B Begin flecainide

C Begin metoprolol

D Reassure the patient

9 A 67-year-old man has had palpitations for the last 10 years. Recently the episodes have become more frequent and severe. Medical history includes hypertension, diabetes, and hypercholesterolemia. ECG recorded in the office was found to be normal.

Two days ago he came to hospital complaining of dyspnea, chest pressure, and palpitations. He was diaphoretic; the heart rate was 140 per minute, the blood pressure was 100/60 mmHg. Electrocardiogram is shown.

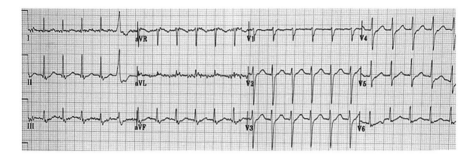

Today during electrophysiologic study anterograde dual AV nodal pathway is demonstrated; however, sustained supraventricular tachycardia (SVT) cannot be induced.

Which one of the following should be done next?

A Repeat electrophysiologic study in 4 weeks

B Prescribe metoprolol

C Ablate the AV nodal slow pathway

D Prescribe amiodarone

10 A 32-year-old woman undergoes electrophysiologic study for recurrent palpitations. The following recording is obtained.

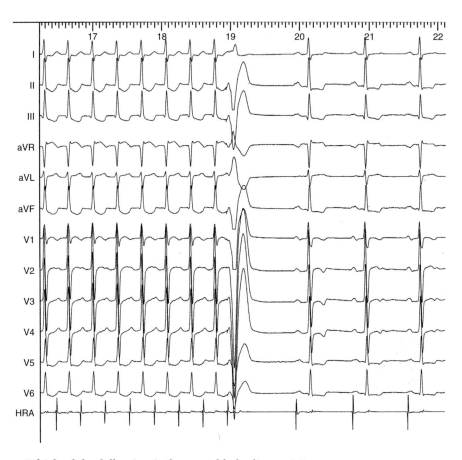

Which of the following is the most likely diagnosis?
A AV re-entrant tachycardia
B Atypical (fast-slow) AV nodal re-entrant tachycardia
C Intra-atrial re-entrant tachycardia
D Typical (slow-fast) AV nodal re-entrant tachycardia

5.6 AV re-entrant tachycardias

1 A 27-year-old female patient presents with AVRT utilizing left lateral AP. There is a variation in the cycle length although the VA interval remains unchanged. The most likely explanation of this observation is:
A Slowing of conduction in AP
B Change in conduction through the AV node due to dual AV node physiology
C Multiple accessory pathways
D Accelerated conduction through His Purkinje system

2 Which one of the following is least likely to present with short RP tachycardia?
   A AVNRT
   B Ventricular tachycardia
   C AVRT
   D Sinoatrial reentrant tachycardia

3 On termination of the SVT the last complex recorded is a QRS. Which one of the following is the most likely mechanism?
   A AVNRT
   B AVRT
   C Atrial tachycardia
   D None of the above

4 His synchronous PVC terminates the SVT without depolarizing the atrium. In which of the following conditions is this phenomenon likely to be noticed?
   A Atrial tachycardia
   B AVNRT
   C Automatic junctional tachycardia
   D AVRT

5 In which of the following conditions is the VA interval likely to be shorter during RV apex pacing than RV base pacing?
   A AV node conduction
   B Septal AP
   C Left posterior AP
   D Atrioventricular connection

6 Which one of the following is likely to present with a constant VA interval with or without His capture during parahisian pacing?
   A Dual AV nodal physiology
   B Septal AP
   C Nodofascicular pathway
   D Atriofascicular pathway

7 Which one of the following is unlikely to cause variable VA interval during AVRT?
   A Intermittent bundle branch block
   B Multiple retrogradely conducting accessory pathways
   C Decremental retrograde conduction through the AP
   D Dual AVN physiology

8 SVT is entrained by RV pacing. On termination of V pacing the response is VAAV. This observation suggests the diagnosis of:
   A Atrial tachycardia
   B AVNRT
   C AVRT
   D Atriofascicular tachycardia

9 SVT is entrained by RV pacing. On termination of V pacing the stimulus to A-VA interval is >85 msec and PPI-TCL interval is >115 ms. These observations suggest the diagnosis of:

A Atrial tachycardia
B Atypical AVNRT
C Atriofascicular pathway
D AVRT

10 Which of the following observations is likely to suggest the presence of antegrade bystander utilization of AP during atrial tachycardia?

A Earliest retrograde atrial activation is through AV junction
B Late PAC advances the whole tachycardia circuit (V and following A)
C PVC delivered at the ventricular insertion site of the AP abolishes the pre-excitation but tachycardia continues
D Ventricles are the integral part of the tachycardia circuit

11 During a wide complex tachycardia it is noted that the atrium and ventricle are an obligatory part of the circuit and retrograde atrial activation is eccentric. These observations suggest presence of:

A Atrial tachycardia utilizing bystander AP
B VT utilizing bystander AP
C Antidromic tachycardia
D Junctional tachycardia

12 PAC delivered during wide complex tachycardia advances the ventricular electrogram and the next atrial electrogram without any change in the atrial activation sequence. These findings are suggestive of:

A AVNRT utilizing bystander AP
B Atrial tachycardia utilizing bystander AP
C Antidromic tachycardia
D Ventricular tachycardia

13 During wide complex tachycardia, a short HV interval is recorded. This finding suggests the presence of:

A Ventricular preexcitation due to bystander AP
B Antidromic tachycardia
C Atriofascicular pathway mediated tachycardia
D BBRVT

14 A 30-year-old male, who is known to have preexcitation, presents to ER with atrial fibrillation of 1 hour duration. The ventricular rate is 130–170 bpm. The patient is hemodynamically stable. Which of the following can be safely used to treat AF?

A IV digoxin
B IV verapamil
C IV ibutilide
D IV metoprolol

15 A 19-year-old man who has paroxysmal supraventricular is referred to you for evaluation and recommendation. The patient has had tachycardia since age 10. Electrocardiogram obtained during sinus rhythm is shown. Echocardiogram is normal. At which site, will delivery of radiofrequency result in resolution of the problem?

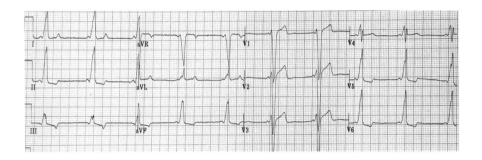

    A Right anterior tricuspid annulus
    B Posteroseptal tricuspid annulus
    C Left lateral mitral annulus
    D Anteroseptal region

16 Surface and intracardiac electrograms recorded during tachycardia are shown in the following tracing.

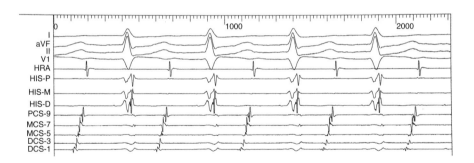

    Which maneuver will help identify the correct mechanism of the tachycardia?
    A Atrial pacing
    B Ventricular pacing
    C Isoproterenol infusion
    D Mapping in the left superior pulmonary vein

17 A 20-year-old male presented with recurrent episodes of palpitations. During electrophysiologic study following arrhythmia was induced. Ablation at which one of the following sites is likely to terminate the tachycardia?

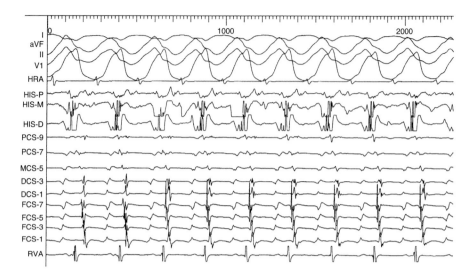

FCS = closely spaced (2 mm) electrograms recorded from CS using femoral approach. DCS, MCS and PCS are recorded from subclavian approach (electrode spacing 10–2 mm).

    A Left lateral mitral annulus
    B LVOT
    C Right lateral tricuspid annulus
    D Right bundle

18 A 50-year-old woman has a long history of paroxysmal tachycardia despite treatment with digoxin, atenolol, and flecainide. She underwent electrophysiologic study and radiofrequency ablation (tracing A). Two months later she had a recurrence of the tachycardia. Electrophysiologic study was repeated (tracing B).

Tracing A

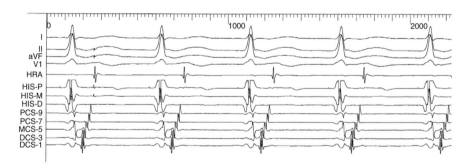

Tracing B

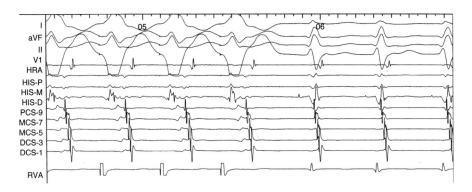

Which of the following best describes the mechanism(s) of the tachycardias?
A The patient had atypical AVNRT and now has typical AV nodal reentrant tachycardia
B The patient had AVRT utilizing the anteroseptal accessory pathway and now has atrial tachycardia
C The patient had AVRT utilizing the LLAP and now has typical AVNRT
D The patient had permanent junctional reciprocating tachycardia and now has atypical AV nodal reentrant tachycardia

19 A 15-year-old female fainted in a physician's office while the blood was being drawn. There is no previous history of syncope, chest pain, or palpitations. ECG rhythm strip recorded in the physician's office is shown below.

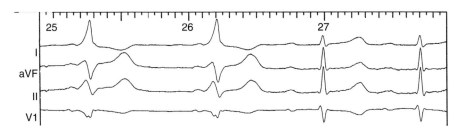

What will be your recommendation?
A Consider electrophysiologic study and RF ablation
B Begin procainamide
C Begin Metoprolol
D Reassure the patient

20 A 44-year-old man is referred to you because he has had three episodes of palpitations in the past year. Each episode began suddenly, lasted up to 30 minutes, and was associated with severe lightheadedness. The patient has not had syncope, dyspnea, or chest pain, and he has no family history of heart disease. The findings of the physical examination are normal. Electrocardiograms recorded a few minutes apart are shown in tracings A and B.

Tracing A

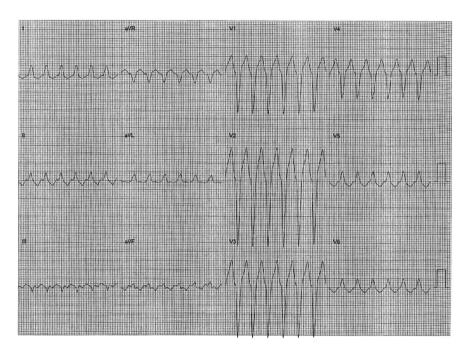

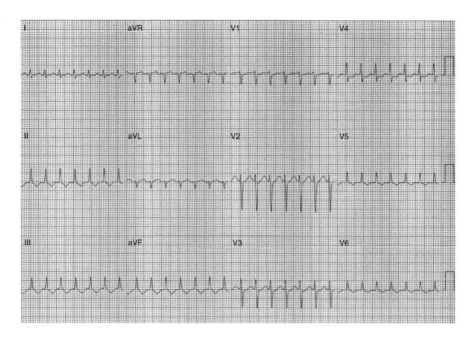

Tracing B.
What is the most likely diagnosis?
A AVNRT
B Atrial tachycardia
C AVRT
D RVOT-VT and atrial tachycardia

5.1 Atrial flutter[1-5]

- Atrial flutter is due to re-entry (Box 5.1).
- Typical atrial flutter is a macrore-entrant tachycardia around the tricuspid annulus.
- Classical atrial flutter is confined to right atrium where the impulse travels up the atrial septum and then travels inferiorly down the right atrial free wall to re-enter the atrial septum through the isthmus (Figure 5.1).
- Atrial flutter produced by this mechanism is called typical atrial flutter. It has also been called common or counterclockwise atrial flutter. A 12-lead ECG during typical atrial flutter produces negative "sawtooth" flutter waves[1] in leads II, III, and aVF (Figure 5.2).
- If the impulse travels in the opposite direction down the atrial septum and through the isthmus to travel up the right atrial free wall it is called *reverse typical atrial flutter* or clockwise atrial flutter. A 12-lead ECG during reverse typical atrial flutter produces positive flutter waves in leads II, III, and aVF.
- Isthmus is an area of slow conduction between tricuspid valve annulus, and inferior vena cava. The Eustachian ridge, which extends to the posterior wall of the coronary sinus ostium is an integral part of this isthmus and contributes to the slow conduction. The isthmus is an integral part of the circuit in typical atrial flutter Fractionated electrograms could be recorded from the area of slow conduction (Figure 5.3).
- Entrainment occurs when pacing at shorter cycle length results in acceleration of the flutter. On termination of pacing flutter resumes without change in its cycle length.
- Entrainment can be manifest when fusion occurs or it can be concealed when paced complexes are identical to spontaneously occurring flutter complexes (Figure 5.4).
- Concealed entrainment of typical flutter occurs when pacing from the isthmus. If the post-pacing interval is the same as the flutter cycle length, this would suggest that the flutter is isthmus-dependent.
- Incisional atrial re-entry is seen in patients with right atrial free wall incisions fallowing cardiac surgery. The re-entrant circuit travels around the line of block caused by the incision
- In left atrial flutter the area of slow conduction is between one or more of the pulmonary veins or the mitral valve annulus. It may occur spontaneously or fallowing ablation for atrial fibrillation where an attempt to isolate pulmonary

---

Box 5.1 Classification of atrial flutter

1 Typical atrial flutter
2 Reverse typical atrial flutter
3 Incisional scar related atrial flutter
4 Left atrial flutter

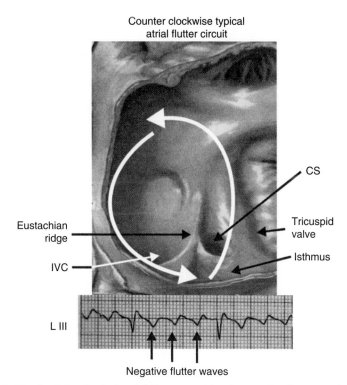

Counter clockwise typical
atrial flutter circuit

Figure 5.1 Circuit of the classical atrial flutter resulting in negative flutter waves in LII, LIII and aVF. CS = coronary sinus ostium. IVC = inferior vena cava.

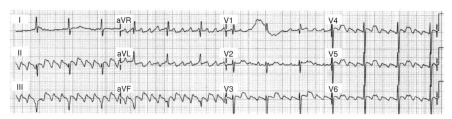

Figure 5.2 Typical atrial flutter.

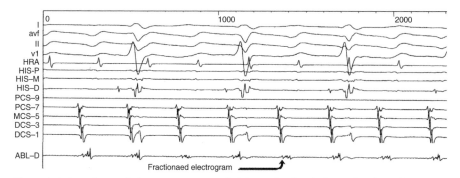

Figure 5.3 Fractionated electrograms recorded from the distal electrode of an ablation catheter located between tricuspid annulus and anterior wall of the coronary sinus.

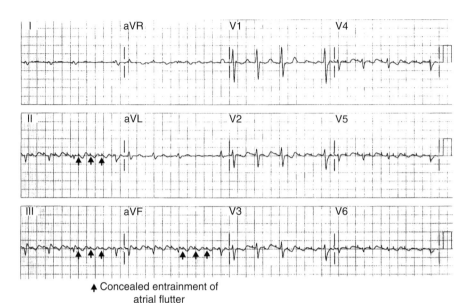

▲ Concealed entrainment of
atrial flutter

Figure 5.4 Pacing from the medial segment of the flutter isthmus results in concealed entrainment. Paced atrial complexes are identical to spontaneously occurring typical counterclockwise flutter waves. Short stimulus to F interval suggests that the capture is located at the exit site of the flutter isthmus.

veins may result in corridor of slowly conducting tissue between mitral annulus and pulmonary veins.
- Left atrial flutter may also result from the gaps in ablation lines in the left atrium.
- Atrial flutter often presents with the same symptoms as atrial fibrillation. The atrial rate is typically between 250 and 350 bpm, with resultant 2:1 or 4:1 atrioventricular conduction block. Diagnosis is made on 12-lead ECG. The blocked flutter waves may not be readily apparent on 12-lead ECG, because they may be masked by the QRS complex. The presence of a regular, narrow complex tachycardia at 150 bpm should raise suspicion of atrial flutter.
- Persistent atrial flutter with rapid ventricular response may result in tachycardia mediated cardiomyopathy.
- During atrial flutter atrioventricular node (AVN) conduction is often 2:1.
- If the flutter waves are not clearly visible, increase in AV block by vagal maneuvers or pharmacologic agents such as adenosine may clarify the diagnosis.
- Use of class IC drugs may slow atrial rate and allow most of the atrial impulses to pass through the AVN thus increasing the ventricular rate.

Treatment[2,3]

- The risk of thromboembolic events from atrial flutter is the same as with atrial fibrillation. Therefore, the recommendations for anticoagulation with atrial flutter are the same as with atrial fibrillation[4].
- New onset flutter of short duration can be treated by:
  1 Intravenous ibutilide if serum potassium is >4.0 mEq/L, QTc is less than 440 ms and left ventricular function is normal.
  2 Single oral dose of flecainide (300 mg) or propafenone (600 mg).
  3 Cardioversion 25–50 J can achieve cardioversion to sinus rhythm.
  4 Overdrive atrial pacing using high outputs.
- IV ibutilide may prolong QT interval and may induce Torsades de Pointes. Patient should be monitored for the half life of the drug (4 h) fallowing administration of the drug[5].
- Cardioversion should be considered if patient is hemodynamically unstable[6].
- Beta-blockers or calcium channel blockers can achieve rate control[7, 8].
- For paroxysmal or chronic atrial flutter radio frequency ablation of the isthmus is the treatment of choice. These patients should be anticoagulated for 4 weeks prior to cardioversion or ablation. Alternatively if the transesophageal echocardiogram is negative for intracardiac blood clots immediate cardioversion can be performed after starting anticoagulation.
- Oral antiarrhythmic drug therapy to maintain sinus rhythm is not very effective.

Atrial flutter ablation

- In a typical flutter the activation in right atrium occurs in a counterclockwise direction. This produces negative saw tooth pattern in L2, L3 and aVF. It produces positive flutter waves in V1 and negative flutter waves in V6 (Figure 5.1).
- In a clockwise flutter the pattern is reversed.
- Flutter wave travels along the broad area of the anterolateral wall of the right atrium. It then enters the narrow and slowly conducting isthmus area. Anterior boundary of the isthmus is tricuspid annulus (TA) and posterior boundary includes inferior vena cava (IVC), Eustachian ridge (ER) and coronary sinus (CS) os. In some patients the wave front after emerging from the isthmus may divide in to two exits traveling anterior and posterior to the CS os. In other patients continuation of the Eustachian ridge in to posterior lip of CS os prevents posterior exit. Thus the wave front only travels between TA and ER.
- The wave front then emerges in low right atrium and ascends along the interatrial septum. Block along the crista terminalis prevents the impulse from entering anterior trabeculated segment of the atrium. This prevents the collision with the reentrant wave.
- Principal of ablation for re-entrant tachycardia with an area of slow conduction bounded by two anatomical barriers is transaction of the circuit with lesion extending from one fixed barrier to the next.
- In typical atrial flutter that area is the narrow isthmus between TA annulus and IVC and/or ER and CS os.

- Entrainment mapping should be used to confirm that the isthmus is an integral part of the flutter circuit. Sometimes a typical electrocardiographic pattern may be present in non-isthmus dependent atrial re-entrant tachycardias.
- Flutter is entrained by pacing at the isthmus (6 or 7:00 clock position of TA in left anterior oblique view) at a cycle length 20 ms shorter than flutter cycle length.
- The following features are suggestive of entrainment with concealed fusion and indicate that the flutter is isthmus dependent.
  1 Long interval from pacing stimulus to the onset of the flutter wave.
  2 No change in flutter wave morphology on surface ECG.
  3 No change in endocardial activation pattern along the tricuspid annulus.
  4 Post pacing interval equals tachycardia cycle length.
- The width of the isthmus may vary from 2 to 4 cm. It may contain fibrous thebesian valve and pectinate muscles. In some patients the narrowest portion of the isthmus is towards the septum between anterior lip of CS os and TA.
- Three-dimensional mapping helps identify electro anatomically characteristics of the flutter circuit.
- During ablation sheaths may be needed to maintain proper orientation and tissue contact.
- Goal should be to create an ablation line between TA to IVC.
- Larger lesions can be achieved by using large tip or irrigated tip ablation catheter[9].
- Transient isthmus block during RF application may terminate atrial flutter, but complete and permanent block across the isthmus is essential for cure.
- Termination of atrial flutter during ablation and subsequent noninducibility are not reliable markers for ablation success.
- Bidirectional block across the isthmus should be demonstrated by pacing from low lateral right atrium and from CS.
- RF energy can be applied during atrial flutter or during CS pacing. Block across the isthmus will change the activation sequence along the lateral aspect of the right atrium when pacing from CS.
- Pacing from the lateral aspect of the isthmus, before isthmus block, results in negative P waves in inferior leads as activation proceeds through the isthmus to CS os and atrial septum. After the successful ablation the P wave morphology in inferior leads becomes positive and bifid, as activation along the septum is no longer possible.
- Split potential on the ablation line where the interval between the two potentials exceeds 100 ms during CS pacing, is also suggestive of block across the isthmus.
- When assessing block across the isthmus long pacing cycle lengths should be used. Shorter cycle lengths may result in slowing of conduction and appearance of a block (pseudo block).
- Incomplete block across the isthmus may result in "leak" across the isthmus on pacing from the lateral or medial aspect. Site of such leak is generally located on adjacent to TA, lip of the Eustachian ridge, at the anterior wall or base of the deep subeustachian sinus, large pectinate muscle in the isthmus.

- Gaps can be identified during CS pacing or during flutter by identifying narrowly split or single electrograms along the ablation line interposed by widely separated double potentials.
- Electroanatomical three-dimensional mapping may help in identifying the "leaks" of conduction across the isthmus.
- Intracardiac echocardiography may help identify right atrial landmarks such as crista, CS os.
- Acute success rate of flutter ablation is 90% and reoccurrence rate of 5–10%.
- In patients who present with paroxysmal atrial flutter/atrial fibrillation, ablation of the atrial flutter may make treatment of atrial fibrillation more manageable.
- If antiarrhythmic drug therapy organizes atrial fibrillation into atrial flutter, a hybrid approach of flutter ablation and continued antiarrhythmic drug therapy may be effective in maintaining sinus rhythm.
- RFA should be considered a first-line therapy for symptomatic AFL.
- Bidirectional conduction block (BCB) in the inferior cavotricuspid isthmus (CTI) should be demonstrated.
- Cryoablation is inferior to RF ablation for the treatment of atrial flutter as evidenced by the higher recurrence rate of common AFL.

5.2 Atrial tachycardias[4,9]

- Five percent of all supraventricular tachycardias (SVT) in adults can be attributed to atrial tachycardia (Figure 5.5). Electrocardiographically it is characterized by atrial rate of less than 240 bpm and presence of isoelectric interval between P waves.

Focal atrial tachycardia
- Atrial tachycardia could originate from any one of the following sites.
  1 Along the crista terminalis
  2 Pulmonary veins superior more common than inferior
  3 Coronary sinus ostium
  4 Mitral and tricuspid annulus
  5 AVN fast pathway region
  6 Superior vena cava (SVC)
  7 Left atrial appendage.
- Electrophysiologic mechanism of the atrial tachycardia can be re-entry, abnormal automaticity or triggered activity (Table 5.1).
- Focal tachycardias are characterized by centrifugal spread of electrical impulse from a single focus.
- Activation covers less than 20% of the tachycardia cycle length.
- Localization of the focal atrial tachycardia can be achieved by three-dimensional electroanatomical mapping.
- Some focal atrial tachycardia origin sites may produce misleading activation results. These sites include:
  1 RSPV focus could be mistaken for superior right atrium
  2 SVC focus may be mistaken for right atrial tachycardia.

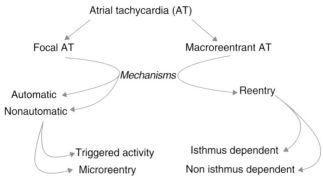

Figure 5.5 Classification of atrial tachycardia.

Table 5.1 Characteristics of the different mechanisms of focal AT.

	Automatic AT	**Triggered activity**	**Microre-entrant AT**
PES	No response	CL dependent	Reproducibly initiates and terminates AT
Isoproterenol for induction	Yes	No	No
Entrainment	No	No	Yes
Warm up Cool down	Yes	No	No
Response to adenosine	No*	Yes	Yes
Response to propranolol, verapamil	Propranolol	Propranolol, verapamil	Verapamil
Vagal maneuvers	No response	Terminates AT	No response

AT = atrial tachycardia. PES = programmed electrical stimulation. *yes if AT is induced by isoproterenol.

3 Focal atrial tachycardia arising from the left side of the interatrial septum.
4 Epicardial focus and Marshall's ligament. Tachycardia arising from these sites may be difficult to ablate due to epicardial origin and can be mistaken for tachycardia arising from left pulmonary vein or atrial appendage.
Major drawback of the above observations is the overlap of responses.

Clinical presentation
• Patients present with palpitation, dyspnea, dizziness or chest pain.
• Rapid firing of the focal atrial tachycardia may induce atrial fibrillation, thus patient may present with atrial fibrillation.

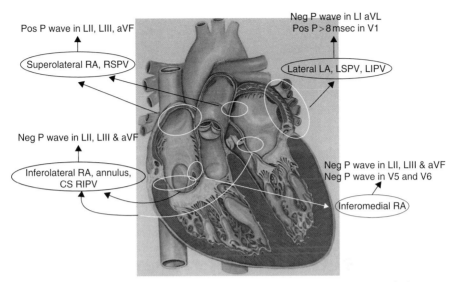

Pos P wave in LII, LIII, aVF

Superolateral RA, RSPV

Neg P wave in LI aVL
Pos P > 8 msec in V1

Lateral LA, LSPV, LIPV

Neg P wave in LII, LIII & aVF

Inferolateral RA, annulus, CS RIPV

Neg P wave in LII, LIII & aVF
Neg P wave in V5 and V6

Inferomedial RA

Figure 5.6 Site of origin of focal atrial tachycardia and respective P wave morphology.

Electrocardiographic characteristics of focal atrial tachycardia[8,10]:

- In focal atrial tachycardia P waves are separated by isoelectric line.
- P wave morphology may help identify the approximate site of origin of the atrial tachycardia (Figure 5.6).
- Commonest location of right atrial tachycardia in patients with structurally normal heart is crista terminalis. P wave morphology is positive in LII, LIII and aVF.
- Presence of anisotropy and automaticity in the cells of crista terminalis may facilitate the occurrence of the tachycardia in this location.
- Tachycardias arising from the atrioventricular annulus or coronary sinus os account for approximately 20% of all atrial tachycardias.
- The criterion of a negative P wave in leads I and aVL indicating a left atrial appendage (LAA) atrial tachycardia focus was associated with sensitivity of 92.3%, specificity 97.3%, positive predictive value 92.3%, and negative predictive value 97.3%.
- Atrial tachycardia with AV block may be a manifestation of digoxin toxicity, regardless of the serum digoxin level.
- In focal automatic atrial tachycardias the first P wave is identical to the subsequent P waves during the tachycardia and the rate generally increases gradually (warms up) over the first few seconds. In comparison, intraatrial re-entry or triggered-activity atrial tachycardia is usually initiated by a P wave from a premature atrial complex (PAC) that differs in morphology from the P wave during the tachycardia.
- The atrial to ventricular relationship is usually 1:1 during ATs, but Wenckebach or 2:1 AV block can occur at rapid rates, in the presence of AVN disease, or in the presence of drugs that slow AVN conduction.

- The presence of AV block during a supraventricular tachycardia (SVT) strongly suggests atrial tachycardia, excludes atrioventricular re-entrant tachycardia (AVRT), and renders atrioventricular nodal re-entrant tachycardia (AVNRT) less likely.
- Atrial tachycardias usually have a long RP interval, but the RP interval can also be short, depending on the degree of AV conduction delay (i.e., PR interval prolongation) during the tachycardia.
- Cristal atrial tachycardias (atrial tachycardias arising from the crista terminalis) are characterized by right-to-left activation sequence resulting in P waves that are positive and broad in leads I and II, positive in lead aVL, and biphasic in lead V1.
- A negative P wave in lead aVR identifies cristal ATs with 100% sensitivity and 93% specificity.
- High, mid, or low cristal locations can be identified by P wave polarity in the inferior leads.

Electrophysiologic characteristics of atrial tachycardia
- Changes in A-A cycle length that precede changes in H-H cycle length, strongly favor atrial tachycardia.
- Changes in H-H intervals that precede and predict subsequent A-A intervals with constant VA time, argue against an atrial tachycardia mechanism.
- Ventricular pacing during atrial tachycardia with successful capture of the atrium, if it demonstrates VAAV response on termination of ventricular pacing, is suggestive of atrial tachycardia.
- Attention must first be directed to whether or not the tachycardia has, in fact, been entrained.
- Pseudo VAAV response can be seen if the VA conduction is through slowly conducting accessory pathway.
- Pseudo-VAAV responses can occur due to failure to capture the atrium and a variable tachycardia cycle length that fortuitously correspond to the pacing cycle length at the end of the drive train.
- Endocardial activation occupies only a small fraction (less than 50%) of the tachycardia cycle length (CL) during focal atrial tachycardia with major portions of the tachycardia CL without recorded activity. In contrast, atrial activation occupies most (~90%) of the tachycardia CL during macrore-entrant AT.
- Microre-entrant atrial tachycardia is easy to initiate with a wide range of atrial extrastimulation (AES) coupling intervals (A1–A2 intervals).
- The initiating AES coupling interval and the interval between the initiating AES and first beat of atrial tachycardia are inversely related. The first tachycardia P wave is different from subsequent P waves; the first P wave is usually a PAC or AES that is necessary to start the AT. No delay in AH or PR interval is required for initiation, although it can occur. AV block can also occur at initiation.
- Triggered atrial tachycardias can be initiated by AES or (more commonly) atrial pacing. Initiation frequently requires catecholamines (isoproterenol). There is usually a direct relationship between the coupling interval or pacing CL initiating the atrial tachycardia and the interval to the onset of the atrial tachycardia and the early CL of the atrial tachycardia.

- Automatic atrial tachycardias cannot be reproducibly initiated by AES or atrial pacing. The first tachycardia P wave occurs late in the cardiac cycle and is therefore not associated with atrial or AVN conduction delay. The first tachycardia P wave and subsequent P waves are identical; the atrial tachycardia does not require a PAC to start.
- The tachycardia CL tends to progressively shorten (warm up) for several beats until its ultimate rate is achieved. No delay in the AH interval is required for initiation, although it can occur.

Ablation for atrial tachycardia[4]

- Atrial tachycardia arising from the atrial septum (right or left) or triangle of Koch may require electrophysiologic study and multielectrode or three dimensional mapping for precise localization prior to ablation.
- Dense mapping in the area of interest, using 3D sequential mapping system may help in precise localization of the focal atrial tachycardia. Incomplete mapping may result in erroneous results and failed ablation[4].
- If the earliest activation appears to be on the right side of the interatrial septum but activation time from the onset of the P wave is less than 15 ms, the earliest site appears to be near Bachmann bundle, or narrow monophasic P wave is present in V1, consider further mapping on the left side of the interatrial septum.
- Tachycardia arising from the right superior pulmonary vein may be mistaken for right atrial tachycardia. When multiple sites in posterior superior right atrium register same activation time, it is likely that the tachycardia is arising from right superior pulmonary vein.
- Presence of diffuse area of activation near the left superior pulmonary vein (LSPV), left inferior pulmonary vein (LIPV) and the posterolateral mitral annulus, may suggest an epicardial focus.
- Focal ablation site can be further confirmed by the presence of fractionated electrograms, negative unipolar atrial electrogram or transient termination of the tachycardia during mechanical pressure from the ablation catheter.
- Atrial tachycardia should be differentiated from AVRT and atypical AVNRT. (Table 5.2).
- Target for ablation is the earliest activation preceding P wave by more than 30 ms; 30 to 50 W of energy is delivered for 30 to 60 s.
- Acceleration of the tachycardia and termination within 10 s of RF application is a sign of successful outcome.
- Ablation in the lateral wall of the right atrium, crista terminalis may result in phrenic nerve damage.
- Ablation from atrial septum, Koch's triangle carries the risk of AV block. Titrating energy delivery from 5 to 40 W and closely monitoring AV conduction may avoid occurrence of AV block.
- Ablation of the atrial tachycardia arising from the annulus requires documentation of the small A and larger V electrogram at the site of ablation.
- If ablating in venous structures (CS veins, SVC), lower power may be required
- Success rate from RF ablation of the focal atrial tachycardia is 90% and recurrence rate of 10%.

Table 5.2 Differential diagnosis of SVT.

	AVRT	AVNRT	Atrial tachycardia	Atypical AVNRT
Features that Suggest	Pre-excitation on baseline EKG	Induction dependent on critical AH interval	AV block during SVT	AV Block during tachycardia
	Increase VA >20 ms with BBB	Dual AVN physiology	Earliest atrial activation away from AV groove	HA V pace minus HA SVT of >−10 msec
	Eccentric atrial activation during SVT	Septal VA <70 ms	VA dissociation during rapid V pacing	VA dissociation during SVT with rapid V pacing
	Extra nodal response to His Pacing	Concentric activation of A during SVT	A activation during V pacing different then SVT	Earliest retrograde A in atrial septum
	On cessation of A pacing first VA same as subsequent VA	On cessation of A pacing first VA same as subsequent VA	On cessation of A pacing first VA variable	On cessation of A pacing first VA same as subsequent VA
	Eccentric activation of A during V pacing same as SVT	Concentric activation of A during V pacing same as SVT	VA block CL during V pacing longer than SVT CL	SA-VA >85 ms PPI-TCL >115 ms *
	AV response on termination of V pacing	AV response on termination of V pacing	AAV response on cessation of V pacing**	AV response on termination of V pacing
	Atrial pre-excitation with PVC when His refractory	No atrial pre-excitation with PVC when His refractory	No atrial pre-excitation with PVC when His refractory	No atrial pre-excitation with PVC when His refractory
	SVT terminates with A	SVT terminates with A	Tachycardia terminates with V not A	SVT terminates with A
	HA is constant during tachycardia	HA is constant during tachycardia	HA may be variable during tachycardia	HA may be variable during tachycardia
	Termination by PVC when His is refractory without retrograde A	Shortening of VA with BBB if HV prolongs	Shortening of VA with BBB if HV prolongs	AH during A pacing >40 ms longer than AH SVT

Table 5.2 (*Continued*)

	AVRT	AVNRT	Atrial tachycardia	Atypical AVNRT
Features that Exclude	Septal VA <70 ms	Increase VA with BBB	Termination with AV block	Increase VA with BBB
	AV block during SVT	Termination by PVC when His refractory	Induction dependent on critical AH interval	Termination by PVC when His refractory
	No VA conduction at baseline	Earliest atrial activation away from AV groove	Atrial pre-excitation with PVC when His refractory	Earliest atrial activation away from AV groove
	VA block CL during V pacing longer than SVT CL	Atrial pre-excitation with PVC when His refractory	On cessation of A pacing first VA same as subsequent VA	Atrial pre-excitation with PVC when His refractory
	A activation different during V pacing then SVT	Eccentric activation of A during V pacing same as SVT	Termination by PVC when His refractory without atrial activation	Eccentric activation of A during V pacing same as SVT
	VAAV response on cessation of V pacing	VAAV response on cessation of V pacing	Eccentric activation of A during V pacing same as SVT	VAAV response on cessation of V pacing

Entrainment of AVNRT during right ventricle pacing SA is measured from last pacing stimulus to last retrogradly entrained HRA electrogram. VA = VA interval during tachycardia. PPI (post-pacing interval) is measured from last pacing stimulus to first return cycle on right ventricle electrogram. TCL = tachycardia cycle length.

- Predictors of lower success rate or recurrences include:
  1 Left atrial septal tachycardia.
  2 Multiple focal origin.
  3 Older patients.

Atrial tachycardias arising from aortic valve sinus of Valsalva (SOV)

- The noncoronary SOV is adjacent to the right and left atria, whereas the right and left SOV abut the ventricular septum and aortic outflow tract.

Electrophysiologic criteria for the diagnosis of left atrial tachycardia

- P-wave configuration different from that recorded during sinus rhythm and atrial activation sequence supporting a nonsinus node origin;

- Tachycardia induction and maintenance independent of AV nodal conduction;
- Exclusion of accessory pathways, AVN re-entry, sinoatrial re-entrant tachycardia, and atrial flutter (cycle length <280 ms) as arrhythmia mechanisms.
- Left atrial appendage atrial tachycardia exhibits a positive P wave in leads II, III, aVF, and V1 and a negative P wave in leads I and aVL.

Focal atrial tachycardia with multiple foci

- Associated arrhythmias in patients with focal atrial tachycardia with more than one focus are atrial flutter/fibrillation, followed by AVNRT and AVRT.
- Given episode of atrial tachycardia has a single morphology P-wave. Different episodes may present with different morphology of the P waves. This differs from multifocal atrial tachycardia where a single episode may manifest with three or more different morphologies of the pulmonary vein.
- Patients who have a focal AT with more than one focus have greater cardiovascular comorbidity than did those with a single focus.
- Hypertension, ischemic heart disease, and dilated cardiomyopathy are common comorbidities in patients who had a focal AT with more than one focus.
- Left atrial focus, cardiovascular comorbidity, and shortest tachycardia cycle length are independent predictors of focal AT with more than one focus.
- Focal AT with more than one focus is commonly associated with left atrial involvement.

Repetitive automatic and repetitive focal atrial tachycardias

- This is probably a manifestation of enhanced automaticity,
- It occurs in patients with structural heart disease, who develop an acute event, such as a myocardial infarction, pulmonary decompensation, sepsis, alcohol intoxication, hypokalemia, hypomagnesemia, hypoxia, stimulants, cocaine, and theophylline.

Multi-focal atrial tachycardia (MAT)

- MAT is characterized by multiple P wave morphologies (three or more separate P-wave morphologies) with continuous variation in PR interval and marked irregularity of the rhythm.
- This may be the result of pacemaker arising in different atrial locations, but a single focus with different exit pathways or abnormalities in intraatrial conduction can produce identical electrocardiographic manifestations.
- MAT is usually caused by enhanced automaticity.
- MAT occurs in patients with severe respiratory disease and pediatric populations.
- Synonyms include chaotic atrial tachycardia, multifocal atrial rhythm, and wandering atrial pacemaker.

Macrore-entrant atrial tachycardia

- Macrore-entrant tachycardia can be classified into isthmus or nonisthmus dependent types of atrial tachycardia (Figure 5.7).
- Activation and recording of the fractionated electrograms identifies the area of slow conduction (Section 5.1).

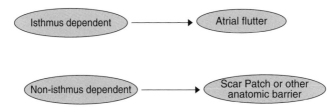

Figure 5.7 Classification of macrore-entrant AT.

- Pacing for concealed entrainment from the isthmus at cycle length 30 ms shorter than atrial tachycardia cycle length results in acceleration of the tachycardia to pacing cycle length without any change in the morphology of the P waves recorded on surface ECG. On termination of pacing, the post pacing interval is same as the tachycardia cycle length. The sensitivity and specificity of this maneuver for the diagnosis of re-entrant isthmus dependent tachycardia is approximately 90%[5,11].
- Typical flutter is an atrial macrore-entrant arrhythmia, rotating clockwise (CW) or counterclockwise (CCW) around the tricuspid annulus.
- Any other atrial re-entrant arrhythmias, regardless of the atrial cycle length, are classified as atypical atrial flutter.
- Focal atrial tachyarrhythmias, regardless of atrial rate, are considered as atrial tachycardia.
- Macrore-entrant circuits tend to have a stable cycle length with little beat-to-beat variability.
- Recognition of macrore-entrant circuits is made by mapping of the chamber of interest where the entire cycle length can be accounted for by the timing of intracardiac electrograms.
- Transient entrainment of macrore-entrant arrhythmias demonstrates that the post-pacing interval is similar to the tachycardia cycle length at widely separated regions and helps to localize the cardiac tissues that are part of the circuit.

Microre-entrant atrial tachycardia
- Both microre-entrant and focal mechanisms (triggered activity or abnormal automaticity) demonstrate a centrifugal pattern of activation and attempts to transiently entrain the tachycardia typically show a post pacing interval similar to the tachycardia cycle length in only a small region.
- Microre-entry and focal mechanisms often demonstrate considerable variability in tachycardia cycle length.
- Small re-entrant circuits are associated with fractionated electrograms that are of small amplitude. It is this finding that is most useful for differentiating a small re-entrant circuit from a true focal mechanism.
- With a quadripolar catheter, the timing of activation on the proximal and distal electrode pairs often spans at least 50% of the tachycardia cycle length for microre-entrant arrhythmias.

- In contrast, focal mechanisms are characterized by relatively similar activation times for electrograms recorded. The electrograms are often of high amplitude with little fractionation.
- Distinction between microre-entrant and focal atrial tachycardia can be difficult in the presence of significant scar that results in delayed conduction from a focal source producing fractionated electrograms that are "innocent bystanders" rather than integral components of a small re-entrant circuit.

Atypical atrial flutter with no previous cardiac intervention
- Atypical atrial flutter (AFL), in patients who have not had cardiac surgery or a prior catheter ablation procedure, is rare.
- Left atrial flutter should be considered as atypical.
- Incidence of atypical right atrial flutter is 5%.
- Lower loop re-entry (LLR) incorporating the cavotricuspid isthmus (CTI), and counterclockwise AFL is the most common pattern.
- Bidirectional conduction block in the CTI eliminates all LLR flutters.
- Upper loop re-entry (ULR), a non-CTI-dependent AFL is rare. This mechanism is characterized by a CW flutter loop, with early breakthrough in lateral annulus and collision of activation fronts over the CTI.
- Left septal AFL has been described in patients taking antiarrhythmic drugs such as amiodarone for treatment of atrial fibrillation (AF), it may be due to slowing of electrical conduction, which then allows stable flutter circuits to persist.
- The AFL circuits can be entrained, with postpacing intervals matching the AFL cycle lengths, from sites on the left side of the interatrial septum, and may manifest as CW as well as CCW loops.
- On the surface electrocardiogram CCW and CW septal AFLs manifests as prominent positive or negative atrial flutter wave respectively in lead V1, whereas the limb leads demonstrated flat P wave morphology.

Left atrial flutter[12,13]
- Activation sequence mapping in these patients shows large electrically silent areas located in posterior or anterior left atrium free wall as well as pre-existing zones of block, usually more than one per patient, in various different locations.
- Some of these macrore-entrant circuits may be perimitral, and the others may manifest various different mechanisms with pathways winding around the electrically silent areas and the zones of conduction block.
- Small areas of re-entry and multiple-loop circuits are less common.
- More than one catheter ablation session may be required for effective control of the left AFL in one third of patients.

Surface electrocardiogram (ECG) during AFL
- The surface ECG during LLR (Lower loop re-entry) tends to be similar to the pattern observed during the CCW AFL, except for the decrease in the atrial cycle length and the decrease in the amplitude of the terminal voltage in the inferior limb leads.

- In ULR (Upper loop re-entry), the surface ECG pattern resembles that observed during CW CTI-dependent AFL. This finding would be expected because the collision of the two wavefronts of ULR in the CTI does not result in any change in the activation sequence of left atrium, the septum, and the caudal–cranial activation of the lateral right atrium.
- The AFLs dependent on septal macrore-entrant loops manifests with prominent voltage in V1, and flat voltage in the limb leads.
- ECG patterns observed during left AFLs may be quite variable, and unlike the focal left ATs, negative polarity P waves in limb leads 1 and aVL are present only in a minority of macrore-entrant AFLs.
- In patients presenting with AFL after surgical or transcatheter procedures for treatment of atrial arrhythmias or for correction of congenital heart disease, surface ECG patterns may be different from the usual ones associated with typical CCW or CW, CTI-dependent AFL, but may still be associated with a mechanism that is CTI-dependent
- Some left atrial or septal flutter loops may mimic the surface ECG patterns of typical CCW or CW CTI-dependent AFL, if there is a pre-existing line of conduction block in the CTI.

PostMAZE atypical AFL
- Focal atrial tachycardias are rare.
- AFLs may be CTI-dependent right AFLs, even though the surface ECG pattern may not suggest this mechanism.
- Left atrial macrore-entry is a common underlying mechanism after the surgical MAZE procedure.
- May present with double loop re-entry.
- These AFLs can be treated by radiofrequency (RF) ablation.
- Characteristics of postMAZE AFL may be different in patients undergoing a primary antiarrhythmic MAZE procedure with an epicardial approach from those patients who are undergoing maze procedure as a concomitant therapy doing mitral valve replacement.
- At different institutions where the MAZE procedure may be performed using a different lesion set, other mechanisms underlying postMAZE atypical AFL may be observed.
- The incidence of postMAZE atrial tachyarrhythmias is approximately 10%.

Post-catheter ablation atypical AFL
- The incidence of iatrogenic post-catheter ablation atrial tachyarrhythmias has been rising with increasing use of left atrium catheter ablation and pulmonary vein isolation to treat AF.
- The mechanism of these tachyarrhythmias may be left atrial macrore-entrant circuits.
- Patients with postablation AFL tend to be more symptomatic compared with their symptoms during AF because of poor rate control during AFL.
- Left AFL, shortly after catheter ablation procedure, may subside over time, spontaneously or with the use of antiarrhythmic drugs.

- If antiarrhythmic drugs fail and other ablation procedure may be required.
- The incidence of postablation atypical AFL is higher in patients with chronic AF compared with paroxysmal AF. Left atrium size tends to be larger in patients with chronic AF
- Linear RF ablation attempts are frequently carried out in the roof of the LA, between the left inferior pulmonary vein and the mitral annulus (unlike CTI, there is no universally accepted mitral isthmus location), and elsewhere in the left atrium.
- Presence of bidirectional conduction block should be validated by appropriate pacing maneuvers; Zones of slow conduction without complete conduction block may promote AFL.
- During catheter mapping of atypical postablation AFL, both atria should be mapped, and both activation sequence mapping and entrainment mapping should be performed.
- Performing and interpreting the actual activation sequence during AFL may be limited by difficulties associated with assigning accurate local activation times to low-amplitude, complex, fractionated electrograms.
- If the re-entry is confined to a small area of the left atrium, activation sequence mapping may erroneously suggest a focal mechanism.
- Entrainment mapping may be limited by high capture threshold over large areas previously subjected to RF energy.
- Macrore-entry may include perimitral circuits, septal circuits, and others associated with breaks in the previously attempted lines of conduction block.
- There may be simultaneous multiple circuits present in the same patient the mechanisms may switch back and forth between different circuits complicating the interpretation of activation and entrainment mapping.
- Seemingly different mechanisms may share common pathways.
- Even with complex underlying mechanisms, and technical difficulties catheter mapping and ablation remains an effective and often curative method for treatment of post–catheter ablation atypical AFL.

Atypical AFL in surgically corrected congenital heart disease

- After surgical correction of congenital heart disease the atria are scarred and dilated for example after the Mustard operation or Fontan procedure.
- CTI-dependent AFL remains a common arrhythmia after surgical correction of pulmonic stenosis and tetralogy of Fallot although surface ECG pattern may not be typical.
- Multiple circuits and mechanisms are common.
- Activation and, entrainment, mapping may demonstrate the presence of large low-voltage regions harboring various AFL circuits.
- Recurrence of atypical AFL with a different mechanism after effective elimination of one mechanism is common.

Entrainment mapping[13]

- Entrainment mapping can be used to determine if the tachycardia is originating from right or left atrium.

- During entrainment, the difference between the postpacing interval (PPI) and the tachycardia cycle length (TCL) is an indicator of the conduction time between the pacing site and the re-entrant circuit.
- The criterion for determining whether a pacing site is located inside the re-entrant circuit is the difference between the PPI and the TCL. If the difference is <20 to 30 ms, the pacing site probably is located inside the re-entrant circuit.
- Further the distance from the pacing site to the re-entry, the longer is the PPI–TCL difference.
  - If the PPI–TCL ≤ 50 ms in high right atrium (HRA) and proximal coronary sinus (PCS), it is suggestive of right atrial flutter.
  - If the PPI–TCL ≤ 50 ms in HRA but >50 ms in PCS, it is suggestive of lateral RA tachycardia.
  - If the PPI–TCL ≥ 50 ms in HRA and PCS, it is suggestive of left pulmonary vein tachycardia.
  - If the PPI–TCL ≥ 50 ms in HRA and <50 ms in PCS and distal coronary sinus (DCS) consider left atrial flutter utilizing mitral annular isthmus.
  - If the PPI–TCL ≥ 50 ms in HRA and <50 ms in PCS and >50 ms in DCS consider right pulmonary vein or septal tachycardia.
- Computerized three dimensional mapping allows recording of the isochronal maps of the tachycardia circuit[14].
- Scar related macrore-entrant right atrial tachycardias have been characterized as atypical atrial flutter.[13,15,16]
- Scar related atrial tachycardia may require higher energy and temperatures for successful ablation. This could be accomplished by large/irrigated tip catheter [17].
- Combination of the electroanatomical and electrophysiologic mapping improves ablation outcome[4].
- As opposed to focal atrial tachycardia, atrial activation during macrore-entrant tachycardia occupies 90% or more of the TCL. Earliest and latest activation tend to be adjacent.
- Left atrial macrore-entrant tachycardia is characterized by the following:[8]
  1 Negative P waves in LI and aVL.
  2 Area of slow conduction between mitral annulus and anatomic barrier which could be pulmonary vein, scar or atrial appendage.
  3 Post pacing interval in the right atrium is >40 ms longer than the tachycardia cycle length at three or more sites including cavotricuspid isthmus thus excluding right atrial flutter or macrore-entrant tachycardia.
  4 Cycle length variation in the left atrium precedes the right atrium.
  5 Right atrial activation accounts for less than 50% of the tachycardia cycle length during sequential catheter mapping.
- Macrore-entrant tachycardias are common after surgical repair procedures such as Mustard and Senning, Fontan or repair of tetralogy of Fallot.
- Identification and elimination of areas of slow conduction between the scars or scars and anatomical barriers is preferred approach during radiofrequency ablation.

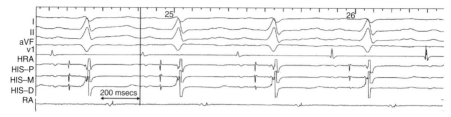

Figure 5.8 Electrogram to onset of P wave 200 ms.

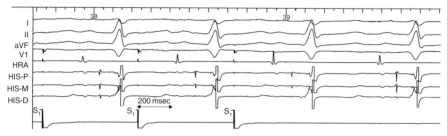

Figure 5.9 Stimulus to onset of P wave 200 ms. Tachycardia is entrained without change in activation or P wave morphology.

- Incisional (scar related) re-entry may occur following:
  1 Surgery for congenital heart disease.
  2 Following partially successful MAZE procedure
  3 Following catheter based ablation for AF.
- Fallowing a patch repair of the ASD the isthmus for re-entrant tachycardia may be between the patch and CS.
- Atriotomy scar-related macrore-entrant tachycardia may occur from the scar that extends from the atrial appendage to inferoposterior right atrial free wall. Incision typically does not extend to inferior vena cava or TA producing a narrow isthmus.
- Entrainment with concealed fusion can be demonstrated from the entry, mid portion or the exit site of this isthmus.
- The following observations are likely to identify the optimum site for successful ablation (Figures 5.8 and 5.9).
  1 PPI is the same as TCL.
  2 Earliest electrogram precedes the onset of surface P wave by more than 50 ms.
  3 On pacing from the site of the earliest electrogram, at cycle length 20 to 30 ms shorter, results in concealed entrainment.
  4 Interval from the electrogram to the onset of P wave is same as the interval from the stimulus to the onset of P wave.
- Electroanatomical mapping can identify the activation pattern and scar by using voltage map and sites for ablation.
- To guide RFCA, conventional strategies are based on bipolar local activation time (LAT) mapping and the presence of a QS configuration of the unipolar electrogram for predicting a successful ablation site.
- Reversed polarity of adjacent bipolar electrograms can be used to guide ablation.

- Hypothesis is that the excitation wavefront propagates radially from the breakthrough site producing the reversal of electrograms as wavefront propagates in opposite directions as demonstrated in the presence of accessory pathways and focal atrial tachycardias.

5.3 Atrial fibrillation[15]

- AF is a multifaceted cardiac arrhythmia manifesting with different etiologies, gene expression, mechanisms, and response to treatment. There is a known correlation with thyrotoxicosis, hypertension, diabetes, heart failure, and AF. Other types include "lone" AF, vagotonic AF or adrenergic AF, not associated with any structural heart disease or any of the comorbidities.
- Mechanistically AF could be focal most often arising from pulmonary vein, or macrore-entrant or multiple wavelet type.
- Autonomic mechanisms operative in triggering and maintaining AF may differ between structurally normal atria and remodeled atria.
- AF is associated with increased inward-rectifier current I_{K1}. MicroRNA-1 (miR-1) reciprocally regulates inwardly rectifying potassium channel (Kir)2.1 expression. miR-1 levels are reduced in human AF, possibly contributing to up-regulation of Kir2.1 subunits, leading to increased Up-regulation of inward-rectifier currents I_{K1}.
- 1% or more than 2 million Americans are afflicted with atrial fibrillation.
- Approximately 30% of AF patients have parents with a history of AF, suggesting a genetic predisposition
- 7% over 80 years of age may have AF.
- Heart failure affects 2% of the population.
- The two conditions may occur in the same patients, perhaps as a result of common risk factors.
- 41% of people with heart failure have AF at some stage, and 42% of patients with AF have heart failure.
- Cumulative 20-year AF incidence rates are higher for pulse pressure >61 mmHg.
- The incidence of AF is 1% per year.
- 6% of patients following an acute myocardial infarction develop atrial fibrillation.

Risk factors for AF include
- Other cardiovascular illnesses such as myocardial infarction or heart failure.
- Aging.
- Inflammatory response to disease or injury.
- Genetic abnormalities.
- Obesity.
- Sleep apnea.
- Hyperthyroidism.
- Alcohol consumption.
- Hypertension.

Morbidities associated with AF

- Risk of death increases twofold in patients with AF.
- Quality of life with symptomatic AF tends to be lower than that for patients without AF. The risk of stroke increases fivefold.
- Atrial fibrillation with persistent rapid ventricular response may result in tachycardia mediated left ventricular dysfunction.
- There may be increased risk of ventricular arrhythmias especially in the presence of previous scars and left ventricular dysfunction.
- Untreated atrial fibrillation may be associated with cognitive impairment.

Mechanism of structural remodeling of the atrium during atrial fibrillation

- Persistent AF is associated with atrial structural remodeling due to interstitial fibrosis.
- Peroxisome proliferation-activated receptors (PPARs) are ligand-dependent transcription factors important in cellular metabolism lipid transport, such as regulation of brown fat differentiation.
- PPAR-γ activation has been shown to limit the inflammatory response.
- Activation of PPAR-γ by the drug pioglitazone is associated with attenuation of atrial fibrosis and subsequent fibrillation.
- Heart failure and myocardial infarction are associated with an inflammatory response that results in infiltration of immune cells such as monocytes and macrophages into the atrial tissue from the endocardial surface into the subendocardial region where they produce and secrete inflammatory cytokines.
- Cytokines alter the balance of matrix metalloproteinases (MMPs) and their endogenous inhibitors, the tissue inhibitors of MMPs. This imbalance leads to expansion of the extracellular matrix.
- Cytokines initiate and support the transformation of resident fibroblasts into reactive myofibroblasts, leading to systemic inflammatory response.
- Myocytes respond to cytokines by activating the hypertrophic signaling cascades and initiating inside-out signaling via the integrins, which stimulates collagen production and deposition.
- Activation of tumor necrosis factor-α (TNF-α), interleukin (IL)-1β, IL-6, and transforming growth factor-α (TGF-β) receptors leads to activation of gene programs that upregulate the formation and deposition of collagen via the myofibroblasts.
- Pioglitazone belongs to a family of drugs described as insulin enhancers, the thiazolidinediones.
- These drugs increase the reactivity to insulin in cases of insulin resistance by activating PPAR-γ.
- Activation of PPAR-γ inhibits the production of inflammatory cytokines by monocytes. Pioglitazone may decrease atherosclerosis and attenuated Parkinson's disease and a number of other inflammatory-based diseases
- Pioglitazone, outside of its role in increasing insulin sensitivity, causes an overall immune suppression.

Electrical remodeling of the atrium

- Electrical remodeling is characterized by shortening of the atrial refractory period.
- Stimulation of the vagal nerves shortens the atrial action potential duration (APD) and the effective refractory period (ERP) and increases dispersion of atrial repolarization, thus creating an arrhythmogenic substrate for AF. These effects are mediated via activation of the atria-selective $I_{K,ACh}$ channels.
- Suppression of $I_{K,ACh}$ may leave sympathetic modulation of AV-conduction unopposed, leading to enhanced impulse conduction to the ventricles.
- In atrial fibrillation I_{CaL} is reduced. This results in shortening of APD and refractory period.
- Shortening of refractory period may persist after recovery from AF and predispose to reoccurrences.
- Atrial dilatation and stretch may result in decrease of refractory period.
- Shortening of ERP, APD, increase in dispersion of refractoriness, and change in conduction velocity perpetuates AF.
- Human atrial repolarization uses I_{Kur}. I_{to} and I_{Kur} are decreased in AF resulting in shortening of refractory period.

Atrial anatomy

- The interatrial septum is formed largely by the primary septum, representing the floor of the oval fossa, and secondary septum, which is a superior infolding of the atrial walls.
- Appendage forms the anterior atrial wall.
- This part is distinguished from the remainder of the atrium by the pectinated nature of its walls, with the terminal crest, or crista terminalis, marking the border with the smooth-walled systemic venous component.
- The myocardium of this venous component surrounds the orifices of the superior and inferior caval veins and the coronary sinus, with sleeves of myocardium extending into the venous lumens at their junctions with the atrium.
- The sinus node is located at the junction of the superior caval vein with the right atrium.
- The vestibule of the right atrium, also smooth walled, inserts into the leaflets of the tricuspid valve at the atrioventricular junction
- The left atrium, in contrast, has a significantly larger body. The appendage is smaller with pectinate muscles are confined within it.
- The larger part of the left atrial cavity is smooth walled.
- The pulmonary venous component forms the atrial roof, typically with one vein entering at each of the four corners, there may be variations in the location of venous orifices. Myocardial sleeves extend from the atrial roof for short distances along the veins, being longer on the superior than on the inferior veins.
- These sleeves are composed of working atrial myocardium, albeit with intermingling myocytes arranged in circumferential and longitudinal fashion.
- The identity of the working atrial myocardium of the morphologically right as opposed to the left atrium is established by the expression of genes responsible for left-right asymmetry.

- Pitx2c is one of these genes.
- During the fetal period, pacemaking activity and expression of Hcn4 become restricted to the developing sinus node, recognized by its expression of the T-box transcription factor Tbx3.
- Atrial fibrillation could be due to persistent rapid firing from the single focus termed as focal driver or it could be maintained by multiple wavelets after being initiated by premature atrial beats called focal triggers.

Pericardium
- The human heart has two pericardial layers, the visceral pericardium (which is closely applied to the epicardial surface of the heart) and the parietal pericardium.
- The pericardial reflections on the heart form two distinct sinuses that allow mapping of the epicardial surface of the heart.
- The transverse sinus allows passage of catheters from the left to the right side of the epicardial surface of the heart in between the great arteries.
- The oblique sinus allows for mapping the posterior/inferior wall of the left ventricle and the posterior left atrial wall (including the ligament of Marshall).

Classification of AF
Atrial fibrillation can be classified in to following categories:

1 Paroxysmal AF: starts and stops spontaneously.
2 Persistent AF: requires electrical or pharmacologic cardioversion to terminate an episode.
3 Permanent chronic AF: persists in spite of therapeutic intervention or based on a decision not to restore sinus rhythm.

- Lone AF can either be paroxysmal, persistent or chronic. It is defined as atrial fibrillation occurring in patients less than 60 years of age who have no associated cardiovascular diseases.
- Paroxysmal AF often progress to chronic AF. Conversion and maintenance of sinus rhythm becomes increasingly difficult with chronic AF.
- Chemical and electrical cardioversion for maintenance of SR is easier in AF of short duration.

Neurohumoral changes during atrial fibrillation
- Atrial natriuretic factor (ANF) increases due to atrial stretch and dilation.
- Elevated ANF decreases after cardioversion.
- ANF may shorten ARP.
- Acetylcholine-mediated AF is facilitated by isoproterenol, which decreased the threshold of acetylcholine concentration for AF induction and increased AF duration.
- Abbreviation of APD by acetylcholine permits rapid rates of excitation, which leads to intracellular calcium (Cai) accumulation. If this is coupled with a long pause such as that occurring after termination of AF, a large Ca

release from the sarcoplasmic reticulum could induce late phase 3 early after-depolarizations.

- Elevated Cai activates the forward mode of the sodium/calcium exchanger, resulting in early after-depolarizations and triggered activity.
- Factors that may participate in the generation of atrial fibrosis/inflammation/ oxidative stress, include angiotensin II, TGF-β1, mitogen-activated protein kinase (MAPK), platelet-derived growth factor (PDGF), PPAR-γ, Janus kinase (JAK), Rac1, nicotinamide adenine dinucleotide phosphate (NADPH) oxidase, signal transducers and activators of transcription (STAT), calcineurin.

Genetics and AF

- In familial AF multiple family members are affected.
- It is not uncommon to find AF in only one parent or first-degree relative (30% of a Framingham Heart Study subgroup with AF had at least one parent with AF).
- Majority of AF is "nongenetic" lone AF and AF with comorbidities.
- KCNQ1 is the pore-forming α-subunit of the I_{KS} potassium channel that opens slowly in response to depolarization of the membrane and is important in the repolarization of cardiac action potentials (APs).
- S140G mutation in *KCNQ1* has been linked to AF.
- Mutation causes a gain of function of the I_{KS} channel such that the channels lose voltage dependence and remain open at all physiological voltages.
- In response to a voltage change, the potassium current flowing through the mutant channels changes rapidly, behaving similarly to the background KCNQ1–KCNE2 potassium current.
- Thus S140G mutation is likely to initiate and maintain AF by reducing APD and shortening the ERP in atrial myocardium.
- Familial AF has been related to mutations leading either to a gain of function (genes *KCNQ1, KCNE2, KCNJ2, KCNH2 KCNA5* Kv1.5) or to a loss of function (gene *SCN5A*) of sodium channels.
- Gain of function mutation of potassium channel also results in short-QT syndrome.
- Sodium channel *SCN5A* mutation as in Brugada syndrome and in progressive cardiac conduction defect has higher prevalence of the atrial arrhythmia.
- LQT-3 may be associated with AF. The causative mutation was Y1795C identified on the *SCN5A* gene encoding the cardiac sodium channel.
- Sodium blocker flecainide may be useful in acute treatment for AF.
- Mutation in the natriuretic peptide precursor A gene *NPPA*, which encodes ANP may be associated with AF, association between a defect in a circulating hormone and susceptibility to AF.
- Brugada syndrome caused by *SCN5A* loss-of-function mutations have also been shown to have an increased incidence of AF, ranging from 20 to 39%.
- Consistent with a loss of sodium channel function, these patients had slower AV conduction, longer atrio-His and His–ventricular intervals, and longer refractory period of the AV node compared with normal controls.

- Thus, it is possible that certain *SCN5A* mutations give rise to AF in the atrium and a cardiomyopathy phenotype in the ventricle, supporting the notion that ventricular and atrial tachyarrhythmias associated with *SCN5A* mutations may be allelic disorders.
- Gain-of-function mutation in *SCN5A* can give rise to a mixed phenotype of LQTS and familial lone AF.
- Reduced ARP predisposes to atrial arrhythmias including AF.
- Gain-of-function mutations in genes encoding subunits of cardiac potassium channels responsible for generating I_Ks (KCNQ1/KCNE2) and I_{K1} (KCNJ2), decrease action potential duration.
- Prolongation of ARP would be a reasonable therapeutic target.
- AF locus has been mapped to chromosome 1p36–p35 and identified a heterozygous frameshift mutation in the gene encoding atrial natriuretic peptide (ANP).
- High concentrations of circulating chimeric ANP have been detected in subjects with the mutation. Shortened atrial action potentials may be due to ANP creating a possible substrate for AF.
- *KCNA5* loss-of-function mutations resulting in reduction of I_{Kur} has been identified as a cause of familial AF. Reduction of I_{Kur} results in abbreviation of action potential duration (APD90) in nonremodeled (healthy) atrial cells,

Laminopathies

- An infrequent genetic etiology is mutation in the gene encoding for lamin A/C, LMNA, and the AF is typically associated with a combined cardiac and skeletal myopathy.
- The *LMNA* gene resides on chromosome 1q21 and it encodes for 2 isoforms, lamin A and C, which are generated by alternative splicing.
- Lamins A and C are intermediate-filament proteins that form the nuclear lamina, function as a nuclear scaffold to maintain the structure and size of the nucleus, and are also implicated in transcriptional regulation, nuclear pore positioning, and heterochromatin organization.
- Mutations in nuclear lamins and lamin-associated proteins cause more than 16 distinct human diseases, termed laminopathies.
- Lamin A/C is expressed in multiple cell types, and mutations in *LMNA* result in a range of phenotypes, including premature aging syndromes, types of muscular dystrophy, a subset of lipodystrophies, bone dysplasias, and cardiovascular diseases.
- Cardiac involvements in laminopathies present with progressive atrioventricular block (AVB), dilated cardiomyopathy (DCM), sudden cardiac death (SCD), and infrequently, atrial arrhythmias.
- Cause of heterogeneous phenotypes with variable penetrance remains unclear.
- Cardiac gap junction channels are responsible for rapid electrical communication and coordinated spread of excitation by creating low resistive pathways for the passage of current from myocyte to adjacent myocytes resulting in an efficient and synchronous myocardial contraction.
- These channels directly connect the cytoplasmic compartments of adjacent cells.
- The building blocks of gap junctions are connexin (Cx) proteins.
- In the human adult heart, five Cx proteins have been identified.

- Cx31.9 is expressed predominantly in atrioventricular nodal tissue.
- Cx43 is expressed in both atrial and ventricular tissue.
- Cx45 is expressed in smaller quantities.
- Cx37 is expressed in vascular endothelial cells.
- Cx40 is predominantly expressed in atrial and specialized conduction tissue. It is absent from ventricular myocytes. Cx40 gap junction channels have a very high conductance. High channel conductance and restricted localization of Cx40 to atrial tissue is responsible for mediating atrial tissue conduction velocity.
- There are 21 known human connexin genes, 8 have been identified to cause human disease due to mutation.
- The phenomenon of tissue-specific genetic defects is referred to as somatic mutations. Somatic mutations are the basis of most forms of cancer, but may also be responsible sporadic diseases not related to malignancy.
- Patients with Cx40 mutations may have genetic defect identified from atrial tissue whereas the gene sequence from their lymphocyte DNA may be normal.

Atrial developmental features
- Nkx2–5 establishes the boundary between the working atrial myocardium and the sinus node,
- Hcn4- and Tbx3-expressing cells expand from the sinus node into the atrium.
- Expression of Tbx3 in the atrium results in expression of pacemaking genes, including Hnc4, in the atrial myocardium.
- Hcn4 contributes to the "funny" current I_f, which is important for the spontaneous activity of the cardiac pacemaker cells.
- A funny current in atrial cells is suppressed by the inward rectifier potassium current I_{K1}, along with the dominant pacemaker current of the sinus node.
- Sinus nodal dysfunction is commonly due to acquired diseases.
- Mutations in *HCN4*, *SCN5A*, and ANiK2 may result in the familial form of sinus node dysfunction.
- Sequence variation on chromosome 4q25 has been found to be associated with an increased risk for AF.
- AF, even gene mutation-associated AF, occurs long after the end of embryonic development. The developmental factors do not directly or solely cause AF.
- Under normal conditions, the myocardium expresses Cx40, with expression of Hcn4 being low or absent. In contrast, when Nkx2–5 expression is reduced, the pulmonary venous myocardial phenotype shifts to become more pacemaker-like, expressing Hcn4 but with a reduced expression of Cx40.
- miR-1 (microinhibitory RNA) regulates Kir2.1 and Cx43 levels in ventricular myocytes and increase in miR-1 levels in pathological conditions may be a trigger for arrhythmias.
- In AF there is a decrease in miR-1 with reciprocal increase in Kir2.1.as compared with ventricular arrhythmias where there is an increase in miR-1.
- Melanocyte-like cells have been noted in the heart. The melanin synthesis enzyme dopachrome tautomerase (DCT) is involved in intracellular calcium and reactive species regulation in melanocytes.

Natural history

- In 30% of patients persistent AF progresses to permanent AF.
- Patients who progress to persistent form of AF tend to be older, more often have heart failure and valvular heart disease, and have a larger left atrium.
- Approximately half of individuals who experience an initial episode of AF will go on to develop recurrent AF, typically within the first 2 years of follow-up.
- Patients with "lone AF" or AF in the absence of other risk factors and in younger patients are less likely to progress.
- Despite the use of antiarrhythmic therapy in patients who do experience recurrent AF, more than half of patients will develop persistent AF.
- Two thirds of patients who develop persistent AF despite antiarrhythmic therapy go on to develop permanent AF.
- Newly detected AF is associated with significantly higher rates of death.
- AF is associated with an increased risk for mortality as well as significant morbidity, including bothersome symptoms, exacerbation of heart failure, and thromboembolic events
- A particular harbinger of poor outcome is the new diagnosis of AF in patients with congestive heart failure (CHF).
- Blood pressure (BP) is strongly associated with incident AF, and systolic BP is a better predictor than diastolic BP.

Clinical presentation

- Most common symptoms are fatigue, reduced exercise tolerance, dyspnea and palpitation, although most episodes of AF remain asymptomatic.
- Tachycardia from atrial fibrillation can exacerbate angina or CHF.
- Irregular rhythm is consistent with but not diagnostic of AF. Other conditions, such as sinus rhythm with frequent supraventricular or ventricular ectopic beats, sinus arrhythmia, or MAT, can cause irregular pulse. An electrocardiogram is necessary to confirm the diagnosis. Absence of P waves is characteristic of AF. Extremely rapid ventricular response may appear regular.
- AF with rapid ventricular response and aberrant ventricular conduction can result in a wide complex tachycardia which may be mistaken for ventricular tachycardia [2].
- Obesity and the magnitude of nocturnal oxygen desaturation, due to obstructive sleep apnea, are independent risk factors for AF in individuals <65 years of age.
- The overall incidence of post-coronary artery bypass graft (CABG) AF is 24%,
- Incidence of post-CABG AF is highest in the first 4 days after surgery. It may result in worsening of heart failure, stroke, prolong hospitalization.
- AF may be associated with dementia.

Treatment[13,12]

- The goals of therapy for AF are elimination of symptoms and improvement in quality of life; prevention of complications such as thromboembolic events, rate control to avoid tachycardia-mediated cardiomyopathy; and, possibly improvement in survival.

- Antiarrhythmic drug that blocks ion channels, beta receptors, as well as I_{KAch} would be more effective than beta-blockers or ion channel blockers alone in controlling AF. Amiodarone, which blocks multiple ion channels and receptors is an effective drug for AF control.
- If the patient is hemodynamically unstable immediate cardioversion should be considered.
- Rate control can be achieved by AVN blocking drugs [3,6,18]
- Digoxin is least effective in controlling the rate especially in physically active patients.
- Beta-blockers and/or calcium channel blockers are effective AV node blocking agents[19].
- Calcium channel blockers are preferred in patients with bronchial asthma. Aim should be to achieve ventricular response between 80 to 100 bpm.
- AVN blocking agents should be avoided in the presence of ventricular pre-excitation. Amiodarone could be used in this setting because it prolongs the refractory period of accessory pathway.
- Duration of AF and risk factors for thromboembolic complication determine the need for anticoagulation. AF increases the risk of stroke eightfold[4].
- Risk factors for thromboembolic events in the presence of AF include:
  1 Age > 65 years.
  2 Hypertension.
  3 Left ventricular failure.
  4 Enlarged left atrium.
  5 Diabetes mellitus.
  6 History of transient ischemic attacks (TIA).
  7 Valvular heart disease.
- The CHADS2 (Congestive heart failure, Hypertension, Age, Diabetes, Stroke [Doubled]) score evolved from the Stroke Prevention in AF (SPAF) risk stratification scheme, and was validated in the National Registry of Atrial Fibrillation cohort as well as in a pooled analysis of patients treated with aspirin.
- American College of Cardiology/American Heart Association/European Society of Cardiology (ACC/AHA/ESC) guideline risk schema evolved into the CHA2DS2-VASc score (Cardiac failure or dysfunction, Hypertension, Age 75[Doubled], Diabetes, Stroke[Doubled]-Vascular disease, Age 65–74 and Sex category [Female]) score, which was validated in a European cohort of 1084 subjects who were not anticoagulated at baseline.
- The Framingham and CHADS2 schemes are point-based scores, the Framingham is based on a mathematical formula that assigns point values to age, gender, systolic blood pressure, diabetes, and previous stroke or transient ischemic attack, and the CHADS2 is based on 1 point for congestive heart failure, hypertension, age older than 75 years, and diabetes, and 2 points for previous stroke or TIA.
- CHADS2 score is defined as scores of 0 low risk, 1 intermediate risk, and 2 high risk.
- The Framingham score is defined as score 0 to 7 low risk, 8 to 15 intermediate risk, and 16 to 31 high risk.

- The CHA2DS2-VASc score includes additional categories: score 0 low risk, 1 intermediate risk, and 2 as high risk.
- Evidence that anticoagulation with warfarin prevents thromboembolic complication is supported by the following studies:

1 Benefit of anticoagulation versus placebo: SPAF trial[20].

- It was concluded that aspirin or warfarin significantly reduces events when compared with placebo. SPAF is not a comparison of aspirin with warfarin.
- Retrospective analysis suggested a lack of benefit of anticoagulation for patients younger than 60 years.

2 Benefit of warfarin over aspirin: Atrial Fibrillation, Aspirin, Anticoagulation (AFASAK) trial[10]

- There was substantial reduction of thromboembolic events with warfarin versus aspirin or placebo (2% per year versus 5.5% per year).
- There was no significant difference in mortality. The bleeding rates were 6% per year with warfarin, 1% per year with aspirin or placebo.
- This study supported the conclusion that warfarin is superior to aspirin and placebo in preventing thromboembolic events among a largely elderly population.

3 The Boston Area Anticoagulation Trial for Atrial Fibrillation (BAATAF)[8]

- There was significant reduction in events in warfarin treated group (0.4% per year versus 2.98% per year in the control group, an overall 86% reduction).
- Increased mortality was noted in the control group.
- There was no significant difference in bleeding events.
- It was concluded that warfarin is superior to placebo in reducing thromboembolic events and mortality.

4 SPAF-II trial[14]

- SPAF-II demonstrated higher event rates in high risk patients over 75 years old. This is reduced with warfarin anticoagulation.
- Increased risk for bleeding was noted.

5 Aspirin in low-risk patients: SPAF-III trial

- SPAF III supports the use of aspirin for thromboembolic prophylaxis in low risk patients and suggests that patients with prior hypertension may be at sufficient risk to justify anticoagulation with warfarin.
- Warfarin remains underused within the outpatient setting. Nontherapeutic INR levels are associated with increased risk of stroke, bleeding, and thromboembolism compared with therapeutic INR levels.

6 Dabigatran and RE-LY trial

- Compared with warfarin, 150 mg dabigatran is associated with lower rates of stroke and systemic embolism but similar rates of major hemorrhage.
- Dabigatran etexilate is a prodrug that is converted to the active direct thrombin (factor IIa) inhibitor dabigatran. This conversion is independent of cytochrome P-450, making drug–drug and drug–diet interactions less likely.
- Dabigatran is excreted by the kidneys.
- Dabigatran is administered in fixed doses without laboratory monitoring of anticoagulation intensity.

- Participants had at least 1 risk factor for stroke (previous stroke or transient ischemic attack or systemic embolism, left ventricular ejection fraction <40% or symptomatic heart failure [New York Heart Association class II or higher in the last 6 months], hypertension, age ≥75 years, or age 65 to 74 years with either diabetes mellitus or coronary artery disease).
- Exclusion criteria in RE-LY included a prosthetic heart valve or hemodynamically significant valvular heart disease, disabling or recent stroke, recent or pending surgery, recent or known bleeding disorders, uncontrolled hypertension, need for anticoagulation of disorders other than AF, planned ablation or surgery for AF, reversible causes of AF, severe renal dysfunction (creatinine clearance <30 mL/min), active liver disease, or pregnancy.
- Rates for the primary outcome of all stroke (ischemic or hemorrhagic) or systemic embolism were lower in a group receiving Dabigatran etexilate, 150 mg twice daily.
- At this dose there was no increase in major bleeding.
- In the warfarin group, target INR was achieved 64.4% of the time.
- Dyspepsia occurred more frequently with dabigatran compared to warfarin.
- Myocardial infarction was more frequent with dabigatran the increase in myocardial infarction seen in RE-LY was not statistically significant in the dabigatran groups.
- Dabigatran did not cause hepatotoxicity.
- Drug discontinuation rates were higher in the dabigatran groups compared with warfarin. There was no difference in mortality with dabigatran compared with warfarin.
- There is no specific antidote for dabigatran, which has a half-life of 12 to 17 hours. Supportive therapy for severe hemorrhage may include transfusions of fresh-frozen plasma, packed red blood cells, or surgical intervention if appropriate.
- Because of the twice-daily dosing and greater risk of nonhemorrhagic side effects with dabigatran, patients already taking warfarin with excellent INR control may have little to gain by switching to dabigatran.
- Dabigatran etexilate is indicated for the prevention of stroke and systemic embolism in patients with nonvalvular AF.
- A dose of 150 mg twice daily is recommended in order to work for patients with a creatinine clearance >30 mL/min, whereas in patients with severe renal insufficiency (creatinine clearance 15–30 mL/min) the approved dose is 75 mg twice daily.
- There are no dosing recommendations for patients with creatinine clearance <15 mL/min or patients on dialysis.

Rivaroxaban and ROCKET-AF study
- Rivaroxaban (xarelto) oral direct factor xa inhibitor has been approved for the treatment of atrial fibrillation to prevent of thromboembolic complication in nonvalvular AF.
- Dose is 20 mg daily if renal functions are normal.
- In patients with left ventricular hypertrophy and new-onset AF, there is an increased risk of ischemic stroke clustering during the initial presentation.

Early and aggressive anticoagulation should be initiated in patients with left ventricular hypertrophy and new onset AF.

- In AF with CHF a strategy of rhythm control does not reduce the rate of death from cardiovascular causes, as compared with a rate-control strategy.

Rate control versus rhythm control

The issue of treating patients with AF with rate control agents versus using anti-arrhythmic drugs to maintain sinus rhythm has been addressed by two clinical trials.

Affirm[15]

- The Atrial Fibrillation Follow-up Investigation of Rhythm Management (AFFIRM) trial: patients were randomized between a strategy of rate control with beta blockers and calcium channel blockers targeted to a resting heart rate of 80 bpm versus rhythm control using antiarrhythmic drugs.
- There was a nonsignificant trend toward higher total mortality in the rhythm control group, the study's primary endpoint.
- Prespecified subgroup analysis demonstrated a statistically significant mortality benefit with rate control for patients above the age of 65. There was no significant difference in the incidence of stroke (roughly 1% per year); the majority (73%) of ischemic strokes occurred in patients who had discontinued warfarin or had an INR < 2.0.
- These findings support the recommendation that anticoagulation be continued in patients even if atrial fibrillation is successfully suppressed.
- AFFIRM demonstrated no advantage to a rhythm control strategy for recurrent atrial fibrillation, and suggests a rate control strategy may be superior in patients older than 65 years.
- Patients enrolled in this study were minimally symptomatic and relatively old (mean age approximately 70 years).
- These results do not apply to patients with symptomatic AF.
- Higher mortality in rhythm control group may be due to proarrhythmic effects of antiarrhythmic drugs rather than due to maintenance of sinus rhythm.
- The results cannot be extrapolated to younger patients whose quality of life is impaired by symptomatic AF.
- A small annual survival benefit of sinus rhythm over AF is likely to become clinically significant in younger patients followed for 2 to 3 decades than in older patients followed for 3 to 5 years, as in AFFIRM.

Race

- The RACE (Rate Control versus Electrical Cardioversion for Persistent Atrial Fibrillation) showed no significant difference in cardiovascular death or thromboembolic events, but 83% of all thromboembolic events occurred in patients who had discontinued warfarin or had an INR < 2.0.
- The study demonstrated no significant advantage to a rhythm control strategy for the management of persistent atrial fibrillation. Any benefits derived by rhythm control may have been neutralized by the proarrhythmic effects of the antiarrhythmic drugs.

- A rate control strategy is an acceptable approach to management of patients with atrial fibrillation, particularly if they are asymptomatic and elderly.
- Rhythm control should be considered for patients with symptomatic atrial fibrillation. This strategy should also be considered in minimally symptomatic young patients with atrial fibrillation.

Spironolactone and sodium nitroprusside[16]
- Spironolactone is an aldosterone receptor blocker with powerful antifibrotic properties. It has the potential of decreasing AF by reducing the scarring in the atrium.
- Nitric oxide (NO), with its antiapoptotic and anti-inflammatory effects, is involved in many biologic processes.
- Sodium nitroprusside (SNP) is a potent nitric oxide donor.
- Use of SNP has been shown to reduce the incidence and duration of postoperative AF following coronary artery bypass surgery.

Anticoagulation for conversion to sinus rhythm
- If AF is of less than 48 hours in duration, cardioversion can be attempted.
- The presence of AF for more than 48 hours necessitates 3–4 weeks of therapeutic anticoagulation prior to conversion, unless transesophageal echocardiography (TEE) demonstrates absence of clot in the left atrium and its appendage.
- Regardless of whether a TEE is performed, systemic anticoagulation is required for 3 weeks following cardioversion in all patients with atrial fibrillation of greater than 48 hours duration.

The ACUTE trial[17]
- Patients were assigned to TEE followed by DC cardioversion (if no intracardiac clot was found) versus conventional therapy consisting of 3 weeks of anticoagulation before DC cardioversion.
- All subjects (TEE group and conventional therapy group) received therapeutic anticoagulation for 4 weeks after cardioversion.
- At 8 weeks (from the time of enrollment), there was no significant difference in primary endpoint of cerebrovascular accident, TIA, and peripheral embolus.
- Fewer bleeding events were noted in the TEE group.
- The risk of thromboembolic events is higher in the first 3–4 weeks immediately following conversion to sinus rhythm.
- This may be due to atrial stunning, a term describing the observation of reduced atrial systolic function following conversion to sinus rhythm.
- Atrial stunning can allow relative stasis of blood within the atrium, potentially resulting in thrombus formation.
- Patients should receive anticoagulation with warfarin for 3 weeks following conversion to sinus rhythm even if they are in a low risk category for thromboembolic events.
- Patients with the indications for chronic anticoagulation with warfarin mentioned above (valvular heart disease, age above 65, prior thromboembolic event, hypertension, heart failure, coronary artery disease or diabetes) should receive long-term anticoagulation following cardioversion.

DC cardioversion

- Emergent electrical cardioversion is indicated if the patient is hemodynamically unstable as a result of tachycardia.
- Cardioversion is performed with a biphasic defibrillator.
- Amiodarone and sotalol facilitate successful electrocardioversion, which can be achieved in a stepwise fashion. Upon achievement of successful electrocardioversion, amiodarone is superior to placebo, and sotalol has a lesser effect.
- Antiarrhythmic drugs had no effect on the total number of energy step use in patients who had successful electrocardioversion.
- Calcium channel blockers had no influence on the success rate in achieving sinus rhythm. Successful electrocardioversion was associated with lower BMI and AF history ≤1 year. Lower energy use was associated with biphasic shocks, lower BMI, and AF duration ≤1 year.

Rectilinear biphasic defibrillation

- During biphasic defibrillation there is change in the polarity of the waveform during delivery of energy.
- Biphasic defibrillation allows for similar current delivery (which is the most important variable for achieving cardioversion) with lower energy.
- Number of shocks required to achieve cardioversion is also reduced.
- Biphasic defibrillation is superior to monophasic defibrillation.

Chemical cardioversion[21]

- Ibutilide, a substituted methane sulfonamide derivative, is an intravenous Class III antiarrhythmic agent indicated for rapid conversion of AF or atrial flutter to normal sinus rhythm.
- Unlike other class III antiarrhythmic agents that block outward potassium currents, ibutilide exerts its actions by promoting the influx of sodium through slow inward sodium channels.
- Ibutilide prolongs the action potential duration, thereby causing a mild slowing of the sinus rate and AV conduction. These effects are in contrast to class I antiarrhythmic agents, which inhibit the influx of sodium.
- Clinically, ibutilide converts AF or flutter to normal sinus rhythm without altering BP, heart rate, QRS duration, or PR interval.
- Ibutilide can be used for cardioversion alone or as an adjuvant to facilitate DC cardioversion, particularly when initial DC cardioversion is unsuccessful.
- Ibutilide is administered by intravenous infusion.
- The pharmacokinetics of ibutilide show considerable intersubject variability.
- Systemic clearance is approximately equal to liver blood flow (29 mL/min/kg), and protein binding is about 40%.
- Metabolism occurs in the liver by omega-oxidation with sequential beta-oxidation to eight metabolites.
- Only one metabolite possesses class III antiarrhythmic effects that are similar to those of ibutilide, however, the plasma concentration of this metabolite is less than 10% of that of ibutilide.

- Excretion of ibutilide and its metabolites occurs via the urine and feces. Approximately 82% of a 0.01 mg/kg dose may be excreted in the urine, with 7% as unchanged drug. About 19% may be excreted in the feces.
- The elimination half-life of ibutilide is about 6 hours, with a range of 2–12 hours.
- Ibutilide is administered intravenously 1mg over 10 minutes for patients weighing >60kg. Usually does is 0.01mg/kg.
- Ten to fifteen% of patients with new onset AF may convert to sinus rhythm with ibutilide alone.
- When cardioversion is performed after the administration of ibutilide, the success rate may approach 100% and the amount of energy required may also be less.
- Patients should be monitored for 4 hours after administration of ibutilide.
- Risk factors for ibutilide induced ventricular arrhythmias include prolonged QT, depressed left ventricular function (ejection fraction <0.30), hypokalemia, or hypomagnesemia.

Maintenance of sinus rhythm[11,22]
- Antiarrhythmic therapy is indicated for patients with symptomatic AF.
- Rate control alone can be used for elderly minimally symptomatic patients.
- For moderate to severe left ventricular systolic dysfunction the agent of choice is amiodarone. Dofetilide can be used.
- All other antiarrhythmics are relatively contraindicated in patients with LV dysfunction because of the potential for proarrhythmias.
- For patients with ischemic heart disease and preserved left ventricular systolic function, sotalol may be useful because of its beta-blocker effects.
- Disopyramide can be used in patients suspected of having AF due to increased vagal tone.
- Class IC agents such as flecainide and propafenone can be used in patients without ischemic heart disease and normal LV wall thickness and function.
- These agents can be administered daily for maintenance of sinus rhythm.
- They can also be used on an as needed basis for acute conversion of symptomatic paroxysmal atrial fibrillation.
- 300 mg of flecainide or 600 mg of propafenone can be administered orally[3].
- Beta-blockers or calcium channel blockers should be administered 30 to 60 minutes prior to administration of the antiarrhythmic agent to prevent accelerated AV conduction.
- First trial of this approach should be performed while the patient is being monitored.
- Treatment of lone AF with Class IC agents can result in conversion to atrial flutter because of prolongation of ARP and slowing of conduction velocity.
- This "Class IC atrial flutter" can be treated with ablation of the right atrial cavotricuspid isthmus followed by continuation of the Class IC drugs.
- Class III agents include amiodarone, sotalol and dofetilide.

Amiodarone[11,23]
- Evidence supporting the efficacy of amiodarone comes from the Canadian Trial of Atrial Fibrillation (CTAF) trial.

- At 1-year follow-up, 69% of patients treated with amiodarone were in sinus rhythm compared to 39% of individuals treated with sotalol or propafenone.
- Amiodarone was associated with a higher discontinuation rate due to side effects that were not statistically significant.
- There was no significant difference in total mortality between the groups.
- Amiodarone has multiple adverse reactions; patients receiving amiodarone need monitoring of pulmonary function tests (carbon monoxide diffusion test), thyroid function, liver function and ocular examination for corneal deposits.
- Although, there is no FDA indication for amiodarone in AF this is most commonly prescribed antiarrhythmic agent for treatment of AF.
- Amiodarone can be initiated as an outpatient, usually at 400 mg per day for a period of 2 to 4 weeks then decreasing the dose to 200 mg per day.

Dofetilide[24]
- It requires in-hospital initiation and monitoring for arrhythmias.
- Safety of dofetilide in patients with heart failure is supported by the Danish Investigations of Arrhythmia and Mortality on Dofetilide in Congestive Heart Failure (DIAMOND-CHF)[25] Study. Patients with left ventricular ejection fractions <35% were enrolled. The dofetilide dose was 500 µg bid. It was adjusted to 250 µg bid for creatinine clearances between 40–60 mL/min and 250 µg qd for patients with creatinine clearance of <40 mL/min. Patients with creatinine clearance of less than 20 mL/min were excluded.
- There was no significant difference in total mortality.
- Retrospective analysis of the results demonstrated that 12% of patients with atrial fibrillation in the treatment arm converted to sinus rhythm, compared to 1% in the placebo arm, with a significant reduction in the subsequent development of atrial fibrillation.

Sotalol
- It should not be given to patients with renal dysfunction, left ventricular hypertrophy, prolonged QT intervals, bradycardia, or electrolyte abnormalities (hypokalemia).
- Nodally active agents should be stopped or dose should be decreased before initiation of sotalol because of risk of bradycardia from beta-blocking properties seen at 40 mg bid. The class III antiarrhythmic effect (action potential prolongation) appears at 120 to 160 mg bid.
- Sotalol should be initiated in hospital while monitoring for proarrhythmias and prolongation of the QT interval.
- Sotalol can be administered as follows:
  (a) 80 mg tid for 1 day.
  (b) Then 120 mg bid on second day.
  (c) Then 160 mg bid on third day.
  (d) Discharge on 120 mg bid, with increase to 160 mg bid if needed.

Quinidine verapamil combination:
- Verapamil is a blocker of cardiac L-type calcium channels.

- Verapamil slows AV nodal conduction, and may prevent excessive calcium influx into the ventricular cardiomyocyte suspected of causing early after-depolarizations and triggering Torsades de Pointes.
- It causes constipation.
- This combination of effects is almost a mirror remedy of the problems identified with quinidine.

Newer agents

- Ultrarapid delayed rectifier outward potassium channels (I_{Kur}) is present in atria, but not in the ventricles. I_{Kur} blockers may provide specific therapy for the management AF.
- Selective atrial sodium channel blockers, such as ranolazine, maybe effective in suppressing AF.
- The atrial selectivity is caused by differences in the AP characteristics and biophysical properties of atrial and ventricular sodium channels.
- Late Na channel blocker ranolazine may have a role in the treatment of AF.

I_{Kur} and AF

- Natural flavone acacetin from the traditional Chinese medicine Xuelianhua suppresses I_{Kur} and the transient outward K^+ current and prolonged action potential duration and effective refractory period in human atrial myocytes. The compound blocked the acetylcholine-activated K^+ current.
- Inhibition of I_{Kur} may promote AF in nonremodeled atria. The contribution of I_{Kur} in AF may be relatively small because I_{Kur} density is reduced with the acceleration of activation rate. I_{Kur} density is also reduced in cells isolated from atria of patients with chronic AF.
- Ultrarapid delayed rectified potassium current (I_{Kur}), carried by Kv1.5 channels encoded by the *KCNA5* gene, is present in atria, but not in the ventricles.
- Block of I_{Kur} can provide the substrate for development of AF in healthy canine atria, presumably via abbreviation of APD and ERP.
- Clinical AF is commonly associated with atrial fibrosis, inflammation, or oxidative injury.
- Oxidative stress may induce inflammation and both of these factors may promote atrial structural remodeling (i.e., interstitial fibrosis, fibroblast proliferation, accumulation of collagen, dilatation, and hypertrophy). Pro-AF actions of atrial structural remodeling are largely related to conduction disturbances that promote re-entrant arrhythmias. Triggered activity may be involved.
- Interventions that reduce structural remodeling, inflammation, and/or oxidative stress, such as angiotensin-converter enzyme (ACE) inhibitors, angiotensin II receptor blockers (ARBs), or statins, have not been shown to reduce the occurrence of AF.

Postcardioversion atrial stunning

- The reversion of AF or atrial flutter to sinus rhythm with internal or external cardioversion, pharmacological therapy, or radiofrequency ablation of atrial flutter is associated with transient persistence of mechanical dysfunction of the left atrium and LAA known as stunning.

- Stunning may be responsible for the risk of thromboembolic complications, failure of improvement in cardiac output and exercise tolerance, and increased risk of recurrence after restoration to sinus rhythm.
- Stunning is a form of tachycardia-mediated atrial cardiomyopathy that develops in response to persistent atrial arrhythmia.
- Abnormalities in calcium cycling, atrial myolysis and fibrosis may be responsible for the development of stunning.
- Pacing and use of isoprenaline or calcium have been shown to reverse atrial mechanical stunning.
- AF often recurs in the first weeks after cardioversion.
- Electrical remodeling may be responsible for this phenomenon. AF shortens the atrial action potential and refractory period.
- The atria "recover" from electrical remodeling in 2–4 weeks after cardioversion to sinus rhythm.
- The main electrophysiologic effect of many antiarrhythmic drugs is prolongation of the atrial AP.
- Hence, action potential-prolonging therapy aimed at preventing recurrent AF after cardioversion possibly could be limited to a few weeks after cardioversion.
- Amiodarone or sotalol may facilitate successful electrocardioversion. Upon successful electrocardioversion, amiodarone is superior to placebo, and sotalol has a lesser effect in maintaining sinus rhythm.
- Calcium channel blockers had no influence on the success rate in achieving sinus rhythm.
- Successful electrocardioversion likely in patients with
  1 Lower BMI.
  2 AF history ≤1 year.
- Lower energy is needed in
  1 Biphasic shocks.
  2 Lower BMI.
  3 AF duration ≤1 year.

Proarrhythmia
- Although majority of proarrhythmic side effects occur in the first days or weeks after initiation of treatment. Proarrhythmia is a constant threat during antiarrhythmic drug therapy. Risk factors for proarrhythmia include:
  1 Female gender.
  2 Left ventricular hypertrophy.
  3 Prolonged baseline QT interval, and abnormal prolongation of the QT interval after exposure to the potentially proarrhythmic drug.
  4 Bradycardia.
  5 Hypokalemia.
  6 Transient reductions in hepatic and renal function.
  7 Abnormalities of drug metabolism (e.g., abnormal function of cytochromes).
  8 Abnormal pharmacokinetics (e.g., altered expression or function of p-glycoprotein) may markedly increase serum drug levels.

Pill-in-the-pocket treatment approach to convert recent-onset AF

- Antiarrhythmic drug therapy can be used to acutely terminate recent-onset AF in the first hours of the arrhythmia.
- This treatment concept requires that the patient recognizes and treats recurrent AF without medical assistance.
- A single dose of flecainide (300 mg) or propafenone (600 mg) is administered as soon as AF recurs. This approach may terminate more than 90% of the episodes.

Nonpharmacologic options in the management of AF

Radiofrequency (RF) ablation[25]

- Arrhythmias are produced by abnormality of impulse generation or impulse propagation. RF ablation seeks to eliminate these abnormalities.
- When the RF current passes through the tissue it produces heat which is proportional to the power density within tissue. It is an alternating current.
- Maximum heating occurs at the tip of the electrode and it diminishes as the distance from the tip increases. Increase in the radius (distance) from the tip will decrease the heat by fourfold. For this reason depth and volume of the tissue that is affected by heat is small (2 mm). Deeper tissue heating is due to heat conduction.
- Commonly used radio frequency is 300 to 1000 kHz. Lower frequency may produce muscle stimulation. At higher frequency mode of heating changes from resistive to dielectric.
- RF energy is delivered in a unipolar fashion from catheter tip to the dispersive patch electrode placed on the skin.
- The surface area of catheter electrode is 12 mm^2 and the surface area of patch electrode is 100–250 cm^2. This results in increase power density and heating at catheter tip.
- Catheter tip electrodes with large surface area or when the catheter tip is cooled by irrigation, allows lower system impedance and delivery of higher power. This results in deeper and larger lesion.
- The temperature is measured at the catheter tip it does not reflect actual tissue temperature which may be high.
- Very high tissue temperature results in heat expansion of the tissue, crater formation and may produce steam pop.
- Amount of power and duration of the energy delivery would depend on the catheter characteristics (for 4 mm tip 50 W for 60–90 s, for 8 mm tip catheter 50–70 W 30–60 s, and for irrigated tip catheter 15–45 W for 15–30 s)
- Rise in temperature at deeper tissue level may continue if high power or temperature settings are used producing thermal latency even after termination of energy delivery.
- Radio frequency generated heat produces coagulation necrosis of the myocytes. Healing by fibrosis is complete by 8 to 12 week.
- Primary benefit of catheter ablation of AF appears to be improvement in symptoms, quality of life, decrease in left atrial size, improvement in left ventricular ejection fraction, and New York Heart Association (NYHA) functional class.

- Catheter ablation should be considered for patients with AF who have failed one or more trials of anti-arrhythmic therapy.
- Best results (up to 85% success) have been achieved in patients with lone or paroxysmal AF. Lower success rates (50–70%) have been reported in other subsets of AF patients.
- Lower success rate is noted if the AF has been present for more than a year, left atrial size is >6 cm, patients age >75 years.
- Potential complications include PV stenosis, stroke, left atrium esophageal fistula and pericardial effusion and tamponade.
- Approach to AF ablation could be classified as elimination of the triggers, substrate or autonomic facilitators (parasympathetic ganglion).
- The long-term safety of discontinuation of anticoagulation in patients with AF who have remained in sinus rhythm after catheter ablation has not been demonstrated.
- Catheter ablation should not be considered in asymptomatic individuals with AF simply to avoid long-term anticoagulation with warfarin.
- Recurrent organized left atrial tachycardia after PV isolation may be due to macro re-entrant circuits in the left atrium.
- CFAEs (continuous fractionated atrial electrograms) are defined as: (1) atrial electrograms with 2 deflections or more, and/or perturbation of the baseline with continuous deflection of a prolonged activation complex over a 10-second recording period; (2) atrial electrograms with a very short cycle lengths (≤120 ms) averaged over a 10-second recording period.
- After a successful ablation of cavotricuspid isthmus for atrial flutter, 50% of these patients may present with AF.
- The endpoint is antral ablation to isolate the PV in patients with paroxysmal and chronic AF, with more extensive ablation of antral CFAEs in the latter.
- Combined approaches have been adopted, using (1) pulmonary vein isolates (PVI), (2) ablation of CFAEs, (3) left atrial linear lesion deployment.
- The MI (mitral isthmus) line joins the mitral annulus to the pulmonary vein either anteriorly or laterally. Creating a complete line of block is challenging because of tissue thickness, anatomic complexity, catheter instability, and myocardial sleeves connecting the left atrium to the CS.
- In patients with persistent AF, PVI results in a significant decrease in both PV and non-PV areas of CFE.

Elimination of the triggers
- It was noted that AF is initiated by rapidly firing triggers located in PV.
- This may manifest as frequent PACs or clearly discernible atrial activity in the form of atrial tachycardia at the onset of AF or during AF.
- These foci arise from the myocardial muscular sleeve that extends few centimeters into the PV.
- Initial approaches included identification of PACs with earliest activation and elimination of these foci within pulmonary vein. Possible risk of pulmonary vein stenosis shifted the focus to ablation outside the orifice of the pulmonary vein in a quadrantic fashion.

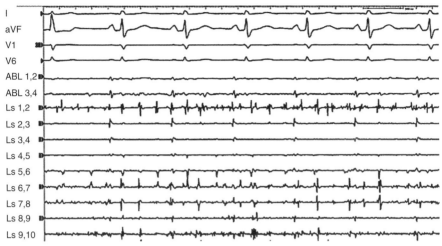

Figure 5.10 Intracardiac electrogram obtained after isolation of the right superior pulmonary vein showing fibrillation within the vein recorded by the ring catheter (LS 1–10), whereas the atria remain in sinus rhythm

Pulmonary vein isolation using RF ablation in left atrium

- In this approach attempt is made to isolate all the four PV orifices from the left atrium. It reduces the probability of the PV stenosis.
- Rationale is that PACs (triggers) could arise from any of the four PV.
- It may also produce compartmentalization and "debulking" of the left atrium.
- Drawback of this approach includes reoccurrences, creation of the isthmus that may predispose to atrial tachycardia[26].
- Esophageal perforation fallowing posteromedial left atrial or right superior PV ablation may occur. This is a serious and often fatal complication.
- Presently, the approach for catheter ablation of paroxysmal atrial fibrillation (PAF) involves electrically isolating the pulmonary veins (either individually or in pairs of ipsilateral veins) by placing circumferential RF lesions in the left atrial antrum surrounding the veins (Figure 5.10).
- Using this strategy, long-term arrhythmia-free rates of ≥70% have been reported.
- Recurrence of PAF is associated with recovery of PV conduction.
- PV electrical isolation, not just circumferential ablation, represents an end-point for catheter ablation of PAF.
- In the setting of long-lasting persistent AF, PV isolation alone can eliminate AF in at least 60% of patients with long-term AF control and in more than 80% when previously ineffective antiarrhythmic agents are added to the treatment regimen.
- Electrical isolation is confirmed with exit block to and from the pulmonary vein
- Carina or isthmus region between PV regions may add to the difficulty of isolating the pulmonary veins.

Identification of the pulmonary vein potentials
- Ectopic impulses triggering AF, originate predominantly from the PV.
- Electrical isolation of the PV from the left atrium is performed to eliminate these triggers from the PV. In addition to the initiating role of the PV, these structures are also critical as a substrate for maintaining AF.
- Near the ostium of the PV, both high and low frequency potentials may be recorded. The former represent local myocardial activation (PV potentials) and the latter represent far field atrial potentials, the amplitudes of which are usually smaller than those of PV potentials.
- Far field atrial potentials from the left atrium appendage are commonly observed in the anterior portion of the left PV ostia, because of their proximity to the appendage.
- Such potentials can be distinguished from PV potentials by pacing techniques: both the PV and appendage are activated at the same time during sinus rhythm, while pacing at the appendage advances the far-field appendage potential to within the stimulus artifact and delays the PV potentials relative to the stimulus artifact. Conversely, pacing from within the pulmonary vein advances the PV potential and delays the left atrial potential relative to the stimulus artifact.
- Other regions may also contribute to far-field potentials, such as the posterior or inferior left atrium, and pacing from there can distinguish such potentials in a similar manner.
- To avoid PV stenosis and eliminate ostial foci, the preferential ablation site is approximately 1 cm proximal to the ostium, except for the anterior rim of the
- Sudden prolongation of PV potential cycle length may be observed, representing modification of the left atrium–PV connection by RF energy delivery.
- Currently, PV antrum isolation with or without additional linear lesions probably represents the most accepted ablation strategy
- Continuation of Coumadin at a therapeutic INR at the time of PVI without use of heparin or enoxaparin for bridging is a safe and efficacious periprocedural anticoagulation strategy.
- Warfarin, rivaroxaban or dabigatran remain the simplest, reliable method of anticoagulation.
- Reduction in creatinine clearance affects dosing and use of LMWH, rivaroxaban, and dabigatran.
- Cardioversion for AF can be considered if serial INR are therapeutic for 4 consecutive weeks.
- Thrombus formation is associated with thrombin activation, not prevented by warfarin, continued use of heparin during AF ablation procedures is recommended.

Ligament of Marshall[27]
- The ligament of Marshall is an epicardial vestigial fold that marks the location of the embryologic left SVC.
- It contains the nerve, vein (vein of Marshall), and muscle tracts.

- The proximal portions of the muscle tracts connect directly to the coronary sinus myocardial sleeves. The distal portions of the muscle tracts extend upward into the pulmonary vein region.
- Ligament of Marshall is located between the left atrial appendage and left PV.
- The ligament of Marshall contains sympathetic nerve trunks as well as sympathetic ganglia. It also is richly innervated by parasympathetic nerves.
- AF arises more frequently from the distal portion than the proximal portion of the ligament of Marshall.
- Ectopic atrial tachycardia arises more often from the proximal portion of the ligament of Marshall, especially in locations near the coronary sinus (CS).
- The P-wave morphology associated with vein of Marshall ectopic activity is characterized by an isoelectric P wave in leads I and aVL, positive in leads II, III, aVF, and V2–V5, and similar to that seen with ectopic beats arising from the left pulmonary veins.
- Ligament of Marshall vein can be identified by CS angiogram,

Elimination of the substrate
- Identification and elimination of the fractionated electrograms may result in termination of the AF during the procedure.
- Fractionated electrograms may be recorded from left atrium around PV, left atrial appendage or interatrial septum. In the right atrium the fractionated electrograms could be recorded from crista terminalis, orifices of the vena cava, the orifice of the coronary sinus or up to 2 to 3 cm within the coronary sinus.
- Like PV, muscular extension in to proximal coronary sinus may produce rapidly firing automatic foci responsible for initiating AF.

Modification of autonomic substrate
- The posterior wall of the left atrium is richly innervated by vagal (parasympathetic) fibers.
- Parasympathetic stimulation produces bradycardia and shortening of the atrial refractory period. These electrophysiologic changes are conducive to initiation and maintenance of AF, termed as vagally induced AF.
- Vagally induced AF occurs during sleep and may be responsible for the atrial arrhythmias that occur during sleep apnea.
- During ablation of the vagal neural terminals, located in the posterior wall of the left atrium, bradycardia or junctional rhythm may occur.
- It may be necessary to tailor these three approaches when using ablation as the therapeutic modality in the management of AF. For example a paroxysmal AF in a young patient with structurally normal heart where focal tachycardia or premature beats are identified as the initiator of the AF may benefit from elimination of that focus.
- Targeting ganglionated plexuses at or near the left atrium–PV junction of the human heart may have antifibrillatory effects.
- AF triggers and drivers in the PV and posterior left atrial wall may be modulated by the autonomic nervous system.

- The noradrenergic and cholinergic nerves may be localized in and around the PV without any area of discrete adrenergic or cholinergic predominance.
- Presence of interstitial cells of Cajal within the left atrial musculature provides a potential substrate for automaticity
- Three epicardial subplexuses are the sole source of the PV neural network. The extrapulmonary segments of the PVs do not receive input from the bronchial plexus.
- Epicardial ganglia predominantly are located on the inferior portion of all four PV, whereas free nerve endings, which morphologically seem to be sensory, aggregate subendothelially on their anterior surface.
- The largest number of PV-related cardiac AChE-positive neural structures are located on the inferior surface of the roots of both the LIPV and right inferior pulmonary vein (RIPV), as well as on the anterior surface of the root of right superior pulmonary vein (RSPV) and posterior surfaces of the roots of both LIPV and RIPV.
- The roof ablation line joins the superior PVs, whereas the mitral isthmus line is performed between the inferior PV and the mitral annulus.
- Termination of AF may require right atrium ablation in 20% of patients.
- Termination of chronic AF may require PV isolation, electrogram-based ablation, and linear ablation.
- Chronic AF lasting >5 years is more difficult to terminate by RF application
- AF cycle length of less than 140 ms may be associated with poor outcome following RF ablation.
- Single procedure success for catheter ablation for paroxysmal AF is estimated between 60 and 70%.
- In patients with recurrent AF following catheter ablation, PV reconnection is present in 79% to 100%. It has been noted following surgical Cox MAZE approach to PV isolation.
- Additional ablation of CFAEs after APVI does not appear to improve clinical outcomes in patients with long-lasting persistent AF.
- AAD treatment for the first 6 weeks after AF ablation is well tolerated and reduces the incidence of atrial arrhythmias and the need for cardioversion or hospitalization.
- In patients hospitalized for heart failure AF at the time of hospitalization is common but is not an independent risk for long-term adverse outcomes, including death or rehospitalization.
- Delayed enhancement magnetic resonance imaging (DE-MRI) can be used to visualize RF-induced scarring postablation
- RF-induced scar appears to have formed by 3 months postablation. At 24 hours postablation, DE-MRI enhancement appears consistent with a transient inflammatory response rather than stable LA scar formation.

Intracardiac echocardiography (ICE) technology
- Two forms of ICE transducer technology, mechanical and phased array are in clinical use.
- Mechanical ICE transducers have a single ultrasound crystal mounted at the end of a nonsteerable catheter (6–9Fr). An external motor drive unit

rotates the crystal within the catheter to provide an imaging plane that is circumferential and perpendicular to the catheter's shaft.

- The imaging frequency of mechanical ICE systems is 9 to 12 MHz. These frequencies provide high-resolution near-field imaging but poor remote tissue penetration. Usable field of view for ablation procedures extends only 6 to 7 cm from the transducer.
- Phased-array ICE imaging uses a 64-element transducer on the distal end of an 8Fr or 10Fr catheter.
- The imaging frequencies are adjustable from 5 to 10 MHz. The wedge-shaped image sector extends to depths of 12 cm in a plane that is in line with the shaft of the catheter.

Patient selection for AF ablation
- Symptomatic AF
- Failure of one or more antiarrhythmic drugs Catheter ablation may have better efficacy than antiarrhythmic
- Catheter ablation of AF can be considered in patients who have hypertensive heart disease, coronary artery disease with or without prior revascularization, congestive heart failure and atrial septal defect repair with a pericardial or synthetic material.
- Although age is not a limiting factor for catheter ablation of AF success rate may be lower in older patients with chronic AF of more than 1 year's duration. Ablation therapy should be individualized in older patients, taking into consideration their overall physical health, lifestyle preferences, longevity, and risk of complications.
- A left atrial diameter <50 to 55 mm predicts a higher probability of a successful outcome. A dilated left atrium is associated with electroanatomic remodeling, and may decrease the probability of a successful outcome.
- Chronic AF of long duration may be associated with a higher probability of recurrence after ablation. In patients with paroxysmal AF the duration of AF does not appear to be a predictor of outcome.

Surgical ablation
- In patients with AF who require cardiac surgery for other reasons, such as coronary artery disease or mitral valve disease, concomitant intraoperative therapy for AF could be considered.

The ideal candidate for catheter ablation of AF
- Has a symptomatic episode of paroxysmal or chronic AF
- Has not responded to one or more antiarrhythmic drugs
- Does not have severe comorbid conditions or significant structural heart disease
- Is younger than 70 years
- Has a left atrial diameter <50 to 55 mm
- For chronic AF, has had AF for <1 year.

Relative and absolute contraindications for AF ablation

1 Significant obstructive carotid artery disease.
2 Intractable CHF.
3 Severe aortic stenosis or hypertrophic cardiomyopathy with left ventricular outflow tract obstruction.
4 Nonrevascularized left main or three-vessel coronary artery disease.
5 Severe pulmonary arterial hypertension.
6 Severe pulmonary disease because of the impact of pulmonary vein stenosis.
7 Patients who cannot be anticoagulated both during and for at least 2 months after the ablation procedure should not be considered for catheter ablation of AF. Because the risk of thromboembolic events both during the procedure and in the early postoperative period may be prohibitive in the absence of systemic anticoagulation.
8 Presence of left atrial appendage thrombus or a recently implanted left atrial appendage occlusion device.
9 High risk patients or elderly who are not a candidate for open heart surgery should such intervention may be warranted because of cardiac perforation or catheter entrapment.
10 Catheter ablation of AF is likely to be of little or no benefit in patients with end-stage cardiomyopathy or massive enlargement of the left atrium (>6 cm); or who have severe mitral regurgitation or stenosis and are deemed inappropriate candidates for valvular intervention.

POST ASD repair

- AF and atrial flutter are the most common cardiac arrhythmias associated with atrial septal defects (ASD) in adult patients. The incidence could be as high as 52% in patients ages 60 years or more.
- Pre-existing atrial flutter or AF and patient age more than 40 are two independent predictors for postoperative recurrence of atrial tachyarrhythmias (mainly AF).
- Early surgical ASD closure before 25 years of age results in survival similar to that in the normal population and freedom from postoperative atrial tachyarrhythmias, mainly atrial fibrillation.

Complications of AF ablation[28]

- As ablation strategies have evolved toward antral or left atrial ablation away from the ostia of the veins, the incidence of pulmonary vein stenosis has decreased.
- Pericardial tamponade, retroperitoneal hematoma, groin complications, and phrenic nerve palsy, thromboembolic complications and atrioesophageal fistula remain major complications.
- The incidence of severe complications ranges from 1 to 4%.
- Thromboembolic events have become infrequent with the use of aggressive periprocedural anticoagulation regimens.
- Atrioesophageal fistulas are rare (<0.5%) and should remain very infrequent with increased awareness of the risk of esophageal injury.

- Patients with a prosthetic mitral valve can be challenging because of the risk of catheter entrapment.
- Transseptal catheterization in patients who have undergone closure of a patent foramen ovale or atrial septal defect with a percutaneous closure device may pose additional risks.
- The risk of complications, particularly pericardial tamponade and thromboembolic events, may be higher in elderly patients.

Thromboembolic complications
- Thromboembolism is responsible for development of cerebrovascular events, although air embolism has rarely been implicated.
- Several factors can promote thrombogenicity during the procedure, including nature/burden of AF, patient characteristics, presence of spontaneous echo contrast, deployment of multiple intracardiac catheters via long sheaths in the left atrium, and ablation-related char formation and tissue disruption
- Intracardiac thrombi can be identified by using phased-array intracardiac ultrasound. These tend to form on the circular mapping (Lasso) catheter, long sheaths, and rarely at the edge of endocardial lesions.
- Presence of spontaneous echo contrast is the strongest predictor for development of intracardiac thrombi, and maintaining ACT levels >300 s can minimize thrombus formation.
- In the event that intracardiac thrombi cannot be retrieved and/or becomes dislodged in the left atrium, the procedure should be stopped, and thrombolytics may need to be administered.
- If the patient develops a stroke despite all the precautions, then, depending on the time course of the event, administration of tissue plasminogen activator (TPA) may be considered. Thrombolytic use can increase the risk of bleeding at sites of vascular access.
- Magnetic resonance imaging may demonstrate higher incidence of asymptomatic cerebrovascular events in patients undergoing AF ablation.

PV stenosis
- Flow-limiting and/or severe PV stenosis (>70% reduction in diameter) occurs infrequently (1%–3%).
- With the technique of lesion delivery on the atrial aspect of the PV ostia, the occurrence of PV stenosis has been reduced.
- PV stenosis progresses insidiously, and patients can present with a variety of respiratory complaints, including cough, hemoptysis, dyspnea, pleuritic chest pain, and wheezing.
- One third of patients with severe PV stenosis remain asymptomatic., especially when only one vein demonstrates stenosis.
- Spiral computed tomographic angiogram and/or magnetic resonance imaging are the best tools for diagnosis. Caliber tends to remain relatively stable beyond 3 months after ablation.
- In the absence of symptoms, there is no consensus on the best treatment strategy, and late resolution of symptoms without any intervention can occur. Balloon

angioplasty with or without stenting has been shown to achieve satisfactory results (reduction in stenosis and augmentation of flow), although about half of these patients may develop restenosis requiring repeat intervention.

- Development of PV stenosis can be prevented by antral isolation.
- Modest augmentation of acute PV flow velocities (~10–50 cm/s) can be anticipated across the ostia of isolated PVs. An increase in PV flow velocity to >100 cm/s should raise concern and force a reassessment of ablation strategy. Flow velocities ≥158 cm/s (estimated pressure gradient ≥10 mmHg) are associated with a risk for significant late PV stenosis.

Esophageal injury
- In patients undergoing catheter-based endocardial ablation, the incidence is approximately 0.01%, although this likely represents an underestimate due to underreporting.
- The mechanism underlying fistula formation is thermal injury to the anterior esophageal wall following ablation along the posterior left atrium wall. The esophagus lies in close proximity to the posterior left atrium, the distance between the esophageal mucosa and the left atrium endocardium is <10 mm
- The clinical picture can mimic acute pericarditis, pneumonitis, sepsis, seizures, stroke(s), myocardial infarction, massive gastrointestinal bleeding and circulatory collapse.
- Most common presenting symptoms were neurologic deficits and hematemesis.
- Chest pain suggestive of pericarditis is the most common complaint and may occur as early as 3 days after the procedure.
- Neurologic deficits can take up to 3 weeks to manifest.
- The diagnosis can be confirmed by a transthoracic echocardiogram, magnetic resonance imaging, or computed tomographic scan, especially when combined with water-soluble contrast.
- Transesophageal echocardiography, esophagogastroduodenoscopy, or any other form of esophageal instrumentation should be performed with a great deal of caution
- Air insufflations during esophagogastroduodenoscopy can cause massive air embolization, resulting in diffuse strokes, myocardial infarcts, and damage to other end organs.
- Surgical intervention is preferred. Mortality remains high (≥50%). Surgical intervention is directed at repairing separately the posterior left atrium and the esophageal wall.
- Best strategy is to avoid injury to the esophagus during posterior LA ablation. This may be difficult for the fallowing reasons:
  1 Anatomic variability in the esophageal location.
  2 Lack of temporal stability in the esophageal course.
  3 Inability to optimize energy delivery that can transmurally interrupt atrial tissue without damaging the esophagus.

- Factors that contribute to the development of esophageal fistula include
  1 Small atrial size.
  2 Use of large catheter tips
  3 Power >50 W during energy delivery to the posterior wall (with an 8-mm tip catheter and >30 W with irrigated RF energy).
  4 Overlapping lesions in the posterior LA.
- Use of phased-array intracardiac ultrasound, can provide online assessment of esophageal location relative to the posterior left atrium.
- Postulated mechanism include injury to the esophageal vasculature that leads to an ischemic lesion that progresses to erosion, initial thermal injury followed by progressive lesion enlargement promoted by reflux of stomach acid bathing the lesion.
- Patients undergoing RFCA of AF may develop pathologic acid reflux after ablation. Patients may have pre-existing asymptomatic reflux prior to ablation.
- AF and gastroesophageal reflux disease share risk factors of obesity and advanced age.
- Calcium channel blockers and nitrates, commonly used in the AF population, can promote reflux by reducing lower esophageal sphincter tone.
- Ablation procedure itself could aggravate reflux. Patients are supine for an extended period of time.
- Ablation can potentially interrupt vagal efferent fibers along the surface of the esophagus. Injury to vagal efferents has been postulated as the cause of gastroparesis reported after ablation.
- Acid erosion may result in progression of esophageal injury to atrioesophageal fistulas.
- Routine administer of proton pump inhibitors to patients undergoing catheter ablation of AF is recommended.
- Monitoring the proximity of the esophagus to ablation sites, monitoring esophageal temperature, and reducing ablation energy in proximity to the esophagus, may potentially reduce the risk of esophageal injury.
- Hypotension and dehydration should be avoided. If right atrial pressure is <10 mmHg prior to trans-septal left heart catheterization, the patient should be hydrated with intravenous fluids.
- Hydration and normal perfusion may increase the potential convective heat loss through blood flow within the esophageal vasculature during energy delivery.
- The esophagus receives a rich blood supply from multiple sources (inferior thyroid arteries, bronchial arteries, thoracic aorta, left gastric and inferior phrenic arteries). It also has a dense venous plexus connecting the portal and systemic circulations.

Pericardial effusion
- Pericardial effusion (PE) is commonly observed in patients undergoing AF ablation. Development of cardiac tamponade is <1%.

- The causes of PE in patients undergoing AF ablation are:
  1 Cardiac perforation by various catheters.
  2 Trans-septal puncture.
  3 Aggressive anticoagulation.
- The low incidence of cardiac tamponade despite the high prevalence of PE is the perhaps due to small size of the effusion.
- Hypotension and diaphoresis, should be suspected to be due PE unless proven otherwise.
- Diagnosis of PE:
  1 Fluoroscopic assessment of the cardiac silhouette.
  2 Cardiac echocardiography using either the transthoracic and/or substernal approach.
  3 Intracardiac phased-array echocardiography.
- The management of PE is determined by its relative size and hemodynamic effect.
  1 Trivial PE ($\leq$3mm), if recognized early during the AF ablation, should be monitored continuously but does not warrant termination of the procedure.
  2 PE that exceeds 3mm, the procedure should be terminated, and anticoagulation should be reversed and temporarily withheld (6–12 hours). In the majority of cases, such conservative measures alone are sufficient.
  3 Pericardiocentesis is indicated for PE >8mm and/or smaller PE manifesting signs of cardiac tamponade.
  4 An indwelling catheter is required for a short interval after initial drainage to confirm that the bleeding has stopped and that no effusion is reaccumulating.
  5 In the event of persistent and rapid reaccumulation, exploration by thoracotomy may be required.
- The development of PE and subsequent tamponade can be prevented by attention to various aspects of the ablation procedure:
  1 Cannulation of the CS.
  2 Maintaining the Brockenbrough needle within the dilator before and immediately after successful transseptal puncture.
  3 Minimizing inadvertent ablation catheter deployment in the left atrium appendage.
  4 Avoiding "pops" and endocardial tissue disruption during lesion creation by monitoring power delivery, impedance rise, and intracardiac bubble formation.
  5 Periodically monitoring the pericardial space by phased-array intracardiac ultrasound for early detection.
  6 Monitor cardiac silhouette.
- Potential sites of cardiac perforations include:
  1 Left atrial appendage.
  2 Thin walled right ventricular apex.
  3 Right ventricular outflow tract.
  4 The transseptal puncture.
  5 Lesions associated with steam pops may lead to cardiac perforation.
- First detectable sign of a significant pericardial effusion is the decrease in left heart border motion in the left anterior oblique (LAO) projection.

- Patients with prior cardiac surgery who previously had their pericardium opened are at reduced risk for pericardial tamponade.
- If the patient has been administered heparin, protamine (1.5 mg per 1000 units of heparin given, maximum dose 50 mg, typically after a 1-mg test dose) can be administered.
- If the international normalized ratio is elevated fresh-frozen plasma or preferably recombinant factor VII infusion.
- Pericardial access using subxiphoid approach should be considered.

Left atrial tachycardia
- The incidence of organized atrial tachyarrhythmias in patients who have undergone AF ablation is approximately 10%.

Aortic root injury/fistula
- This complication results from anterior trans-septal puncture.
- It is likely to occur in patients with large and distorted atrial chambers and/or dilated aortic root.
- It can be prevented by demarcating the aortic root fluoroscopically (positioning a pigtail catheter or guidewire in the aortic root and/or placing a catheter across the His-bundle region, which sits opposite the aortic root).
- Phased-array intracardiac ultrasound provides online assessment of transseptal needle placement and adjacent structures may help to further reduce this risk.
- The sheath should not be advanced until the position of the tip of the needle is determined to be in the left atrium.

Phrenic nerve injury
- The phrenic nerve is in close proximity to the right superior PV.
- It could be damaged if the lesions were targeted more distally in this vessel.
- The current strategy of ostial/proximal PV ablation has reduced the occurrence of this adverse event.
- Stimulation of the phrenic nerve and diaphragm by high-output pacing (10 mA, 2.0-ms pulse width) around the right superior PV ostium identifies the location and proximity of the nerve. This area should be avoided from the ablation site.
- SVC isolation as a part of the AF ablation procedure can increase the risk of phrenic nerve injury. The nerve lies in close proximity to the lateral right atrium–SVC junction.
- SVC ablation should be limited to patients who clearly demonstrate triggers from this structure.
- Energy delivery should be avoided/minimized in the lateral aspect of the SVC–right atrium junction where the phrenic nerve course has been identified using pacing techniques.

Left phrenic nerve (LPN)
- The nerve descends on the fibrous pericardium along one of three courses:
  1 Over the anterior surface of the left ventricle
  2 Over the lateral margin of the left ventricle (most common)
  3 Posteroinferior direction of left ventricle

- The endocardium of the roof of the left atrial appendage can be few millimeters away from the LPN.
- LPN is especially at risk when procedures are performed in the vicinity of the left atrial appendage and high left ventricular wall.
- Right phrenic nerve is in proximity to the SVC and the RSPV.

Catheter entrapment in the mitral valve apparatus
- The Lasso (circular) catheter could be entrapped in the mitral valve apparatus during AF ablation, resulting in valve injury that requires valve replacement.
- The risk of this complication can be minimized by preventing anterior displacement of the Lasso catheter during the ablation.
- Catheter position can be monitored using fluoroscopy (ensuring that the Lasso catheter remains behind the CS on the right anterior oblique fluoroscopic projection), intracardiac ultrasound and characteristics of the electrograms recorded from the catheter.

Gastric injury
- This is a relatively rare complication.
- Acute pyloric spasm and gastric hypomotility has been observed following posterior left atrial lesions.
- The clinical presentation included abdominal pain and distension within 48 hours of the procedure.
- It may be due to thermal injury of the periesophageal vagal innervations.
- Recovery is spontaneous. Some patients may require laparoscopic/ endoscopic interventions.

SVC ablation complications
- In addition to phrenic nerve injury, SVC isolation can rarely result in sinus node injury.
- It is uncommon because the sinus node is a large structure.
- In patients with sinus node dysfunction it may result in bradycardia.

Complications during creation of the mitral isthmus line
- Delivery of RF energy within the CS may result in damage/occlusion of the left circumflex coronary artery, perforation of CS and development of stenosis.
- These complications can be prevented by decreasing the duration of the lesion, using lower power (~20–25 W) and temperature (≤50°C).

Autonomic dysfunction
- Ablation in the vicinity of PVs may produce transient profound bradycardia, hypotension, and sinus arrest.
- Thermal stimulation of the vagal nerve fibers triggering a Bezold–Jarisch-like reflex may be responsible for this phenomenon.

- Terminating energy delivery results in resolution of this reflex, some patients may require temporary ventricular pacing to counteract the bradycardia/hypotension.
- Transient elevation of resting heart rates (inappropriate sinus tachycardia) may persist for as long as 1 month after PV isolation.
- Parasympathetic withdrawal appears to be the mechanism. It does not warrant treatment, and spontaneous resolution occurs within 1 to 2 months.
- The vagus nerve courses posterior to the left atrium and is vulnerable to injury.
- The manifestations of vagus nerve injury depends on the level at which nerve damage occurs. Ablation of vagus nerve fibers above or at the regions at which they enter the heart will increase the heart rate and reduce AF inducibility.
- Injury to the vagus nerve before its entry into abdomen can result in gastroparesis and pyloric spasm manifested as abdominal bloating, pain, nausea, early or easy satiety, and weight loss.

Other rare complications
- Fluid retention is noted in the initial 2- to 3-day period following the ablation procedure. It may be due to alterations in ANP secretions due to the atrial tissue destruction and the large volume of fluid administered during the procedure.
- Allergic reaction/anaphylaxis reaction to dye or medications.

AVN ablation with permanent pacemaker implantation

- Patients with left ventricular dysfunction or chronic pulmonary disease or those who can not tolerate the doses of AVN blocking agents necessary to achieve rate control or the agents for rhythm control may be candidates for this approach.
- AVN blocking agents may produce negative inotropic effects or bronchospasm in these patients.
- Overall survival of patients undergoing AVN ablation and pacemaker insertion is same as a matched group of patients treated with antiarrhythmic drugs.
- Drawback of AVN ablation and the pacemaker approach include persistence of AF, need for anticoagulation, pacemaker dependence and ventricular dyssynchrony from right ventricular pacing.
- AVN ablation should rarely be performed in young patients with atrial fibrillation.
- PVI may be superior to AVN ablation with pacing in patients with heart failure and AF.

Surgical MAZE procedure

- Incisions are made in the left atrium around pulmonary veins, posterior wall and extended to mitral annulus.
- This procedure can be performed in conjunction with other cardiac surgery such as mitral valve replacement. Success rates are approximately 80 to 90%.
- Epicardial approach, using minimally invasive thoracotomy and microwave, attempts to isolate pulmonary veins.

5.4 Automatic junctional tachycardia

- Automatic junctional tachycardia (AJT; Figure 5.11) is common in infants. It carries high mortality.
- In older patients it has more benign course and is not associated with structural heart disease.
- AJT arises from transitional cells of AV junction and is due to abnormal automaticity. Tachycardia is sensitive to catecholamines.
- Electrocardiogram shows narrow QRS (wide if bundle branch block present) tachycardia. VA block may be present. Sinus capture beats may occur.
- AJT is often irregular and may be mistaken for AF or MAT.
- If the QRS is wide it may be mistaken for ventricular tachycardia.
- Intra-cardiac electrograms show that each QRS is preceded by His and a normal HV interval.
- Initiation termination is spontaneous without critical AH delay.
- AV dissociation is common. The tachycardia is unaffected by atrial or ventricular pacing.
- AJT should be differentiated from non-paroxysmal junctional tachycardia (NPJT), which tends to be slower and regular.
- AJT occurs in the setting of digitalis toxicity, chronic obstructive pulmonary disease, myocardial ischemia, carditis and postcardiac surgery.
- NPJT is believed to be due to triggered activity.
- To differentiate AJT from AVNRT, premature atrial beats are delivered in the region of slow pathway when septal A is committed. This will advance His in AVNRT but not in AJT.
- AV node re-entry tachycardia is initiated by PAC, needs critical AH interval and demonstrates dual AVN physiology.
- Orthodromic nodofascicular tachycardia is often initiated by PACs or PVCs, demonstrates pre-excitation during atrial pacing, occurrence of bundle branch

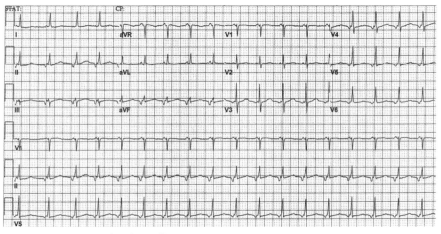

Figure 5.11 Junctional tachycardia.

block results in change in cycle length and advancement of next His or termination of tachycardia with PVC delivered when His is refractory.

Treatment

- In young patients AVN blocking drugs are ineffective. Amiodarone may be more effective.
- Abrupt onset of AV block may occur. Insertion of a permanent pacemaker is recommended.
- If drug therapy fails ablation at the site of earliest activation along the septum or AV node ablation and insertion of permanent pacemaker could be considered.
- In adult patients beta-blockers may be effective.
- AJT may occur following surgery for congenital heart disease. It may last for 1–4 days after surgery.
- Use of inotropic agents such as catecholamines and digoxin, may induce AJT.
- It responds well to IV propafenone, procainamide, or amiodarone.

5.5 AVN re-entry tachycardias[19,29]

- Current evidence, derived from multielectrode recordings and optical mapping studies suggest that the slow pathway is a perinodal tissue.
- Dual AVN physiology is defined as 50 ms increases in A2 H2 for 10 ms decrease in A1A2 interval.
- Fast and slow pathways represent different atrionodal connection as suggested by different sites of earliest retrograde activation during tachycardia or retrograde conduction during ventricular pacing.
- Resetting of the tachycardia by late PAC delivered outside the AVN near posterior right atrial septum or CS also suggests presence of a re-entrant loop.

Fast pathway

- Retrograde earliest atrial activation during AVNRT, suggesting fast pathway insertion site, is located 5 to 7 mm posterior and 8 to 10 mm superior to His bundle electrogram recording. Atrial electrogram at this site may precede atrial activation on His electrogram by 10 to 20 ms. This site is located superior to tendon of Todaro outside the triangle of Koch.
- Retrograde fast pathway activation at posterior superior right atrial septum may demonstrate two components. Initial low frequency component reflects far field atrial potential from left side of the septum.
- Application of RF current superior to tendon of Todaro will eliminate antegrade fast pathway conduction.
- The right side component of fast pathway begins in anterior limbus of fossa ovalis, as atrial cell then becomes transitional cell on crossing tendon of Todaro and insert into common AV bundle distal to compact the AVN.
- This distal insertion may explain why fast pathway has less decremental properties, is less responsive to AVN blocking agents and has greater response to sodium channel blocking agents.

- During decremental atrial pacing block in the fast pathway occurs proximally, closer to anterior limbus of fossa ovalis.
- Earliest retrograde atrial activation during AVNRT may be recorded on the left side of the septum.

Slow pathway

- It is located in posterior septum between tricuspid annulus and coronary sinus ostium.
- The slow pathway connects to the posterior extension of the AVN.
- Retrograde slow pathway activation proceeds from proximal CS to left atrium and across the septum to right atrium. From here it proceeds anteriorly towards the His bundle and posteriorly behind CS ostium and Eustachian ridge.
- CS musculature electrically connects right and left atrium.
- Clinically, the leftward inferior nodal extension can behave as the slow pathway and lead to AVNRT.
- The Eustachian valve and ridge form a line of block that confines SP potential/impulse to within triangle of Koch. This may allow dissociation of slow pathway potential from right atrial electrograms.
- This line of block may explain the late occurrence of slow pathway potential during sinus rhythm when compared with atrial electrogram at His location.
- In sinus rhythm slow pathway activation proceeds from posterior to anterior in the area of triangle of Koch.
- During slow pathwayablation accelerated junctional rhythm occurs with retrograde conduction over fast pathway.
- There may be multiple slow pathways with multiple jumps in AH interval.
- Linear ablation from tricuspid annulus to CS ostium is likely to eliminate most of the Sp conduction.
- After slow pathway ablation presence of A2H2 jump and echo beat may indicates presence of additional slow pathway, which may enter triangle of Koch anterior to CS ostium. These slow pathways may not be capable of causing arrhythmias.
- Subjects without the history of AVNRT may demonstrate dual AVN physiology.
- This may be due to sedation with midazolam and fentanyl, which depresses antegrade and retrograde conduction over fast pathway thus allowing slow pathway conduction to become manifest.
- Isoproterenol speeds up conduction in fast pathway.
- Equal delay in conduction over slow and fast pathway may mask dual AVN physiology.
- A2H2 greater then 200ms may suggest conduction over slow pathway
- Shift in retrograde conduction from fast to slow will change atrial activation sequence.

- The retrograde atrial activation sequences during AVNRT can be
  1 Concentric CS activation, in which the earliest activation is recorded around Koch's triangle outside the CS.
  2 Eccentric, in which the earliest activation is recorded inside the CS distal to the ostium. The earliest sites of the eccentric retrograde atrial activation during the tachycardia and right ventricular pacing can be inferoseptal CS (≤10 mm from the ostium), inferior CS (11–20 mm from the ostium), or inferolateral CS (≥21 mm from the ostium).
- The induced AVNRTs can be classified into a typical (slow-fast) or atypical form
- The tachycardias can be classified as typical when:
  1 A-H interval during the tachycardia is >200 ms.
  2 H-A interval during right ventricular pacing at the tachycardia CL was <70 ms.
  3 Earliest retrograde atrial activation is recorded at the supraseptal right atrium during the tachycardia, and there is no evidence of lower common pathway.
- The tachycardia is classified as atypical when
  1 A-H interval during the tachycardia is either >200 ms or longer (slow–slow form), or shorter than 200 ms (fast–slow form), or variable (irregular atypical AVNRT);
  2 H-A interval during right ventricular pacing at the tachycardia CL is >70 ms
  3 Earliest retrograde atrial activation is recorded at the inferoseptal RA or proximal part of the CS during the tachycardia; and there is evidence for a lower common pathway.

Common or typical AVNRT

- During tachycardia the antegrade conduction is over slow pathway and retrograde conduction over fast pathway.
- It is induced by PAC and rarely by PVC.
- An abrupt increased in AH by 50 ms with PAC before induction is common.
- Lack of increase in AH interval may be due to equal delay in conduction in both pathways.
- AH during tachycardia usually exceeds 200 ms.
- HA interval is short, <50 ms.
- Earliest retrograde atrial activation is superior to tendon of Todaro suggestive of retrograde fast pathway activation
- Short HA interval results in superimposition of P wave on QRS, thus obscuring P waves on surface electrocardiogram. This may result in pseudo R in V1 or pseudo S in inferior leads (Figures 5.12 and 5.13).

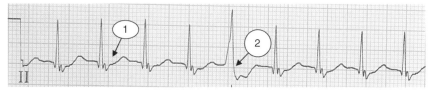

Figure 5.12 AVNRT: Spontaneously occurring PVC (2) does not reset the tachycardia. P waves (1) are noted in terminal portion of the QRS.

- During tachycardia, if there is simultaneous activation of the atrium and ventricles, late PVC may separate atrial and ventricular potentials and help identify the atrial activation sequence.
- Re-entry circuit between atrial ends of fast and slow pathway includes large atrial component, this may explain extremely rare VA block to atrium during AVNRT.
- Late PAC delivered to the atrium that is incorporated in tachycardia circuit may advance next His and reset tachycardia. PACs should be late and reach after retrograde earliest activation by fast pathway.
- Post-pacing interval (stimulus to next A) may be longer than the tachycardia cycle length due to delay in AVN.
- Resetting with shortest post-pacing interval occurs from posteroseptal right atrium and proximal CS.

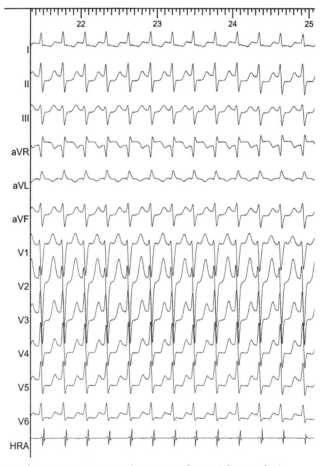

Figure 5.13 Simultaneous activation of atrium and ventricles results in superimposition of P and QRS. P wave location is evident by simultaneous recording of atrial electrograms.

- Retrograde activation of atrial septum occurs through fast pathway, impulse then propagates along the left side of interatrial septum to proximal coronary sinus, CS ostium and posterior end of the slow pathway.
- During decremental right ventricular pacing there is little decremental conduction in lower common pathway.
- HA interval during tachycardia reflects retrograde conduction over fast pathway minus simultaneous antegrade conduction over lower common pathway. HA interval during ventricular pacing reflects retrograde conduction time over lower common pathway and fast pathway.
- HA during tachycardia tends to be shorter than during right ventricular pacing.
- To record retrograde His, right ventricular pacing should be performed near the anterobasal right ventricle septum close to right bundle.
- In the left sided variant of S/F AVNRT the slow pathway is located in posterior mitral annulus. These patients tend to have short HA interval of less than 15 ms. This may be due to a longer lower common pathway.
- During the onset of the AVNRT, block below the AVN may occur resulting in 2:1 conduction.
- Functional infranodal block presumably is initiated by a long–short sequence in the His Purkinje system at the onset of tachycardia. Because of partial penetration of the His bundle during alternate tachycardia cycles, the long–short sequence is perpetuated in the distal His bundle and the functional block continues.
- Premature ventricular depolarization may penetrate and prematurely depolarized the distal His bundle, eliminating the "long" component of the long–short sequence thus eliminating 2:1 conduction.
- In AVNRT, changes in atrial cycle length are preceded by comparable changes in the H-H interval.
- Despite the variability in atrial cycle length, there is a fixed relationship between the QRS complexes and the atrial depolarizations (VA) that fall within the QRS complex.
- A two-for-one phenomenon may occur during programmed atrial stimulation, when there is antegrade conduction of atrial impulse once through fast pathway and the same impulse conducts through slow pathway, resulting in two ventricular electrograms for each atrial electrogram. This may indicate absence of retrograde penetration of slow pathway by antegrade fast pathway (Figure 5.14).
- The presence of more QRS complexes than regular P waves and of group beating with regular irregularity suggest the presence of a dual ventricular response with Wenckebach behavior during normal sinus rhythm.
- Exclusion of tachycardia mechanisms other than AVNRT and diagnosis of AVNRT can be deduced from:
  - Absence pre-excitation during sinus rhythm and atrial pacing.
  - Lack of change in VA interval during tachycardia with occurrence of bundle branch block.
  - Tachycardia does not reset by ventricular extrastimuli delivered while the His bundle is refractory;

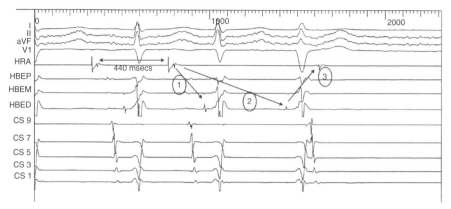

Figure 5.14 PAC at coupling interval of 440 ms results in antegrade conduction through fast pathway (1) fallowed by antegrade conduction through slow pathway (2) thus producing 2 QRS complexes for a single PAC. Same impulse then conducts retrogradely through fast pathway (3).

- Parahisian pacing during sinus rhythm exhibited an exclusive retrograde AV nodal conduction pattern.
- VA interval during pacing from the right ventricular apex is shorter than that during pacing from the right ventricular base.
- Atrial tachycardia can be excluded when a "V-A-V sequence" (not a "V-A-A-V sequence") is observed upon cessation of ventricular pacing associated with 1:1 VA conduction during the tachycardia.
- Tachycardia is reproducibly terminated with ventricular extrastimuli not reaching the atrium is likely to suggest AVRT.
- A diagnosis of AVNRT can be made if an AV re-entrant tachycardia using accessory pathways and atrial tachycardia is excluded by the above-mentioned criteria.

Electrophysiologic assessment[30]
- Begin arrhythmia analysis with the surface ECG: presence of AV dissociation, relative number of As and Vs, and p-wave morphology.
- Dual AVN physiology with SVT argues in favor of AVNRT, but 6% may have AVRT and 8% may have atrial tachycardia.
- Even in patients with manifest ventricular pre-excitation, up to 10% of patients may have AVNRT rather than AVRT as the mechanism of tachycardia.
- SVT can be classified as short or long RP tachycardia.
- Short RP (RP interval less than the PR interval) tachycardia with RP >70 ms includes AVRT, AVNRT, and atrial tachycardia. Long RP tachycardia includes atrial tachycardia, atypical AVNRT, and permanent junctional reciprocating tachycardia (PJRT).
- Next, examine atrial activation sequence.
- Consider diagnostic maneuvers. Some maneuvers make use of differentiating between the parallel activation of the atria and ventricles in AVNRT and the

serial activation necessary during AVRT. Others rely on assessing the presence of more than one route from the A to the V or vice versa.

- Some diagnostic maneuvers are designed to differentiate between septal accessory pathways (APs) and atypical AVNRT. These include
  1 Premature ventricular contraction (PVC) when His is refractory,
  2 Postpacing interval minus tachycardia cycle length (PPI–TCL),
  3 (SA)–(VA).
  4 ΔHA (HAPaced–HASVT), and ΔAH.
  5 PPI–TCL during entrainment of >115 ms is suggestive of AVRNT and shorter interval indicative of septal AVRT. However, that value is not 100% specific, and in some patients the values may fall within a "gray zone."
  6 If the activation sequence of the tachycardia upon discontinuation of ventricular pacing that entrains the tachycardia demonstrates an atrial-atrial-ventricular (A-A-V) pattern, this finding suggests atrial tachycardia. Prior to cessation of ventricular pacing, the atrial rate must accelerate to the ventricular pacing rate.
  7 If entrainment of the tachycardia is not achieved or if the tachycardia stops on termination of ventricular pacing, attempt to induce the tachycardia by ventricular pacing. If the tachycardia is initiated with the V-A-V response, it excludes an atrial tachycardia because the physiology underlying the V-A-V response is identical when there is induction of tachycardia by ventricular pacing as when there is cessation of ventricular pacing that entrained the tachycardia.
- Typical AVNRT or a junctional tachycardia is the most likely diagnosis when a VAV response is observed with a tachycardia that has simultaneous atrial and ventricular activation.

First post-pacing interval after tachycardia entrainment with correction for atrioventricular node delay is for differential diagnosis of AVNRT versus AVRT.

- Although anatomically closer to the AV node, the base of the RV is electrically more distant than the apex of the RV, at which the His Purkinje network directly inserts. The PPI is composed of: 2×(time from pacing site to circuit)+time taken for one revolution of the circuit+decremental conduction in the circuit or between pacing site and circuit.
- Entrainment of the tachycardia is achieved by pacing for 5 to 10 pulses from the RV apex at a cycle length 20 to 40 ms shorter than the TCL. Successful entrainment results in acceleration of the atrial cycle length to the RV pacing cycle length, without a change in the atrial activation sequence and the tachycardia resumes after pacing is terminated.
- PPI is measured from the last right ventricular pacing stimulus to the right ventricle electrogram in the first return beat.
- The post-pacing A-H interval is measured from the last entrained atrial depolarization in the high right atrium to the His electrogram in the first return beat.
- The stimulus-atrial (SA) interval is measured from the last RV pacing stimulus to the last entrained depolarization in the high right atrium.

- TCL, ventriculoatrial (VA) (from the onset of QRS complex and high right atrial electrogram), AV interval, HA interval, and A-H interval should be measured in the tachycardia cycle immediately before pacing.
- Because the postpacing A-H interval is influenced by the previous entrainment and alters the PPI, the increment in AVN conduction time in the first PPI (postpacing A-H interval – basal A-H interval) is subtracted from the PPI–TCL difference ("corrected PPI-TCL difference";)
- Because the HV interval remains constant, the difference between AV intervals (post-pacing AV interval – basal AV interval) can be used if the clear His deflection is lacking.
- Decremental conduction after entrainment most commonly occurs during conduction through the AV node, especially the AVN slow pathway.
- The degree of decrement is dependent on:
  1 Pacing rate,
  2 Functional refractory properties of the AV node.
- Therefore, the PPI and PPI–TCL will prolong if decrement occurs, but the degree of decrement could be different from base compared to apex even though the pacing rates may be same or similar at both sites. this may be caused by changes in autonomic tone affecting anterograde AV nodal conduction.
- PPI–TCL corrects for decrement in the AV node.
- Differential entrainment involves entraining the tachycardia from two sites in the right ventricle – the apex and the base – and comparing the resultant PPIs.
- In the case of AVNRT, the right ventricle apex, where the His Purkinje network directly inserts, is always closer to the tachycardia circuit than is the right ventricle base.
- In the case of AVRT, the apex and base are variably related to the circuit, depending on the actual location of the AP. Because the ventricles are part of the circuit, the times tend to be approximately equivalent.
- PPI–TCL tends to be longer from the base than from the apex in patients with AVNRT, with an average conduction time of 61 ± 22 ms (average >30 ms) versus -3 ± 12 ms in AVRT. This has very high sensitivity and specificity.
- In the presence of left free-wall AP, transseptal conduction time from RV to LV will be the same regardless of an apical or basal pacing site, and both PPIs will reflect that increase identically.
- In any form of AVNRT, the re-entrant circuit is confined above the His bundle, and the ventricle is not an obligatory element of the tachycardia mechanism.
- In contrast, AVRT involves an AP as a component of the retrograde limb, and part of the ventricle is an essential component of the circuit.
- The right ventricle apex is closer to the tachycardia circuit; therefore the PPI approximates the TCL in AVRT compared with AVNRT.
- Longer corrected PPI–TCL values may be observed in patients with ventricular free-wall APs, but even in these patients there is minimal overlap in their maximal corrected PPI–TCL values and the minimal of these values measured for patients with AVNRT.

- Rapid conduction proceeding over retrograde right bundle branch and left bundle fascicles could account for these findings.
- In contrast, in AVNRT the PPI–TCL reflects twice the sum of the conduction time through the His-Purkinje system and the final common pathway of the "nodal" re-entrant circuit.
- The stimulation in inferobasal RV septal sites may increase the differences in PPI–TCL values between patients with orthodromic reciprocating tachycardia (ORT) and those with AVNRT.
- Patients with proposed longer final common pathways, such as those with atypical AVNRT, may show longer corrected PPI–TCL differences than those with typical forms of such tachycardias.
- Stimulus to A (SA) interval during entrainment from the RV is likely to approximate the VA interval in OAVRT more closely when compared with AVNRT.
- SA interval exceeds the VA interval during tachycardia by >85 ms in patients with AVNRT, while it may be less than 85 ms of the VA interval in OAVRT utilizing a septal AP.
- The corrected PPI–TCL is a stronger discriminating criterion than the SA-VA interval, because the PPI reflects bidirectional conduction, whereas the SA interval reflects only retrograde conduction.
- Only variables in the PPI during entrainment from the right ventricle base or apex are
  1 Time from pacing site to the circuit.
  2 Decremental conduction in the circuit or between pacing site and circuit.
- After entrainment of AVNRT, in which the circuit is independent of the ventricles, the difference in PPI from base versus apex will largely be composed of the extra time required to reach the circuit from the base versus the apex.
- The cPPI data indicates that approximately 30 ms extra is required to reach the AVNRT circuit from the base as compared to apex, whereas there is no significant difference in ORT irrespective of the location of the AP.
- This implies that apical and basal pacing sites have approximately equal access and proximity (electrophysiologically) to the circuit in ORT.
- VA index is defined as the difference between VA intervals obtained during apical and posterobasal right ventricular pacing. VA index ≥10 ms (demonstrating that apical pacing took no more than 10 ms longer to reach the atrium) established the presence of a posteroseptal AP.

Slow/slow (S/S) AVNRT

- During this tachycardia antegrade conduction is through the slow pathway as manifested by long AH interval (240 ms or more). Retrograde conduction is also through second slow pathway resulting in long H-A interval with earliest atrial activation at posteroseptal right atrium between tricuspid annulus and CS ostium or within coronary sinus. This atrial activation may precede atrial activation in His electrogram by 30 to 60 ms.
- The VA interval is long and may exceed 70 ms.

- There may be multiple jumps in A2H2 during programmed atrial stimulation indicative of multiple slow pathways. There may be multiple HA intervals during tachycardia during ventricular pacing.
- Half of these patients may also have S/F AVNRT.
- During ventricular pacing retrograde atrial activation may shift from anterior to posterior atrial septum indicating the shift in conduction from fast to slow pathway.
- Tachycardia may be induced by programmed ventricular stimulation resulting in a block in retrograde fast pathway and retrograde conduction over slow pathway.
- S/S AVNRT has longer lower common pathway, which is located posteriorly.
- HA during ventricular pacing tends to be longer than HA during tachycardia in patients with S/S AVNRT.
- HA interval represents retrograde conduction over slow pathway minus antegrade conduction over lower common pathway. Because of the longer lower common pathway HA interval may be short or negative during S/S AVNRT.
- Fast pathway ablation will not eliminate S/S AVNRT.
- Reoccurrence rate is higher after ablation in patients with S/S AVNRT and may require more extensive ablation in posteroseptal right atrium and coronary sinus ostium.
- Supraventricular tachycardia in which earliest atrial activation is recorded near the ostium of the coronary sinus and the AH interval is longer than the HA interval include:
  1 Atrial tachycardia arising in the posterior septum
  2 Atypical slow–slow atrioventricular nodal re-entrant tachycardia (AVNRT)
  3 Orthodromic (AVRT) using a concealed posteroseptal accessory pathway.

Fast/Slow or uncommon type of AVNRT

- It is characterized by short AH (30–180 ms) long HA interval (260 ms).
- Antegrade conduction is over fast pathway and retrograde conduction over slow pathway.
- Earliest retrograde atrial activation is in posteroseptal right atrium or CS ostium.
- On surface electrocardiogram RP interval is longer then PR interval. P waves are inverted in inferior leads
- On termination of the V pacing, where V pacing has successfully entrained AVNRT, PPI – TCL >120 ms and Stim to A minus VA interval of >85 ms suggests the diagnosis of atypical AVNRT and excludes the diagnosis of AVRT utilizing septal accessory pathway (Figure 5.15).
- Atypical fast–slow form of AVNRT is long-RP tachycardia, the HA interval is longer than the AH interval.
- After the last paced ventricular complex if there is an abrupt prolongation of the A-A interval that corresponds to termination of the tachycardia. Presence of this phenomenon excludes atrial tachycardia.
- Termination of the tachycardia by ventricular pacing without pre-exciting the atrium also rules out an atrial tachycardia.

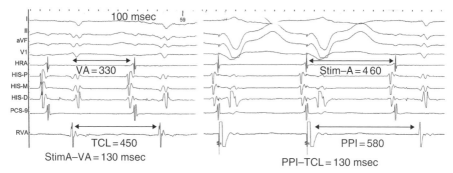

Figure 5.15 Atypical AVNRT response to ventricular pacing.

Definitions

- PPI: Post-pacing interval is measured from the last pacing stimulus to the rapid deflection of the subsequent ventricular electrogram recorded from the pacing site.
- TCL: Tachycardia cycle length is measured as the average of 10 cycles of sustained tachycardia before pacing maneuvers.
- PPI–TCL: TCL is subtracted from the PPI.
- Corrected PPI–TCL (cPPI–TCL): PPI–TCL is corrected for decrement in AV nodal conduction after entrainment by subtracting any increase in the AV interval of the return cycle beat (compared with the AV interval in tachycardia).
- VA interval: The ventriculoatrial interval is measured from the last right ventricular pacing stimulus to the last entrained depolarization at the HRA.
- Differential PPI–TCL and VA interval: The PPI–TCL from the apex is subtracted from the PPI–TCL at the base to give the differential PPI–TCL. Similarly, the differential VA interval is calculated by apical from basal VA values.
- The VA interval as measured by the stimulus-HRA interval is composed of: time from pacing site to circuit + time to conduct to the atrial insertion of the circuit + time to conduct to the HRA + decremental conduction in the circuit, between pacing site and circuit or between circuit and HRA.
- Significant variable in the VA interval during differential entrainment is the extra time required to reach the circuit, that approximately 35 ms extra is required to reach the HRA from the right ventricle base rather than the apex in patients with AVNRT.
- VA interval consists of conduction through the AVN in one direction (via the retrograde fast pathway), it may be less susceptible to the effects of variable autonomic tone, and thus correction for AVN decrement is not required.

Causes of alternating cycle length during AVNRT

- If HA intervals are constant in the presence of variable VA times, the shorter VA intervals may be the result of delayed conduction down the left anterior fascicle resulting in a delayed V rather than more rapid retrograde conduction. This will result in alternating cycle length during tachycardia correlating with alternating HV intervals.
- Alternating A-H interval due to varying conduction through slow pathways.

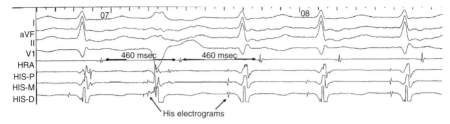

Figure 5.16 His synchronous PVC does not reset atrial electrogram.

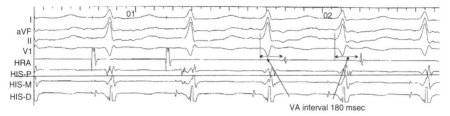

Figure 5.17 Termination of A pacing first VA is similar to subsequent VA intervals.

Differential diagnosis of AVNRT[31] (Table 5.1)

- Single late PVC is delivered 50 ms after the onset of His electrogram and advanced by 10 ms without retrogradely activating His. Advancing of atrial activation without first retrogradely activating the His will suggest the presence of accessory pathway.
- Atrial activation sequence remains unchanged and may advance next His electrogram. In AVNRT His synchronous PVC fails to advance atrial electrogram (Figure 5.16).
- PVCs during SVT should be delivered at the base of right ventricular septum for posteroseptal AP and in parahisian location for anteroseptal AP.
- On termination of atrial pacing the first VA is identical to subsequent VA (Figure 5.17) and on termination of V pacing the response is VAV (Figure 5.18). These observations make the diagnosis of atrial tachycardia unlikely.
- Para-Hisian pacing is performed during sinus rhythm from anterobasal right ventricle, anterior and apical to His recording where high output captures the His resulting in narrow QRS and timing of His is advanced. At lower output His RB capture is lost resulting in wide QRS and delay in timing of atrial activation (equal to the delay in His activation) without change in activation sequence this suggest conduction over the AV node (Figure 5.19).
- With loss of HB RB capture, absence of change in the timing and sequence of atrial activation suggests conduction over AP.
- The His bundle and atria are activated sequentially over the AV node during entrainment of AVNRT from the ventricle but simultaneously during supraventricular tachycardia (SVT).
- They are activated in parallel during AVNRT and sequentially (serial) in AVRT.

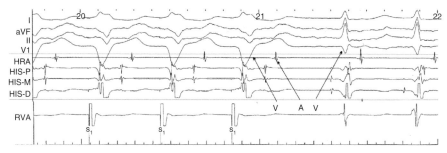

Figure 5.18 Termination of V pacing response is VAV.

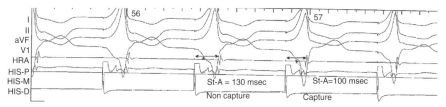

Figure 5.19 Para-Hisian pacing: Stimulus to A is shorter during His capture.

- A ΔHA (HA(entrainment) – HA(SVT)) cutoff value of 0 reliably differentiates AVNRT from AVRT.
- ΔHA values during entrainment from the ventricle are significantly longer during AVNRT than AVRT (31 ± 24 ms vs -38 ± 31 ms).
- ΔHA of 0 has very high sensitivity, specificity. and positive predictive value for correct diagnosis of AVRT.
- In AVNRT, the re-entrant circuit is confined above the His bundle, and the ventricle is not an obligatory part of the tachycardia mechanism.
- In ORT due to AP as a component of the retrograde limb, part of the ventricle is an integral component of the circuit. RV apex is closer to the tachycardia circuit, the PPI approximates the TCL in ORT using an septal AP compared with AVNRT.
- Longer corrected PPI–TCL values may be observed in patients with ventricular free-wall APs, but even in these patients there is minimal overlap in their maximal corrected PPI–TCL values and the minimal of these values measured for patients with AVNRT.
- In AVNRT the PPI–TCL reflects twice the sum of the conduction time through the His-Purkinje system and the final common pathway of the "nodal" re-entrant circuit.
- Stimulation from inferobasal right ventricle septal sites could increase the differences in PPI–TCL values between patients with ORT and AVNRT.
- Patients with atypical AVNRT, showed longer corrected PPI–TCL differences than those with typical forms.
- SA interval during entrainment from the right ventricle likely to approximate the VA interval in ORT compared with AVNRT. Corrected PPI–TCL is a stronger

discriminator than the SA-VA interval, possibly because the PPI reflects bidirectional conduction, whereas the SA interval reflects only retrograde conduction.

Causes of a "pseudo-A-A-V" response

- A "pseudo-A-A-V" response upon the cessation of ventricular pacing may be observed in atypical AVNRT when the AH interval exceeds the tachycardia cycle length.
- Failure to entrain the tachycardia during ventricular pacing;
- Very short His-atrial interval that results in atrial activation that precedes ventricular activation during typical AVNRT;
- Long HV interval during typical AVNRT, which also causes atrial activation to precede ventricular activation.

Diagnosis of AVNRT is made based on the classical criteria

- The absence of an AV accessory pathway is confirmed when:
  1 Ventricular pre-excitation is absent during sinus rhythm and atrial pacing,
  2 VA interval during the tachycardia is not lengthened by an occurrence of bundle branch block,
  3 Tachycardia is not reset by ventricular extrastimuli delivered while the His bundle was refractory,
  4 Tachycardia showed AV block without a tachycardia termination,
  5 Para-Hisian pacing during sinus rhythm showed a retrograde AVN conduction pattern,
  4 VA interval during pacing from the RV apex is shorter than that during pacing from the RV base.
- Atrial tachycardia is excluded when:
  1 V-A-V sequence (not a V-A-A-V sequence) is observed on cessation of ventricular pacing associated with 1:1 VA conduction during the tachycardia.
  2 Tachycardia is induced by ventricular pacing with a V-A-V sequence
  3 Tachycardia is reproducibly terminated with ventricular extrastimuli not reaching the atrium.
- A diagnosis of AVNRT is made if AV re-entrant tachycardia using accessory pathways and atrial tachycardia are excluded by the above mentioned criteria.

Evaluation of the upper and lower common pathways

A functional upper common pathway exists between the re-entrant circuit and atrium when the tachycardia is associated with:
  1 Second-degree VA block,
  2 VA dissociation, and/or
  3 Variable H-A interval during a fixed H-H interval.
- A functional lower common pathway exists between the re-entrant circuit and His bundle when:
  1 Tachycardia is associated with an A-H block without interruption of the tachycardia,
  2 H-A interval is <0 ms during the tachycardia,

3 H-A interval during RV pacing at the tachycardia CL is longer than that during the tachycardia

4 Retrograde Wenckebach CL during RV pacing is longer than the tachycardia CL.

- During tachycardia with simultaneous depolarization of the atrium and ventricle, if a PAC advances the next ventricular complex and resets the tachycardia with the AV interval shorter than the AV interval during tachycardia, then most likely diagnosis would be junctional tachycardia.
- Septal VA interval of <70 ms is too short to support a diagnosis of orthodromic AV re-entry using a septal accessory pathway.
- Shortening of H-H interval before termination of the tachycardia could be due to premature beat.

Treatment
- For immediate termination of the tachycardia, vagal maneuvers, IV adenosine; calcium channel blockers or beta-blockers can be used.
- Ablation of the slow pathway is the treatment of choice.

Ablation for AVNRT[18,32]
- Preferred site of ablation for AVNRT is slow pathway which is located in triangle of Koch.
- The boundaries of the triangle of Koch are delineated by CS os, tendon of Tedaro posteriorly and septal leaflet of the tricuspid valve anteriorly and bundle of His at the apex of the triangle.
- Mean distance from His bundle to the mid portion of the anterior lip of CS os is 15 to 20 mm.
- The fast pathway is located anteriorly in close proximity to His bundle. Slow pathway is located posteriorly near CS os.
- Discrete potentials noted in the posteroseptal right atrium may be due to anisotropic conduction and not due to activation of slow pathway.
- Ablation of slow pathway can be achieved by anatomic or electrogram approach or combination of both.
- Area of interest is identified on fluoroscopic examination between His bundle electrogram and CS os along posteromedial aspect of TA. Multipolar electrograms are recorded at this site. Atrioventricular electrogram ratio should be less than 0.5.
- Electrogram and anatomic approaches should be combined to achieve successful ablation.
- The majority of successful ablation sites are located between TA and CS os. Other sites include within CS os or inferior or superior lip of the CS os.
- Unsuccessful ablation is the result of imprecise mapping or inadequate tissue contact and heating.
- Target temperature should be 45 to 50 °C. Slow junctional rhythm that may last for 15 to 20 seconds may occur (Figure 5.20).
- If junctional rhythm does not occur within 20 seconds of achieving target temperature RF application should be terminated.

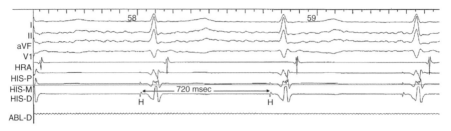

Figure 5.20 Junctional rhythm during RF application to slow pathway.

- Complete AV block may occur in 1% of patients, undergoing slow pathway ablation.
- Monitoring VA conduction during junctional rhythm or prolongation of the PR interval should be performed.
- Complete AV block is unlikely to occur in the presence of intact VA conduction during junctional rhythm. Application of RF energy should be discontinued with the first sign of VA block, slowing of VA conduction or prolongation of the PR interval in conducted sinus beats.
- VA conduction during junctional rhythm may be noted even if there is no VA conduction during ventricular pacing.
- Isorhythmic AV dissociation may mimic intact VA conduction. In the presence of poor fast pathway conduction VA conduction during junctional rhythm may occur and is not a reliable indicator of potential AV block.
- To monitor for intact AV conduction atrial pacing at a fastest rate associated with 1:1 conduction should be performed while observing for the prolongation of the PR interval.
- Isorhythmic AV dissociation may occur during atrial pacing and RF application should be discontinued.
- Forty to 50% of patients may demonstrate residual slow pathway function, as evidenced by single echo beats, even after successful ablation of AVNRT.
- AVNRT may reoccur in 3 to 5% of patients. Most of the recurrences are reported in the first 3 months after ablation.
- Clinically, the leftward inferior nodal extension can behave as the slow pathway and lead to AVNRT. In typical (slow–fast) forms of AVNRT, this would render ablation in the usual inferoseptal right atrium ineffective and may response to the ablation inside the coronary sinus.
- In atypical forms of AVNRT (fast–slow or slow–slow), if the leftward inferior extension serves as the slow pathway conducting retrogradely, then the earliest atrial activation will be recorded in the left, leading to eccentric CS activation.
- Fallowing a slow pathway ablation fast pathway effective refractory period shortens.
- RF ablation should be considered for patients with frequent episodes of symptomatic tachycardia. Slow pathway ablation can be performed in the presence of prolong PR interval. Atypical AVNRT can be successfully eliminated by slow pathway ablation.

- It has the fallowing advantages over the sources of the energy that results in thermal injury to the tissue.
  1 Ability to reversibly demonstrate loss of tissue function with cooling. During cryomapping 90% of the lesions are reversible.
  2 It preserves endothelial lining and tissue architecture with minimal thrombus formation, unlike the hyperthermic injury produced by RF.
  3 Less likely to produce pulmonary vein stenosis, if used for AF ablation.
  4 It is a reasonable strategy in patients with AVNRT who may be at high risk (pre-existing prolong PR interval) anteroseptal or midseptal bypass tracts in whom the risk of damage to the AV node might be high with radiofrequency energy.
- Recurrence rates are lower for RF ablation and higher (8–10%) for cryoablation.
- Cryoablation does not induce junctional acceleration, which is a sensitive marker for successful RF lesions cryoablation impact the assessment of lesion efficacy for AVNRT.
- Cryoablation offers the advantage of cryoadherence, which prevents catheter dislodgment during lesions. In a patient with reproducibly inducible tachycardia on isoproterenol, cryoablation may facilitate lesion delivery during continuous infusion or sustained tachycardia, allowing immediate assessment of lesion efficacy.
- Those with no surrogate markers and difficult-to-induce tachycardia, RF ablation may be preferred because junctional acceleration may be the only indicator of procedural success.
- Patients who have clinically documented SVT and dual AVN physiology but do not have inducible AVNRT at the time of electrophysiologic study may benefit from slow pathway ablation.
- There is increased incidence of catheter induced RV perforation in elderly women. RV catheter manipulation should be minimized.

Nonre-entrant dual AVN pathway tachycardia
- Nonre-entrant dual AVN physiology tachycardia manifests with occasional ventricular pauses and consistent 1:2 AV relationship after the pause, junctional tachycardia is unlikely.
- Phenomenon of repetitive retrograde concealment, or "linking," is common in patients with dual AVN physiology and has been used to explain the mechanism of other forms of nonre-entrant dual AVN pathway tachycardias.
- Nonre-entrant dual AVN pathway conduction can occur even with an underlying AVN conduction abnormality and in the absence of a fast AVN pathway.

5.6 AV Re-Entrant Tachycardia (AVRT)[30,33,34]

- Thirty percent of all SVT are due to AVRT, 10% due to atrial tachycardia and rest due to AVNRT.
- The atria, AV node, His Purkinje system, and ventricles, comprise the circuit

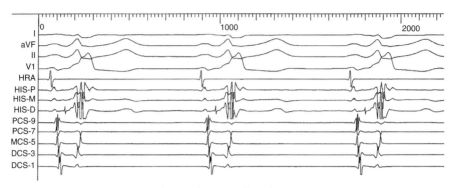

Figure 5.21 Pre-excitation: surface and intracardiac electrograms.

- The ventricles and His Purkinje system are not essential components for AVNRT.
- AP connection can occur anywhere along the mitral and tricuspid annulus except in the region of fibrous trigone where mitral annulus joins aorta.
- Accessory pathway is capable of antegrade or retrograde conduction.
- The presence of antegrade conduction results in short PR interval, slurring on the initial component of the QRS called delta wave and increase in the duration of the QRS. These Electrocardiographic features are due to pre-excitation of the ventricles and if accompanied by tachycardia are characteristic of Wolff–Parkinson–White (WPW) syndrome (Figure 5.21).
- AP with intermittent pre-excitation is incapable of rapid antegrade conduction.
- Concealed AP is capable of only retrograde conduction; there is no pre-excitation at anytime. Retrograde conduction is more reliable as it is easier to activate smaller atrium.
- If AP is located in the lateral wall of annulus, presence of rapid AVN conduction may mask pre-excitation. This can be uncovered by rapid atrial pacing.
- Slowing of AVN conduction may accentuate pre-excitation.
- During orthodromic AV re-entrant tachycardia antegrade conduction is through the AVN and retrograde conduction through AP, resulting in narrow QRS complex tachycardia.
- Antegrade conduction through AP and retrograde conduction through the AVN results in antidromic (wide complex, pre-excited) tachycardia.
- During atrial tachycardia, atrial flutter or AVNRT antegrade conduction may occur through bystander AP. These entities will present with wide complex pre-excited tachycardia. AP is not the part of the re-entrant circuit.
- Atriofascicular tachycardia or the tachycardia utilizing two accessory pathways one for antegrade and other for retrograde conduction will also present as wide complex pre-excited tachycardia.
- A critical distance of ≥4cm between the AP and AVN may be required to support antidromic reciprocating tachycardia, these anatomic constraints could sometimes be overcome by a sufficient degree of slow conduction within the antidromic reciprocating tachycardia circuit, such as combination of anterograde decremental conduction in the AP and retrograde slow conduction in the slow AV nodal pathway.

Clinical presentation
- Common symptoms, during tachycardia are palpitations, chest discomfort, shortness of breath, dizziness or near syncope.
- Tachycardia may be exercise induced.
- Patients have no structural heart disease.

Electrocardiogram
- EKG shows regular narrow complex tachycardia. Functional right or left bundle branch block may occur
- Changes in tachycardia cycle length depend on AVN conduction, which may vary according to autonomic tone.
- AV node blocking agents terminate the tachycardia in AVN resulting in P as a last complex, fallowed by no QRS complex.
- The P wave is located within ST segment. This would be characterized as short RP tachycardia. Lewis lead may help in identification of the P wave.
- In typical AVNRT, P wave is within QRS complex.
- Other tachycardias associated with short RP are atypical AVNRT or atrial tachycardia with prolong PR interval.
- Occurrence of AV block during the tachycardia excludes the diagnosis of AVRT.
- Morphology of the P wave during the tachycardia may help identify the insertion site of the retrogradely conducting AP.
- Prolongation of tachycardia cycle length or ventriculoatrial (VA) conduction with bundle branch block suggests that the mechanism of the tachycardia is AVRT and that AP is located ipsilateral to type of bundle branch block. These changes are not seen in septal AP or if bundle branch occurs in the ventricle contralateral to the location of the AP.
- Electrical alternans of the QRS is not helpful in making the diagnosis of AVRT.
- During pre-excited tachycardia QRS morphology/axis is similar to delta wave seen in sinus rhythm.
- Pre-excited tachycardia may mimic ventricular tachycardia. Structurally normal heart, in a young patient and pre-excitation during sinus rhythm, excludes the diagnosis of VT. Presence of AV dissociation during tachycardia suggests the diagnosis of VT.
- Location of the accessory pathway can be determined by the morphology and the vector of delta wave from surface EKG (Figure 5.1).

Electrophysiologic features of AVRT[26]
- Electrophysiologic study should be performed in a systematic and diligent manner. Attention should be paid to the fallowing points:
  1 Onset and termination of the tachycardia.
  2 Changes in the morphology of the QRS.
  3 Changes in cycle length and its effect on relationship of various electrograms and intervals.
  4 Zone of transition of the QRS.
  5 Changes in conduction intervals with bundle branch block.

  6 Atrial activation sequence

  7 AV relation

  8 Ventricular activation sequence

  9 Identification of His electrogram and its relation to atrial and ventricular electrogram.

  10 Assessment of HV, VA and HA relationship and intervals.

  11 Deliver PVC during narrow complex tachycardia and deliver PACs during wide complex tachycardia.

  12 Para-Hisian pacing.

  13 Intracardiac electrograms should be assessed in light of fluoroscopic location of the recording electrodes.

  14 Effects of various vagal maneuvers and administration of pharmacologic agents such as adenosine or isoproterenol.

- In orthodromic reciprocating tachycardia, the wave front must progress from the ventricle to the atrium. In contrast, in AVNRT, transition from the anterograde to the retrograde pathway does not require intervening depolarization of the ventricle.
- AVRT is a narrow QRS tachycardia with a, normal HV interval preceding each QRS.
- There may be functional bundle branch block during the tachycardia.
- AV block is not compatible with AVRT.
- AH interval may change resulting in variation of cycle length. VA interval remains constant unless there are two AP responsible for retrograde conduction during tachycardia.
- AVRT can be induced by PAC that blocks antegradely in AP and conducts antegradely through AVN with prolong AH interval and arrives retrogradely at AP. This initiates the tachycardia.
- Shortening of AV node refractory period by atropine or isoproterenol may facilitate the induction of tachycardia.
- PVC may induce AVRT by producing retrograde block in His Purkinje system and conduction over AP.
- The shortest VA interval during AVRT is generally greater then 60 ms and QRS to HRA interval of at least 95 ms.
- In the presence of septal AP VA interval during RV pacing tends to be similar to the VA interval during AVRT.
- In AVNRT VA during right ventricle pacing tends to be longer then during tachycardia. In AVNRT there is simultaneous antegrade and retrograde conduction from AV node resulting in short VA interval.
- Atrial activation is eccentric in the presence of lateral AP. AVRT utilizing septal AP demonstrates caudocranial atrial activation in septal region.
- Earliest retrograde atrial activation during AVRT or during ventricular pacing defines the site of AP insertion. Atrial activation during V pacing is identical to the sequence of atrial activation during SVT (Figure 5.22).
- If the occurrence of bundle branch block (BBB) during AVRT results in VA prolongation by 30 ms suggest the presence of ipsilateral AP. VA prolongation with left bundle branch block (LBBB) will suggest left lateral AP.

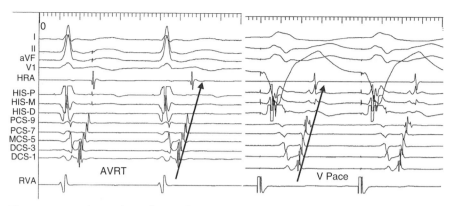

Figure 5.22 During tachycardia atrial activation is eccentric and earliest in DCS. During V pacing retrograde activation is identical to one during tachycardia.

- PVC delivered from right ventricle, during AVRT, is likely to induce functional LBBB because of delayed retrograde activation of LB.
- His catheter maybe used to induce right bundle branch block.
- If, PVC delivered during SVT when His bundle is refractory, advances the atrial electrogram would suggest presence of AP. AV node delay in the next beat may prevent the advancement of the whole tachycardia circuit.
- His-refractory ventricular extrastimuli delivered during the narrow complex tachycardia advances the subsequent atrial timing without a change in activation sequence, suggests that the pathway is participating in the tachycardia.
- PVC delivered during SVT, when His bundle is refractory, if terminates the tachycardia without retrograde activation of the atrium, is suggestive of AVRT utilizing AP (Figure 5.23).
- Left-sided pathway, due to distance from right ventricular pacing site, may not show atrial pre-excitation.
- PVC delivered from base of the heart or close to the AP is more likely to show atrial pre-excitation. Atrial pre-excitation may reveal multiple AP.
- The pre-excitation index is defined as a difference between tachycardia CL and longest coupling interval of right ventricle PVC that results in atrial pre-excitation.
- An index of 75 ms or more suggests presence of left lateral AP. Septal pathways demonstrate an index of less than 45 ms.
- In septal and right-sided AP the VA interval during tachycardia remains same as during right ventricular pacing.
- If the pathway is located on the left side the VA during right ventricular pacing tends to be longer than the VA during tachycardia.
- VA block during V pacing at cycle length longer than the tachycardia cycle length excludes AVRT.
- Administration of adenosine during V pacing may result in transient retrograde AVN block and unmask retrograde conduction through AP.

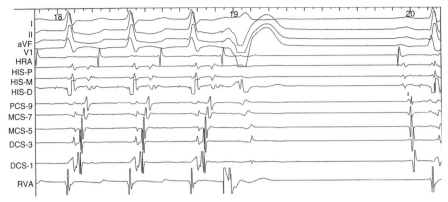

Figure 5.23 Termination of the tachycardia with His synchronous PVC without activation of the atrium.

- If retrograde conduction is through septal AP the VA interval will be shorter with basal than apical pacing site. Opposite will occur if conduction is through His Purkinje AVN because the right bundle inserts into the right ventricular apex.
- A change in atrial activation, during decremental right ventricular pacing, from concentric to eccentric suggests the presence of AP.
- A change in atrial activation could also be due to shift in conduction from retrograde fast to retrograde slow pathway.
- HA during V pacing at tachycardia CL minus HA during SVT of less than –10 ms (for example of –20 to –30 ms) is highly suggestive of AVRT utilizing septal bypass tract. This criterion may be helpful in distinguishing AVNRT from AVRT utilizing septal bypass tract. Although sensitive it may be difficult to utilize if retrograde His during V pacing can not be recorded.
- Lack of decrement in VA interval with decremental V pacing suggests presence of AP.
- V pacing at slower rate at which HPS refractoriness increases more than that of AP may allow conduction over concealed AP.
- In the absence of AP, the VA interval during right ventricular apex pacing will be shorter than VA during right ventricular base pacing.
- During parahisian pacing constant VA interval with or without capture of the His is suggestive of AP.
- On termination of the tachycardia if the last electrogram is A then atrial tachycardia is unlikely. Likely diagnosis includes AVNRT or AVRT that blocks in AV node.
- Cycle length variation during SVT depends on antegrade conduction over the AVN. In AVRT the AH interval may vary depending on whether the antegrade conduction is utilizing fast or slow pathway. The HA (or VA) interval will be constant.
- Variation in VA interval could be due to ipsilateral BBB or multiple retrogradely conducting AP or decremental retrograde conduction through AP.

- Changes in HH interval if precede or predict changes in AA interval, are suggestive of AVN participation in tachycardia circuit and will not occur in atrial tachycardia.
- Constant VA in spite of variability of rate excludes atrial tachycardia.
- If change in A-A interval fallows changes in AH interval then atrial tachycardia is unlikely.
- During PAC if atrial echo beat occurs following His activation, it suggests that AVN is part of the tachycardia mechanism.
- During tachycardia (orthodromic or antidromic) to differentiate if the retrograde limb is fast pathway or septal AP, late PVC should be delivered near His. If this advances the next A, it indicates presence of septal AP.
- The presence of an accessory pathway is confirmed when atrial activation is advanced; however, it does not prove that the accessory pathway is a necessary part of the tachycardia circuit.
- Although uncommon, delayed atrial activation following a PVC introduced when the His bundle is refractory proves the presence of an accessory pathway and its participation in orthodromic re-entrant tachycardia.
- During orthodromic re-entrant tachycardia, a PVC delivered when the His bundle is refractory may result in decremental conduction in the accessory pathway and delay of subsequent atrial activation, instead of advancing atrial activation or terminating tachycardia.

HA interval

- With BBB increase in the VA interval >20 ms is suggestive of AVRT, but this finding will occur in <10% of other supraventricular tachycardia.
- In the presence of LBBB increase in tachycardia cycle length equivalent to the increase in VA interval as measured from surface V lead to the high right atrium suggests the diagnosis of a left-sided accessory pathway.
- Delay in His Purkinje conduction may result in increase in HV interval by up to 30 ms during LBBB. Thus occurrence of LBBB during AVNRT may give misleading information of prolongation of the VA or increase in cycle length.
- It is therefore important to measure HA interval during a BBB instead of the VA interval or the tachycardia cycle length.
- The tachycardia cycle length is the sum of the AH plus HA intervals, whereas the HA interval is the sum of the HV and VA intervals.
- In AV nodal re-entrant tachycardia, the HA interval will not change with BBB with or without HV prolongation.
- In AV re-entrant tachycardia, BBB with an increased HV interval can prolong the tachycardia cycle length without localizing the accessory pathway. Changes in the VA interval with BBB can be deceiving if the HV interval changes.
- Most importantly, HA interval prolongation with BBB is diagnostic of AV re-entrant tachycardia regardless of whether the HA interval increases due to HV or VA prolongation (Figure 5.24). If the HA interval increase is due to the HV interval increase, then localization of the pathway is difficult.

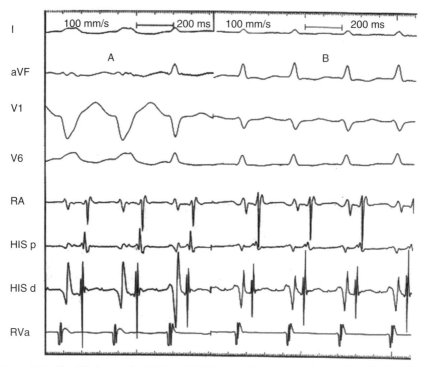

Figure 5.24 The HA interval is 180 ms (HV 80, septal VA 100, tachycardia cycle length 300) during LBBB and 150 ms (HV 50, septal VA 100, tachycardia cycle length 280) during narrow-complex tachycardia. Suggestive of AVRT.

- HV interval prolongation may be due to abnormal right bundle branch conduction thus, the VA interval may prolong because of concealed delay in RB in the presence of LBBB.

Differential diagnosis
- Differential diagnosis of orthodromic re-entrant tachycardia includes atrial tachycardia or AVNRT. Fallowing criteria may be useful in differentiating the mechanisms (Table 5.2).
- Left atrial tachycardia may be mistaken for AVRT utilizing left lateral AP. However in left atrial tachycardia the earliest atrial activation will be away from the mitral annulus and His synchronous PVC will not advance atrial electrogram.
- During tachycardia, with lengthening of AH interval, if there is shortening of the VA interval, it is suggestive of atrial tachycardia and excludes AVRT or AVNRT.
- On termination of the wide complex tachycardia, if atrial pacing at the tachycardia cycle length results in AV block then supraventricular tachycardia with aberrant conduction is unlikely.
- The dual-chamber sequential extrastimulation maneuver consists of an 8-beat drive train of simultaneous AV pacing at 600 ms, followed by an A2 delivered at AVN ERP, followed by a V2 delivered at the drive train cycle

length (600 ms). Repeat drives are then performed with decrements of 10 ms for V2 until VA block is seen.

- This technique identifies slowly conducting APs not revealed with standard pacing maneuvers if the ERP and conduction time of the accessory pathway is similar to the AVN.
- The maneuver uses anterograde concealed conduction to prolong AVN refractoriness much more than that of a concealed AP, thereby allowing the AP to become manifest with the V2.
- Septal APs may have a similar retrograde activation pattern to retrograde AV nodal conduction, especially considering that retrograde atrial activation via the AV node may be slightly eccentric because of left-sided atrial inputs.
- APs that have either slow conduction or decremental properties might be difficult to define with ventricular pacing maneuvers.
- Methods available for clarifying the presence or absence of a concealed AP include assessment of activation sequence and persistence of retrograde conduction during ventricular pacing with adenosine infusion, measurement of conduction time to the atrium during ventricular pacing from the base versus the apex of the heart, and comparison of atrial activation times during para-Hisian pacing at different outputs.
- Both the para-Hisian and basal–apical pacing maneuvers can lead to a false-negative result if an AP has decremental or slow conduction properties.
- The presence of a corrected PPI–TCL <110 ms accurately identified with high reliability those patients with ORT.
- PPI – TCL – (AHpostpacing – AH SVT) = Corrected PPI–TCL
- This discriminant criterion is reliable even for patients with ORT through a septal AP.
- Some Aps are catecholamine sensitive, and isoproterenol may be required to demonstrate retrograde conduction and facilitate tachycardia induction.
  Differential diagnosis of long RP tachycardia includes:
  1 Atypical AVN re-entry tachycardia (AVNRT).
  2 AV re-entrant tachycardia utilizing slowly conducting retrograde accessory pathway.
  3 Atrial tachycardia.
- Comparison of AH interval (in His electrograms) during tachycardia and atrial pacing may help in differentiation. The AH interval during atrial pacing is ±40 ms longer than the AH during tachycardia in patients with atypical AVNRT. In patients with AVRT or atrial tachycardia the difference in AH A pace and AH tachycardia is less than 20 and 10 ms respectively.
- On termination of V pacing during tachycardia stimulus to A minus VA interval of >85 ms and post pacing interval minus tachycardia cycle length interval of >115 ms are suggestive of atypical AVNRT (Figure 5.18).
- Induction of tachycardia by ventricular pacing may be consistent with either ORT or AVNRT but does not exclude AT.
- The concentric atrial activation and relatively long VA timing during tachycardia does not differentiate between perinodal AT, ORT with a septal AP, and AVNRT with a relatively long VA conduction time

- ORT can be excluded if AV dissociation is demonstrated and AT is unlikely if tachycardia terminated without the atrium being affected.

Wolff–Parkinson–White (WPW) syndrome[35]

- The term WPW syndrome describes electrocardiographic pre-excitation accompanied by symptoms of tachycardia. In the absence of symptoms it should be described as WPW pattern.
- Familial WPW syndrome is often associated with glycogen storage cardiomyopathy, a genetic disorder caused by *PRKAG2* gene mutation.
- Familial accessory pathways associated with *PRKAG2* mutation have decrementally conducting properties. Among them are fasciculoventricular pathways and nodoventricular fibers but not atriofascicular fibers.
- The clinical picture of glycogen storage cardiomyopathy includes left ventricular hypertrophy, sinus bradycardia, AV conduction disturbances, and atrial tachyarrhythmias.
- Long-term prognosis may be poor due to the high incidences of sudden cardiac death and heart failure.
- May be wrongly diagnosed as idiopathic hypertrophic cardiomyopathy.
- A missense mutation of the gene that encodes a subunit of the adenosine monophosphate-activated protein kinase (*PRKAG2*) is associated with WPW syndrome
- Incidence of new cases appears to be 4/100 000 per year. The prevalence of WPW electrocardiographic pattern is 0.1 to 0.3%.
- Bone morphogenetic protein (BMP) is important in the development of annulus fibrosus, deletion of *BMP2* bearing microdeletions in 20p12.3 often present with WPW syndrome with variable cognitive deficits and dysmorphic features.
- Females more commonly have right annular APs, and Asians tends to have right anterior APs more frequently than other races. This suggests that the pathogenesis of AP formation may have a genetic component.
- Tachycardia in the absence of pre-excitation which during electrophysiologic study is determined to be due to accessory pathway are labeled as concealed.
- APs are myocardial muscle fibers bridging over annulus and providing electrical continuity between atrium and ventricle.
- Conduction over AP is rate independent. In small number of patients (7%) AP may demonstrate decremental conduction.
- Antegrade decremental conduction is commonly seen over right sided pathways.
- Accessory pathways are classified according to their location on the AV annulus.
- The left free wall location of AP is seen in 50–60%, posteroseptal location in 20–30%, right free wall in 10–20% and anteroseptal is least common.
- Identification of AP potential is help in localization of pathway.
- Antegrade or retrograde conduction block in left lateral and posteroseptal AP occurs on the ventricular insertion side.
- For right sided and septal AP, the site of block appears to be atrium.

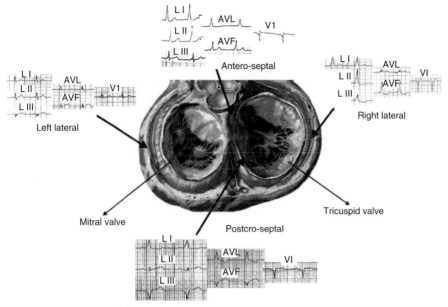

Figure 5.25 Location of the AP and ECG patterns.

- AP may cross the annulus obliquely.
- Multiple accessory pathways are found in 10 to 20% of patients. These are commonly seen in patients with Ebstein anomaly and in those who have been resuscitated from VF.
- Combination of the posteroseptal and right free wall AP is common.
- Not all pathways, found histologically, are functional.

Clinical and electrocardiographic findings in WPW[34]
- Asymptomatic patients with WPW pattern have a benign course.
- 25% of the patients lack retrograde conduction over AP and incapable of producing AVRT.
- 1/3 of patients lose antegrade conduction over AP.
- Once the tachycardia occurs in adult hood, it does not spontaneously resolve.
- Symptoms include palpitations. Syncope does not carry poor prognosis.
- The incidence of sudden death appears to be 1 per 1000 patient years due to AF.
- The degree of pre-excitation depends on relative conduction over AVN and AP. It also depends on distance of the SAN from the AP and conduction time.
- Minimal pre-excitation is often seen in left lateral AP.
- Intermittent pre-exPE implies slow conduction over AP and low risk of sudden death from AF and rapid conduction.
- An increase in sympathetic tone or decrease in vagal tone may enhance AV node conduction and mask pre-excitation. In these patients AP may still be capable of rapid conduction.
- Pre-excitation due to LLAP produces negative delta waves in LI, aVL or V6 and RBBB morphology in V1 (Figure 5.25).

- Activation by right anteroseptal AP produces positive delta wave in L II, L III, aVF with inferior axis and QS pattern in V1 to V3 (Figure 5.25).
- Posteroseptal AP produces superior axis, negative delta wave in inferior leads and rapid transition from V1 to V3 (Figure 5.25).
- Right free wall AP produces positive delta waves in L1, aVL, LBBB pattern and positive delta wave in V1 and left axis (Figure 5.25).

Aortomitral continuity

- Despite being predominantly fibrous in nature, focal atrial tachycardias and left ventricular outflow tract tachycardias may arise from this region. This is possibly due to the cells in the region that exhibit "nodal-like" properties with respect to their response to adenosine and lack of connexin-43 expression.
- Muscle fibers in direct continuity over the fibrous annulus with the left atrial myocardium have been noted.
- In anteroseptal and midseptal pathways, delta wave polarity is positive in aVL and negative in aVR
- Finding of a negative delta wave in both aVL and aVR may be specific to accessory pathways located at the aortomitral continuity. Positive delta waves and QRS polarities were noted in the inferior leads and in leads V4 to V6.
- The QRS morphology on the 12-lead electrocardiogram in WPW depends on the location of the accessory pathway(s) (AP) and the degree of fusion over the normal atrioventricular (AV) conduction.
- Degree of pre-excitation is determined by the site of ventricular insertion of the accessory pathway, AVN conduction time, and atrial conduction.
- When antegrade conduction is over the accessory pathway, the ventricles are activated earlier than from the normal AV conduction system. This results in ventricular pre-excitation.
- Terminal portion of this pre-excited QRS complex is therefore a fusion of antegrade conduction over the accessory pathway and the AVN.
- Although there are a variety of mechanisms of pre-excitation (e.g., fasciculo-ventricular pathways), the commonest is conduction over AV accessory pathway.
- Degree of pre-excitation may vary with heart rate, or it can be intermittent.
- Intermittent loss of pre-excitation implies long accessory pathway effective refractory period, and low risk of sudden cardiac death from rapid pre-excited ventricular rates during atrial fibrillation
- Algorithms facilitate prediction of the location of an accessory pathway, but is limited by the following variables that may produce exceptions and inaccuracies:
  1 Prior myocardial infarction
  2 Ventricular hypertrophy can affect the ECG pattern of pre-excitation.
  3 The orientation and rotation of the heart within the thorax,
  4 ECG electrode position can affect the degree orientation of pre-excitation,
  5 Up to 10% of patients may have more than one accessory pathway, resulting in fusion of pre-excitation patterns or predominance of right-sided conduction because of the proximity to the sinus node.
  6 Intrinsic ECG abnormalities, conduction defects.

- APs can be located anywhere along the AV rings, the 2 most common locations are left free wall and the posteroseptal area.
- Initial 20 ms after the onset of delta wave in particular ECG leads are used. This identifies the delta wave polarity rather than the overall QRS polarity, which may vary from each other.
- Left lateral APs are minimally pre-excited.
- Apparently normal ECG does not rule out an antegrade conducting left lateral AP or a cycle-length-dependent/decremental AP.
- Posteroseptal and right-sided APs tend to have more prominent pre-excitation patterns.

Accessory pathway location

Answer to the following questions may allow the identification of approximate location of APs (Figure 5.25).

Q *Is the delta wave isoelectric or negative in any of these leads I, aVL, or V6?*
- If yes then the accessory pathway is located in either one of two locations;
  1 Left lateral:
     i. No LBBB pattern
     ii. Negative or isoelectric Delta wave in LI, aVL
     iii. Atypical RBBB
        a. Positive delta waves in II, III, aVF- left lateral/anterolateral AP
        b. Negative delta waves in II, III, aVF-left posterolateral AP
  2 Right anteroseptal:
     i. aVL is isoelectric or negative
     ii. LBBB pattern (rS complex in either V1 or V2 with QRS duration >0.1 s)
     iii. QRS axis is downward in the range of +60° or greater

Q *Is the delta wave isoelectric or negative in any of these leads II, III or aVF?*
- If yes then the accessory pathway is located in either one of two locations.
  1 Posteroseptal (right atrial-to-left ventricular connection)
     i. RS or Rs in V1 to V3
     ii. Positive/ isoelectric delta wave in lead II with negative delta waves in III and aVF, right posterior/posterolateral location
     iii. Negative delta waves in all 3 leads (especially lead II, III), suggestive of a true posteroseptal AP near CS orifice
  2 Right lateral
     i. LBBB
     ii. Negative or isoelectric delta wave in aVF positive delta wave in lead II suggests a right lateral AP
- If none of the above plus no LBBB morphology, Rs or RS in V1 and V2, the AP is likely located in the left lateral position.
- If the pre-excitation pattern does not relate to any of the above description, consider the possibility of multiple accessory pathways (may be present in up to 10% of patients), a septal accessory pathway, or another form of pre-excitation such as a fasciculoventricular pathway.
- CS ostium is activated much later than the right atrial annular sites. This activation pattern is unlikely to be present in pre-excitation due to posteroseptal pathway.

- A mismatch between the origin of ventricular pre-excitation and the site of atrial activation during ventricular pacing or orthodromic AV re-entrant tachycardia raises the possibility of multiple APs or an oblique course of the AP.

Electrophysiologic features of pre-excitation

- Decremental pacing from atrium and coronary sinus will determine the antegrade refractory period of the AP. Stimulus to delta interval will be shorter closest to insertion sit of the AP. While ventricular pacing will demonstrate retrograde activation and refractory period of AP.
- For septal AP differential right ventricular pacing from the right ventricle apex and from AP insertion site and para-Hisian pacing may help differentiate conduction over AVN versus AP.
- During parahisian pacing a constant VA during capture and non capture of the His suggests the presence of AP.
- If retrograde conduction is through AVN myocardial capture will show longer VA than His capture.
- Atrial pre-excitation, during SVT, with PVC delivered when His bundle is refractory suggests the presence of AP.
- There are two types of involvement of AP in tachycardia:
  1 AP is an obligatory part of circuit:
     (a) Orthodromic and antidromic AV re-entrant tachycardia.
     (b) Reciprocating tachycardia using multiple accessory pathways.
  2 AP as a bystander:
     (a) Atrial tachycardia, atrial flutter.
     (b) AVNRT.
     (c) VT.
- During AVRT antegrade conduction is over AVN and retrograde conduction is over AP. This results in narrow QRS complex. QRS alternans maybe present.
- Functional BBB during tachycardia may prolong cycle length and the VA interval if the AP is ipsilateral[1].
- ST segment depression during tachycardia is common but it is not related to coronary artery disease.
- Retrograde P wave morphology may help identity location of A.P. Retrograde conduction through posteroseptal AP produces negative P waves in L11, L111 and AVF. Retrograde conduction over left lateral AP produces negative P waves in L1 and aVL.
- Participation of the AVN in tachycardia allows use of vagal maneuvers or AVN blocking agents to terminate the tachycardia. Minor fluctuations in tachycardia cycle length are due to variation in AVN conduction.
- Pre-excitation of the atrium by PVC that is delivered when His bundle is refractory is suggestive of conduction over AP. This does not prove that AP is obligatory participant in the tachycardia.
- Greater the distance from PVC site to AP more premature PVC has to be to produce atrial pre-excitation.
- An abnormal pattern of retrograde activation during tachycardia or during ventricular pacing suggests the presence of AP.

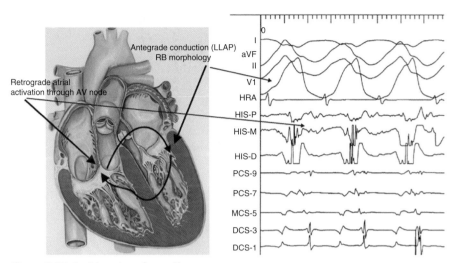

Figure 5.26 Antidromic tachycardia.

- Atypical AVNRT may resemble AVRT on surface EKG; 10–15% of patients with pre-excitation may have dual AV nodal physiology.
- During AVNRT retrograde conduction will be concentric. Retrograde conduction through bystander concealed AP during AVNRT may result in atrial fusion.
- During AVNRT the VA interval in His electrograms tends to be less than 50 ms and His synchronous PVCs do not pre-excite the atrium.
- Differential ventricular pacing and parahisian pacing may help differentiate retrograde conduction over slow pathway and posteroseptal AP.
- RV apex pacing should yield shorter VA interval if retrograde conduction is through slow pathway while pacing from the base will result in a shorter VA if the conduction is through septal pathway.
- Thirty percent of patients with AP may present with AF. Initial arrhythmia may be AVRT which may regress to AF. After ablation of AP spontaneous AF may decrease.
- During AF presence of multiple pre-excited QRS morphologies suggest that multiple AP may exist.
- The shortest pre-excited RR of less than 250 ms may predispose to VF.
- The risk of sudden death is minimal in patients with concealed AP or intermittent pre-excitation.
- Electrophysiologic study and ablation may be considered in asymptomatic patients depending on lifestyle or occupation
- In patients with pre-excitation digitalis and verapamil should not be used as these drugs are known to accelerate conduction over AP.
- Ablation is the treatment of choice for high risk and/or symptomatic patients.

Antidromic tachycardia
- Antegrade conduction is through AP and retrograde conduction is through AVN (Figure 5.26).

- It occurs in 5% of WPW patients. It is rarely seen in patients with septal AP.
- Abrupt lengthening of cycle length during tachycardia may occur due to BBB in retrograde limb of the circuit.
- Differential diagnosis of pre-excited tachycardia includes VT and antegrade conduction over bystander AP during atrial flutter and AVNRT.
- Atrial pacing from AP site will reproduce the QRS morphology identical to tachycardia and also will identify the location of AP.
- AV dissociation during tachycardia will exclude antidromic AVRT.
- Retrograde atrial activation should be through AVN unless antegrade and retrograde conduction are both through AP. Multiple AP may present with pre-excited tachycardia.
- AV node blocking agents and maneuvers will terminate antidromic tachycardia.
- QRS is pre-excited and is identical to that during atrial pacing with conduction over AP.
- There is no His electrogram preceding each QRS. Retrograde His after QRS may be recorded. HA interval during antidromic tachycardia will be similar to HA interval during V pacing.
- Atrial activation is concentric (retrograde conduction through AV node).
- Ventricular activation can be advanced by PAC without involving the AV node. PAC could be delivered near the atrial insertion site of AP.
- If PAC delivered near the AV node simultaneous with atrial activation advances the ventricular electrogram suggests the antegrade conduction is through the AP.
- It may resemble VT. If decremental atrial pacing during sinus rhythm reproduces pre-excitation similar to tachycardia, VT is excluded.
- If atrial pacing during tachycardia advances the QRS without change in morphology it is likely to exclude VT.
- Decremental atrial pacing may produce pre-excitation and as antegrade refractory period of accessory pathway is reached, it may result in normalization of the QRS if antegrade conduction continues through AVN (Figure 5.27).

Bystander AP conduction (Figure 5.28)
- Atrial tachycardia, AVNRT or atrial flutter with 1:1 antegrade conduction through AP should be differentiated from antidromic re-entrant tachycardia where the earliest retrograde activation is in low septal area and is similar to the activation during ventricular pacing if retrograde conduction is through AVN (Table 5.3).
- In atrial tachycardia the site of earliest atrial activation depends on site of origin of tachycardia.
- Adenosine may terminate the tachycardia by blocking retrograde conduction in AVN resulting in QRS that is not followed by A.
- AVNRT with antegrade conduction through bystander AP may result in wide complex pre-excited tachycardia. PVC delivered at the site of antegrade conduction of the AP will block antegrade conduction through AP however AVNRT will continue with narrow complex morphology.
- The HA interval will be shorter during AVNRT with pre-excited QRS due to bystander accessory pathway as opposed to HA interval during antidromic tachycardia in a same patient.

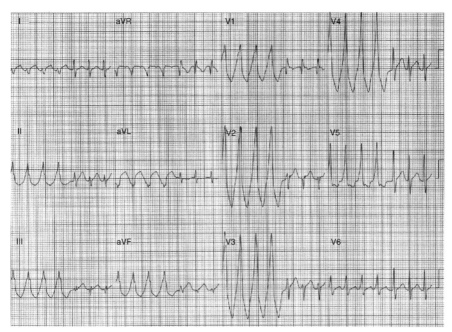

Figure 5.27 Decremental atrial pacing results in pre-excitation as the antegrade ERP of the pathway is reached, it results in normalization of the QRS as the antegrade conduction continues through the AVN.

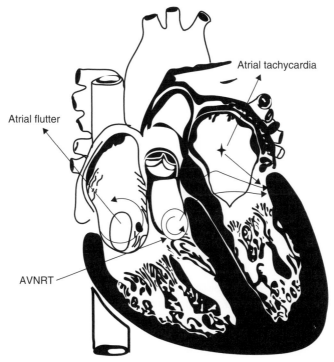

Figure 5.28 Bystander accessory path way.

Table 5.3 Electrophysiologic differential diagnosis of wide complex tachycardia.

SVT aberrancy	VT	Antidromic tachycardia	V pre-excitation due to bystander AP
HV same as in SR	No H preceding QRS	No H preceding QRS	HV shorter than SR
		PAC pre-excite V no change in QRS morphology & no change in His A-A	PAC pre-excites V but does not affect septal A-A excludes Nodoventricular re-entry.
Bifascicular block pattern unusual.	If VT morphology changes from RB to LB without change in H-H interval or CL BB re-entry unlikely. Suggests myocardial VT with penetration of His.	A pacing reproduces QRS morphology	PAC pre-excite V and advances next A excludes AVNRT or AT utilizing bystander AP.
	QRS morphology similar during sinus rhythm and during tachycardia but AV dissociation is present suggestive of BB re-entry or fascicular or His tachycardia.	In atriofascicular tachycardia earliest V at right ventricle apex (RB). No retrograde conduction through atriofascicular pathway	Variable VA with constant AV

- Normalization of the QRS with His extrasystole suggests presence of pre-excitation.
- During bystander pre-excitation the ventricles can be dissociated from the tachycardia.
- In the presence of pre-excitation if there is no retrograde conduction during V pacing, orthodromic tachycardia is unlikely to occur. Antegrade conduction through the AP during atrial pacing and AF should be assessed.

Pathway to pathway tachycardia (Figure 5.29)
1 Atrium and ventricle are obligatory parts of the circuit.
2 Atrial activation is eccentric. Points to the site where the retrogradely conducting accessory pathway is located.
3 QRS is pre-excited. The bundle branch morphology points to the location of antegrade conducting accessory pathway.
   - An AV interval ≥150 ms during pre-excited tachycardia a sensitivity and specific observation with high positive predictive value for AV conduction over a decrementally conducting pathway.
   - AV/TCL ratio of ≥0.55 ms during pre-excited tachycardia has a high sensitivity and specificity and positive predictive value for AV conduction over a decrementally conducting pathway,

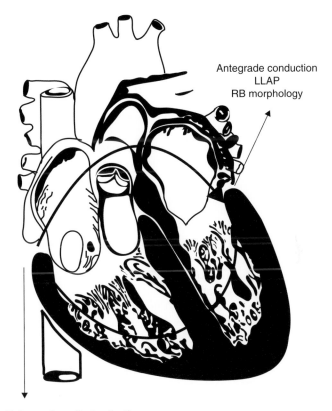

Antegrade conduction
LLAP
RB morphology

Retrograde earliest activation
accentric in right atrium

Figure 5.29 Bypass to bypass taract preexcited tachycardia.

- Wide QRS tachycardia with a LBBB-like morphology and 1:1 ventriculoatrial conduction, the differential diagnosis includes a pre-excited tachycardia using a right-sided AP, which may have rapid or decrementally conducting properties.
- Antidromic tachycardia utilizing atriofascicular pathway has slow conduction and decremental properties. AV interval tends to be longer than the AV interval during antidromic tachycardia using a fast conducting AP.
- Decremental conduction: a minimal increase of 30 ms in accessory pathway conduction during atrial pacing at increasing rates.
- Bystander AV conduction: presence of AV conduction over an accessory AV pathway without participation of this structure in the tachycardia circuit as, for example, in AV nodal re-entrant tachycardia.

Management
- Vagal maneuvers such as Valsalva or carotid sinus massage and AV node blocking drugs such as adenosine beta-blockers or calcium channel blockers are effective in acute termination of tachycardia.

- Drugs that prolong refractory period and conduction over AP such as procainamide, disopyramide and quinidine and drugs that prolong refractoriness in AVN and AP such as flecainide, propafenone, sotalol and amiodarone can be used for chronic treatment of tachycardia.
- Digitalis decreases refractory period of the AP and should be avoided in the presence of pre-excitation.
- Antiarrhythmic drugs may suppress PACs and PVCs thus prevent induction of the tachycardia.
- Adenosine is the drug of choice in acute management of the AVRT. It can be used in patients with hypotension and left ventricular dysfunction. Its half-life is 10 s. Its effectiveness is diminished by theophylline and caffeine.
- Adenosine shortens the atrial refractory period and facilitates occurrence of atrial fibrillation in 10% of patients.
- Intravenous verapamil may take 5–10 minutes to terminate the tachycardia.
- AV node blocking agents should not be used in atrial fibrillation with pre-excitation.
- Infrequent episodes of orthodromic tachycardia can be treated by oral dose of verapamil at the time of occurrence.
- Patients with AF and pre-excited RR interval of less then 250 ms could develop hemodynamic collapse.
- Intermittent pre-excitation implies poor antegrade conduction through the accessory pathway.
- Drug therapy may increase the frequency of the AVRT if it prolongs the antegrade refractory period of the AP without affecting the retrograde conduction or refractoriness.

RF ablation for AVRT
- In symptomatic patients RF ablation of AP is the treatment of choice.
- Most APs travel from the atrium to the ventricle across the AV ring.
- The tricuspid annulus differs from the mitral annulus as outlined below.
  1 Tricuspid annulus is displaced apically.
  2 Larger circumference.
  3 Less fibrous skeleton.
  4 Absence of venous structure along the annulus to map epicardium.
- The AV annulus is identified by the amplitude of the atrial and ventricular electrogram recorded from the mapping/ablation catheter.
- RF ablation could be performed during V pacing. Pathway potentials should be identified.
- Left-sided AP is approached using trans-septal puncture.
- Minimum beat to beat variation in the amplitude of the electrogram indicates firm contact with the tissue.
- Ablation catheter tends to be less stable along the tricuspid annulus and may require use of the preshaped sheath for optimum tissue contact.
- Location of the pathway is identified by shortest local AV (pre-excited) or VA interval and by recording pathway potentials. Ventricular or atrial insertion sites can be identified by ventricular and atrial pacing and earliest atrial or ventricular activation (Figure 5.30).

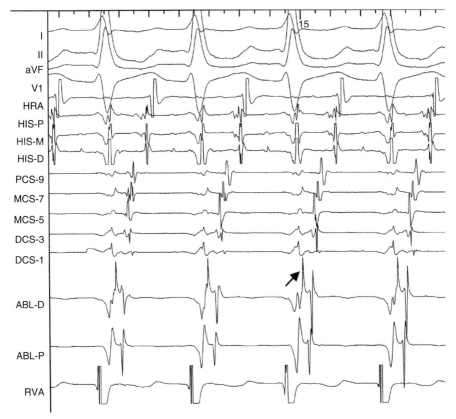

Figure 5.30 Pathway potentials (arrow) recorded from distal ablation electrode.

- Ebstein's anomaly is characterized by apical displacement of the septal leaflet of the tricuspid valve. This results in atrialization of the part of the right ventricle.
- Twenty-five to 30% of patients with Ebstein's anomaly may have AP-mediated tachycardia. These patients are likely to have multiple AP.
- Mapping through right coronary artery may be necessary to localize AP.
- Anteroseptal AP are located in the proximity of the His bundle and are best ablated from ventricular side (large V and small A with bypass potential).
- During ablation of anteroseptal AP, pathway potentials should be prominent and sharper than His.
- The anteroseptal APs could be differentiated from the midseptal APs by two or more positive delta waves in inferior leads, whereas there is significant overlap in electrocardiographic features of midseptal and posteroseptal APs
- Midseptal pathways are located between His electrode anteriorly and CS os catheter posteriorly. Ablation is performed close to ventricular aspect of TA annulus after identifying pathway potential.
- Right posteroseptal APs are located between CS os and tricuspid annulus. Subepicardial left posteroseptal APs are located in proximal CS or in the

cardiac vein structures. Subendocardial pathways are located along the mitral annulus in posterior septum.
- Local ventricular activation precedes the delta wave by 40 to 50 ms.
- Epicardially located pathways produce smaller pathway potentials.
- There may be atrial appendage to ventricular connections. During tachycardia earliest atrial activation is several millimeters away from the annulus.
- Left anterior AP is located at superior medial aspect of mitral annulus.
- Five percent of patients may have multiple APs. These patients tend to have right sided APs
- Reoccurrence of tachycardia after ablation may occur in 6–10% of patients. Complication during procedure may occur in 2–4% of patient.
- Patients with short APERPs and multiple pathways are at higher risk of developing life-threatening arrhythmic events and should be offered prophylactic ablation.
- AP involvement in a tachycardia must be demonstrated before proceeding with pathway ablation.
- Other potential tachycardia mechanisms should be sought in patients in whom the pathway does not appear to be the cause of the symptoms.
- Dyssynchrony due to isolated LBBB or right ventricular apical pacing may result in heart failure.
- Accessory pathway-mediated ventricular pre-excitation with left ventricular dyssynchrony has been suggested as a possible cause of left ventricular dysfunction developmental cardiomyopathy.

Complications of ablation and recurrences of tachycardia
- Tachycardia may reoccur in 5% of patients.
- Complications include cardiac tamponade, thromboembolic events, AV block, and hematomas, and may occur in 2 to 3% of patients undergoing the procedure.

Atypical bypass tract
- The anatomical substrate of tachycardias with characteristics previously attributed to nodoventricular and nodofascicular fibers is actually atrioventricular and atriofascicular AP with decremental conduction properties (i.e., conduction slows at faster heart rates)
- A typical AP in patients with clinical arrhythmias has the following characteristics:
  1 Unidirectional (anterograde only) conduction (with rare exceptions);
  2 Long conduction times; and
  3 Decremental conduction.
- AVRT using a nodoventricular or nodofascicular AP as the anterograde limb generally utilize a second AV AP as the retrograde limb of the re-entrant circuit.
- The atypical AP comprises 3–5% of all AP.
- May present as SVT with a LBBB morphology.
- Ten percent of patients with atypical AP may have multiple bypass tracts.

- Typical, rapidly conducting AV AP may mask the presence of an atypical AP, which may become apparent after ablation of the typical AP.
- Dual AVN pathways are common in patients with atypical APs.
- Atypical APs can also be associated with Ebstein's anomaly.

Nodoventricular bypass tracts (BTs) and nodofascicular BTs

- Nodoventricular BTs arise in the normal AVN and insert into the myocardium near the AV junction.
- Nodofascicular BTs arise in the normal AVN and insert into the RB. These BTs are sensitive to adenosine.

Fasciculoventricular BTs

- Fasciculoventricular BTs uncommon form of pre-excitation (1.2 to 5.1% of atypical APs.

Nodofascicular pathways (Table 5.4)

- First described by Mahaim and Winston as connections between AVN and bundle branch or ventricular myocardium.
- These are characterized by:
  1 Subtle pre-excitation with left bundle morphology and left axis suggestive of right sided connection.
  2 Pathway demonstrates anterograde conduction only.
  3 PAC or atrial pacing increase AH or A-delta interval and enhances pre-excitation.
  4 During tachycardia antegrade conduction is over AP and retrograde conduction over AVN.
  5 Earliest activation occurs at RV apex rather than at the base near the tricuspid annulus.
  6 Demonstration of VA dissociation during tachycardia.

Nodoventricular pathways (Table 5.3)

- May present as pre-excited supraventricular tachycardia with AV dissociation.
- Nodoventricular fibers have associated dual AV nodal physiology, and ablation in the midseptal region, eliminating slow pathway conduction, may be curative.
- HV interval and the degree of ventricular pre-excitation are variable during incremental atrial pacing.
- In response to atrial extrastimulus, progressive AV nodal conduction delay results in shortening of the HV interval with simultaneous increase in degree of ventricular pre-excitation.
- Nodoventricular connections may cause antidromic tachycardia.

Fasciculoventricular connections (FVC)

- They arise from the His bundle or bundle branch and insert into the ventricular septum. They are not capable of sustaining re-entry, do not participate in re-entrant circuits, and are considered an ECG curiosity.

Table 5.4 Nodofascicular/nodoventricular pathways.

	Nodofascicular pathways	Nodoventricular pathway
Pre-excited QRS morphology	Same as for atriofascicular BTs	QRS is wider and atypical LBBB pattern
Site of earliest ventricular activation	At or near the RV apex	Adjacent to tricuspid annulus
Effect of atrial pacing	The degree of pre-excitation is not affected by the site of atrial pacing	The degree of pre-excitation is not affected by the site of atrial pacing
AES from LRA during antidromic AVRT when AV junctional atrium is refractory	The AES does not advance the next ventricular activation	The AES does not advance the next ventricular activation
VH interval during maximal pre-excitation or antidromic AVRT	The VH interval is short	The VH interval is intermediate
Presence of VA block or AV dissociation	May be present	Maybe present

AES = atrial extra stimulus. LRA = lateral right atrium.

- Fasciculoventricular fibers connect the fascicle (or, in rare cases, the most distal part of the AV node) with the ventricular septum and are responsible for ventricular pre-excitation.
- Decremental properties of AV conduction are always preserved, and a constant degree of pre-excitation is observed at any heart rate.
- Fasciculoventricular pathways cannot sustain re-entry and do not cause reciprocating tachycardia, although they can be activated as bystanders in different supraventricular tachycardias.
- It produces minimally pre-excited QRS and a short and fixed HV interval.
- Baseline HV (H-delta) interval during sinus rhythm is less than 35 ms. During decremental atrial pacing HV interval does not change.
- Atrial premature beats cause progressive prolongation of the AH interval without any change in HV interval and QRS configuration. If a closely coupled PAC blocks the fasciculoventricular pathway, it results in a normal HV interval and narrow QRS complex.
- Response to adenosine triphosphate suggests a presence of FVC when prolongation of the PR interval (AH interval) does not change the degree of pre-excitation or complete AV block occurs after the P wave, conducted atrial beats always show pre-excitation.

ECG in FVC
- The delta wave is positive in the inferior leads and in V5 and V6. Delta wave is flat or negative in V1, consistent with a right ventricular insertion.

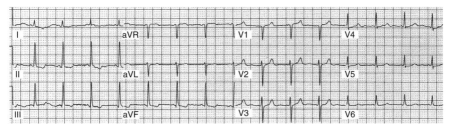

Figure 5.31 ECG in fasciculoventricular connection.

- Mean PR interval is 0.10±0.01s (Figure 5.31).
- QRS, width tends to be narrower in FVC when compared with the pre-excited QRS in the presence of midseptal and anteroseptal BTs is
- Fasciculoventricular pathways may be involved as bystander during AVNRT or AVRT.
- During AVNRT with bystander activation of FVC, a constant degree of pre-excitation is present, His-bundle is activated in an anterograde fashion and an atrial activation sequence during tachycardia is the same as from retrograde conduction over the fast AV node pathway during ventricular pacing.
- Pre-excitation due to fasciculoventricular pathways is benign and requires no therapy.
- Fasciculoventricular BTs are extremely rare.
- True prevalence of this unusual form of pre-excitation may be underestimated due to diagnostic under-recognition.
- The proof of such a pathway relies on
  1 Demonstration of fixed pre-excitation with decremental AVN conduction
  2 Pre-excitation during a His extrasystole
- Because of the close proximity to the native conduction system, re-entry and clinical tachycardia do not occur.
- These nonparticipatory pathways are more intriguing and less clinically relevant.
- Pacing to Wenckebach cycle length may result in AH prolongation with constant HV interval
- On adenosine administration, or carotid sinus massage PR prolongation or complete AV block after the P wave may occur without increase in pre-excitation.
- Forty percent of patients with a fasciculoventricular pathway may have additional accessory atrioventricular pathways
- Fasciculoventricular pathway should be identified so as to avoid targeting it for ablation, which could damage the AV conduction system.

Fasciculoventricular pathway diagnostic criteria
- Baseline HV (H-delta) interval during sinus rhythm is ≤35 ms.
- During decremental atrial pacing HV interval does not change.

- Atrial premature beats cause progressive prolongation of the AH interval but no change in the HV interval and QRS configuration.
- Block in the fasciculoventricular pathway resulting in a normal HV interval and narrow QRS complex.
- In the presence of LV hypertrophy with ventricular pre-excitation due to fasciculoventricular or nodoventricular pathway, should raise suspicion of a γ2-subunit of the adenosine monophosphate-activated protein kinase (*PRKAG2*) mutation.
- LV hypertrophy in patients with *PRKAG2* is caused by glycogen storage in the myofibrils.
- True incidence of *PRKAG2* mutation may be underestimated as patients are misdiagnosed as idiopathic hypertrophic cardiomyopathy.
- Patients with the *PRKAG2* mutation are known to be at high risk for dying from fast AF at an early age (20–30 years) and from complete AV block at a later age.
- Mechanism of death probably is AF with fast heart rate causing ventricular fibrillation.
- The clinical features of glycogen storage cardiomyopathy includes
  1 Left ventricular hypertrophy,
  2 Sinus bradycardia,
  3 AV conduction disturbances, and
  4 Atrial tachyarrhythmias.

Permanent form of junctional reciprocating tachycardia (PJRT)
- PJRT is an incessant long RP tachycardia.
- It may result in tachycardia-mediated cardiomyopathy.
- The electrocardiogram shows negative P waves in inferior lead. Each QRS is preceded by a P wave.
- There is no pre-excitation on surface ECG.
- It is an AVRT utilizing slowly conducting posteroseptal accessory pathway.
- The antegrade limb is the AV node and retrograde limb is slowly conducting posteroseptal accessory pathway, which demonstrates retrograde decremental conduction and is sensitive to vagal maneuvers beta-blockers and calcium channel blockers.
- The long serpiginous course and fiber orientation of the pathway may contribute to slow conduction.
- Slowly conducting left free wall AP may demonstrate similar features.

Electrophysiologic features
- Electrocardiographic features include board and negative P waves in L11, L111, aVF, long RP interval, and transient termination occurs in retrograde limb (Figure 5.32).
- Cycle length may change due to modulation of PR and RP interval.
- Premature beats are not required for initiation of tachycardia.
- Earliest activation, during tachycardia, occurs in posteroseptal region near CS ostium. Retrograde AVN conduction is nonexistent.

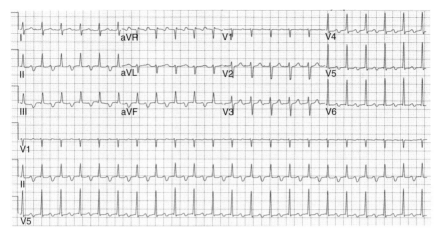

Figure 5.32 PJRT.

- Incessant nature of the tachycardia is due to unidirectional block in limbs, slow conduction and balanced refractoriness.
- It must be differentiated from atypical AVNRT and atrial tachycardia.
- PVC delivered when His is refractory, if advances atrial activation suggests AP.
- Tachycardia occurs spontaneously at a critical sinus cycle length without PACs or PVCs. RP interval is longer than the PR interval.
- QRS complexes are narrow and are preceded by His electrogram and normal HV interval.
- Late coupled PVC may terminate tachycardia by retrograde block in AP.
- Differential diagnosis includes AT arising from posteroseptal region or atypical AVNRT (Tab).
- These pathways are sensitive to adenosine and may not help in differentiating from other tachycardia.
- If a PVC delivered when His bundle is refractory (His synchronous) results in termination of the tachycardia without atrial activation, it excludes the possibility of AVNRT and AT.
- Retrograde conduction through AP is facilitated by isoproterenol.
- PVC may delay atrial activation (post-excitation phenomenon). This occurs if the delay in retrograde conduction exceeds the coupling interval of the PVC, resulting in delayed atrial activation longer then tachycardia CL.
- Drug therapy is ineffective. Ablation is the treatment of choice
- Ablation is guided by earliest atrial activation, during tachycardia, which precedes the onset of the P wave and an AP potential that precedes atrial activation.
- PJRT is characterized by:
  1 Narrow complex tachycardia.
  2 Initiation of the tachycardia is not preceded by prolongation of the PR or AH interval.
  3 1:1 AV relation.

4 RP longer than PR interval.

5 Negative P waves in L2 L3 and aVF.

6 Extra nodal slow and decrementally conducting AP forms the retrograde limb of the circuit.

7 Atrial insertion site is close to or inside CS os.

- The following features suggest the presence of PJRT and make atypical AVNRT less likely.

    1 During tachycardia, PVC delivered when His bundle is refractory results in atrial pre-excitation without any change in activation sequence.

    2 PVC may terminate tachycardia without atrial activation.

    3 Prolongation of the local VA interval.

- Ablation is targeted at earliest atrial activation site during tachycardia.

Atriofascicular re-entrant tachycardia[36–39]

- During tachycardia antegrade conduction is through atriofascicular fibers (also known as Mahaim fibers) and retrograde conduction is through the AVN (antidromic).
- These fibers are capable of only antegrade conduction and have decremental conduction properties.
- The atrial insertion site is in right posterolateral, lateral or anterolateral free wall near the tricuspid annulus.
- Electrocardiographic features include QRS duration <150 ms, QRS axis between 0° and –75°, R wave in lead I, rS pattern in lead V1, and precordial transition beyond lead V4.
- The distal insertion site is right bundle branch.
- Conduction over these fibers, during tachycardia produces ventricular pre-excitation with left bundle morphology.
- Right ventricular apical activation is earlier then basal.
- His Purkinje activation occurs retrogradely as demonstrated by right bundle electrogram preceding His electrogram. Impulse from the right bundle must travel retrogradely to His and antegradely to ventricle simultaneously. This results in simultaneous activation of His and onset of ventricular activation.
- During atrial pacing, progressive AV and AH interval prolongation coupled with a decreasing HV interval results in a greater degree of ventricular pre-excitation with a left bundle branch-like morphology.
- The occurrence of retrograde RBBB during tachycardia will shift His activation to late in the QRS
- PAC delivered during tachycardia, in the RA lateral wall, will advance V and His without activating AVN.
- AP potential can be recorded from right AV groove and successful ablation can be performed from this site.
- Right-sided AP with antegrade conduction will produce ventricle activation at base of right ventricle as opposed to apical activation that occurs with atriofascicular fibers.
- PACs or PVCs can induce atriofascicular tachycardia.
- During tachycardia 1:1 atrium:ventricle relationship must be present

- QRS complexes demonstrate left bundle morphology.
- During sinus rhythm QRS morphology is normal.
- Atriofascicular tachycardia can be differentiated from right ventricular tachycardia by atrial pacing during which QRS morphology will be similar to atriofascicular tachycardia.
- Dual AVN physiology is common in patients with Atriofascicular fibers.
- Antidromic AVRT can be distinguished from atrial tachycardia and AVNRT with bystander AP activation by recording retrograde activation of the His Purkinje system where RB electrogram precedes His bundle electrogram during tachycardia.
- Termination of the tachycardia by single PVC without atrial activation excludes atrial tachycardia.
- Adenosine administration may terminate tachycardia by antegrade block in atriofascicular fibers.
- The following characteristics are noted during electrophysiologic evaluation.
  1 Tachycardia is characterized by LBBB morphology.
  2 The tachycardia has a 1:1 AV relationship, with a central atrial activation sequence and no visible His potential.
  3 Late right atrial extrastimulus delivered while atrial septal refractoriness during pre-excited tachycardia advances ventricular activation without affecting low right atrial septal activation. If ventricular activation is advanced *and the tachycardia is reset* (meaning that the subsequent atrial activation also is advanced), then the atriofascicular AP is part of the tachycardia circuit. Like most diagnostic pacing maneuvers, this one is specific but may not always be demonstrable.
  4 Tachycardia can be entrained from right atrium.
  5 Right atrial pacing from the free wall close to TA results in ventricular pre-excitation, reproducing the QRS complex morphology of the clinical tachycardia.
  6 Shortest stimulus to QRS duration on pacing from TA.
  7 Recording of pathway potentials along the TA.
  8 Pathway demonstrates decremental conduction on right atrial pacing with prolongation of the A to AP potential.
  9 Ventricular insertion site is identified by earliest ventricular activation during pre-excited tachycardia.
- The differential diagnosis of LBBB-morphology tachycardia includes:
  1 Pre-excited tachycardia.
  2 SVT with aberrant conduction.
  3 Ventricular tachycardia (VT).
  4 Bundle branch re-entry VT
- Early sharp intrinsic deflection, does not favor VT.
- The late precordial transition (V5) favors an atriofascicular pathway.
- Late transition is unlikely with antidromic tachycardia due to AV AP.
- ECG may show a minimal pre-excitation pattern in the presence of atriofascicular pathways.
- The increase in cycle length in association with the ipsilateral retrograde BBB is suggestive of an antidromic tachycardia as opposed to VT.

- Presence of nodofascicular, atriofascicular or AV AP may result in bystander conduction from an AV nodal re-entrant tachycardia or atrial tachycardia/flutter and may present as pre-excited tachycardia.
- The mere presence of an atriofascicular AP does not prove the participation of that AP in the tachycardia due to antidromic AV re-entry circuit.
- In up to 10% of cases, the mechanism is atrial tachycardia or re-entrAVNRT, with the atriofascicular AP acting as a bystander for AV conduction

Is it a bystander AP, or is it participating in the tachycardia circuit?

- The following features suggest participation of the atriofascicular pathway in the tachycardia.
  1 During tachycardia, 1:1 VH conduction will be present, with the right bundle branch activated before the His bundle.
  2 A premature atrial beat delivered during atrial septal refractoriness, if advances following ventricular activation with no change in QRS morphology, would suggest participation of accessory pathway as anterograde limb of the tachycardia. It also excludes nodofascicular pathway participation in the tachycardia.
  3 Ventricular electrogram at the right ventricle apex if earlier than the ventricular electrogram at the annulus (His bundle) suggests an atriofascicular tachycardia. Reversal of this pattern during normal sinus rhythm.
  4 While entraining the tachycardia during right ventricular apex pacing the HA interval will not change if atriofascicular pathway is a part of the circuit during tachycardia, ruling out AV nodal re-entrant tachycardia with bystander AP conduction, which would have shown an increase in the HA interval during RV apical pacing.
  5 During pacing from right ventricular apex if atrial rate accelerates to the pacing cycle length implying that the tachycardia has been entrained and the tachycardia resumes on termination of pacing, following features will exclude atrial tachycardia:
      a Atrial activation sequence during pacing is identical to that of the tachycardia.
      b VA linking occurs after pacing.
      c Post-pacing response is A-V An A-V response after overdrive ventricular pacing theoretically could occur in the setting of an atrial tachycardia with a bystander atriofascicular AP because such a pathway (which conducts only anterogradely and may not be penetrated retrogradely by the paced wavefront) may be capable of echoing the last captured atrial activation to the ventricle before resumption of the underlying atrial tachycardia. However, the combination of an identical atrial activation sequence during pacing, reproducible VA linking after pacing, and an A-V response makes atrial tachycardia unlikely.
  6 The PPI if less than 120 ms of the TCL, should distinguish AVNRT from re-entrAVRT, regardless of whether the latter is orthodromic or antidromic. The PPI–TCL difference exploits the greater distance between the right ventricular apex and AVN circuits compared to the distance between the

right ventricular apex and circuits that involve the ventricles (AVRT).indi-cating that the right ventricular apex is close to the tachycardia circuit

7 Stimulus-to-atrial electrogram (SA) interval during pacing, if less than 80 ms of the VA interval during tachycardia, will exclude AVNRT. The SA–VA difference should distinguish AVNRT from AVRT regardless of whether the latter is orthodromic or antidromic. The SA–VA difference exploits the different VA activation relationship during entrainment of AVNRT (V and A activation in series) compared to that during AVNRT (V and A activation in parallel). In contrast, during AVRT (whether orthodromic or antidromic), the VA activation relationship is in series during both the supraventricular tachycardia and during entrainment.

• The pacing maneuver and responses described above should hold true regardless of the type or direction of AV nodal circuit (slow-fast, fast-slow, or slow-slow).

In patients with a pre-excited tachycardia using an atriofascicular pathway, the following situations may affect the tachycardia rate:

1 VA conduction over the His–AV node axis changing into VA conduction over a second AP: When this occurs, the rate change will depend on the location of the ventricular end and the conduction properties of that AP.

2 Retrograde BBB: transient retrograde RBBB may cause a change in the rate of antidromic tachycardia due to changes in the VH interval when using either a single rapidly conducting AP or an atriofascicular pathway as an anterograde limb.

3 Dual AV nodal pathways: when VA conduction occurs over the bundle branch–His-AV node axis, changes in the rate of an antidromic tachycardia may occur when retrograde conduction over a fast pathway changes into conduction over a slow pathway resulting in prolongation of the HA rather than the VH interval.

Differential diagnosis

Atriofascicular pathway
• During pre-excited tachycardia, there is a short V-H interval, early activation of the right ventricular apex, and late activation at the annulus. The atrial insertion is located by finding the accessory pathway potential.

• Decrementally conducting accessory AV pathway connecting the right atrium with the distal part of the RBB.

• In a slowly, decrementally conducting right-sided accessory AV pathway, signs of ventricular pre-excitation are often minimal.

• the distinction between the two types of right-sided accessory AV connection can rapidly be made by measuring the AV interval, and even better the AV/TCL index during the pre-excited tachycardia.

• In atriofascicular pathways, the decremental properties are related to the slow rate of recovery of excitability, which is similar to the fast AV nodal pathway. There is an inverse relationship between heart rate and premature beat inter-vals and conduction time both in atriofascicular pathway and the AV node.

Short decremental AV pathways
- During pre-excited tachycardia, there is a long V-H interval, early ventricular activation at the tricuspid annulus, and late activation at the RV apex.
- Characterized by a delta wave that starts before the end of the sinus P wave because of the proximity of the right atrial end of the pathway to the sinus node

Long decremental right superior AV pathways
- During pre-excited tachycardia, there is late activation of the RV apex and late activation at the tricuspid annulus.
- 12-lead ECG shows normal QRS frontal plane axis between +30 and +60. There is no left-axis deviation.
- Atrial insertion can be located by finding the accessory pathway potential at the right superior area at the tricuspid annulus.

Treatment
- Tachycardia may response to AV node blocking drugs or it can be ablated at atrial insertion site.
- Earliest atrial activation is at retrograde exit site of AV node. Earliest ventricular activation is not near AV groove. These markers cannot help locate atrial insertion site.
- Identification of pathway potential along the AV groove and delivery of energy at that site appears to be the most promising ablation technique.
- Damage to RB may make tachycardia incessant.

References

1 Ghali WA, Wasil BI, Brant R, Exner DV, Cornuz J. Atrial flutter and the risk of thrombo-embolism: a systematic review and meta-analysis. *Am. J. Med.* 2005;118(2):101–107.
2 Feld GK. Radiofrequency ablation of atrial flutter using large-tip electrode catheters. *J. Cardiovasc. Electrophysiol.* 2004;15(10 Suppl):S18–23.
3 Da Costa A, Thévenin J, Roche F, et al. Results from the Loire-Ardèche-Drôme-Isère-Puy-de-Dôme (LADIP) trial on atrial flutter, a multicentric prospective randomized study comparing amiodarone and radiofrequency ablation after the first episode of symptomatic atrial flutter. *Circulation.* 2006;114(16):1676–1681.
4 Lukac P, Pedersen AK, Mortensen PT, et al. Ablation of atrial tachycardia after surgery for congenital and acquired heart disease using an electroanatomic mapping system: Which circuits to expect in which substrate? *Heart Rhythm.* 2005;2(1):64–72.
5 Bottoni N, Donateo P, Quartieri F, et al. Outcome after cavo-tricuspid isthmus ablation in patients with recurrent atrial fibrillation and drug-related typical atrial flutter. *Am. J. Cardiol.* 2004;94(4):504–508.
6 Tanner H, Hindricks G, Kottkamp H. Right ventricular pacing for control of right atrial isthmus block: a new colorful piece in the mosaic. *Heart Rhythm.* 2006;3(3):273–274.
7 Bernstein NE, Sandler DA, Goh M, et al. Why a sawtooth? Inferences on the generation of the flutter wave during typical atrial flutter drawn from radiofrequency ablation. *Ann Noninvasive Electrocardiol.* 2004;9(4):358–361.

8 Anon. The effect of low-dose warfarin on the risk of stroke in patients with nonrheumatic atrial fibrillation. The Boston Area Anticoagulation Trial for Atrial Fibrillation Investigators. *N. Engl. J. Med.* 1990;323(22):1505–1511.

9 Knight BP, Zivin A, Souza J, et al. A technique for the rapid diagnosis of atrial tachycardia in the electrophysiology laboratory. *J. Am. Coll. Cardiol.* 1999;33(3):775–781.

10 Petersen P, Boysen G, Godtfredsen J, Andersen ED, Andersen B. Placebo-controlled, randomised trial of warfarin and aspirin for prevention of thromboembolic complications in chronic atrial fibrillation. The Copenhagen AFASAK study. *Lancet.* 1989; 1(8631):175–179.

11 Roy D, Talajic M, Dorian P, et al. Amiodarone to prevent recurrence of atrial fibrillation. Canadian Trial of Atrial Fibrillation Investigators. *N. Engl. J. Med.* 2000; 342(13):913–920.

12 Garan H. Atypical atrial flutter. *Heart Rhythm.* 2008;5(4):618–621.

13 Jaïs P, Shah DC, Haïssaguerre M, et al. Mapping and ablation of left atrial flutters. *Circulation.* 2000;101(25):2928–2934.

14 Anon. Warfarin versus aspirin for prevention of thromboembolism in atrial fibrillation: Stroke Prevention in Atrial Fibrillation II Study. *Lancet.* 1994;343(8899):687–691.

15 Wyse DG, Waldo AL, DiMarco JP, et al. A comparison of rate control and rhythm control in patients with atrial fibrillation. *N. Engl. J. Med.* 2002;347(23):1825–1833.

16 Cavolli R, Kaya K, Aslan A, et al. Does sodium nitroprusside decrease the incidence of atrial fibrillation after myocardial revascularization?: a pilot study. *Circulation.* 2008; 118(5):476–481.

17 Klein AL, Grimm RA, Murray RD, et al. Use of transesophageal echocardiography to guide cardioversion in patients with atrial fibrillation. *N. Engl. J. Med.* 2001; 344(19):1411–1420.

18 Stern JD, Rolnitzky L, Goldberg JD, et al. Meta-analysis to assess the appropriate endpoint for slow pathway ablation of atrioventricular nodal re-entrant tachycardia. *Pacing Clin Electrophysiol.* 2011;34(3):269–277.

19 Otomo K, Nagata Y, Uno K, Fujiwara H, Iesaka Y. Atypical atrioventricular nodal re-entrant tachycardia with eccentric coronary sinus activation: electrophysiological characteristics and essential effects of left-sided ablation inside the coronary sinus. *Heart Rhythm.* 2007;4(4):421–432.

20 Anon. Stroke Prevention in Atrial Fibrillation Study. Final results. *Circulation.* 1991;84(2):527–539.

21 Hongo RH, Themistoclakis S, Raviele A, et al. Use of ibutilide in cardioversion of patients with atrial fibrillation or atrial flutter treated with class IC agents. *J. Am. Coll. Cardiol.* 2004;44(4):864–868.

22 Camm AJ, Savelieva I. Advances in antiarrhythmic drug treatment of atrial fibrillation: where do we stand now? *Heart Rhythm.* 2004;1(2):244–246.

23 Latini R, Tognoni G, Kates RE. Clinical pharmacokinetics of amiodarone. *Clin Pharmacokinet.* 1984;9(2):136–156.

24 Torp-Pedersen C, Møller M, Bloch-Thomsen PE, et al. Dofetilide in patients with congestive heart failure and left ventricular dysfunction. Danish Investigations of Arrhythmia and Mortality on Dofetilide Study Group. *N. Engl. J. Med.* 1999; 341(12):857–865.

25 Wazni OM, Beheiry S, Fahmy T, et al. Atrial fibrillation ablation in patients with therapeutic international normalized ratio: comparison of strategies of anticoagulation management in the periprocedural period. *Circulation.* 2007;116(22):2531–2534.

26 González-Torrecilla E, Almendral J, García-Fernández FJ, et al. Differences in ventriculoatrial intervals during entrainment and tachycardia: a simpler method for

distinguishing paroxysmal supraventricular tachycardia with long ventriculoatrial intervals. *J. Cardiovasc. Electrophysiol.* 2011;22(8):915–921.

27 Hwang C, Fishbein MC, Chen P-S. How and when to ablate the ligament of Marshall. *Heart Rhythm.* 2006;3(12):1505–1507.

28 Dixit S, Marchlinski FE. How to recognize, manage, and prevent complications during atrial fibrillation ablation. *Heart Rhythm.* 2007;4(1):108–115.

29 Katritsis DG, Becker AE, Ellenbogen KA, et al. Right and left inferior extensions of the atrioventricular node may represent the anatomic substrate of the slow pathway in humans. *Heart Rhythm.* 2004;1(5):582–586.

30 Michaud GF, Tada H, Chough S, et al. Differentiation of atypical atrioventricular node re-entrant tachycardia from orthodromic reciprocating tachycardia using a septal accessory pathway by the response to ventricular pacing. *J. Am. Coll. Cardiol.* 2001;38(4):1163–1167.

31 Ho RT, Mark GE, Rhim ES, Pavri BB, Greenspon AJ. Differentiating atrioventricular nodal re-entrant tachycardia from atrioventricular re-entrant tachycardia by DeltaHA values during entrainment from the ventricle. *Heart Rhythm.* 2008;5(1):83–88.

32 Feldman A, Voskoboinik A, Kumar S, et al. Predictors of acute and long-term success of slow pathway ablation for atrioventricular nodal re-entrant tachycardia: a single center series of 1,419 consecutive patients. *Pacing Clin Electrophysiol.* 2011;34(8): 927–933.

33 Kerr CR, Gallagher JJ, German LD. Changes in ventriculoatrial intervals with bundle branch block aberration during reciprocating tachycardia in patients with accessory atrioventricular pathways. *Circulation.* 1982;66(1):196–201.

34 Fox DJ, Klein GJ, Skanes AC, et al. How to identify the location of an accessory pathway by the 12-lead ECG. *Heart Rhythm.* 2008;5(12):1763–1766.

35 Zhang L-P, Hui B, Gao B-R. High risk of sudden death associated with a PRKAG2-related familial Wolff-Parkinson-White syndrome. *J Electrocardiol.* 2011;44(4):483–486.

36 Tan HL, Wittkampf FHM, Nakagawa H, Derksen R. Atriofascicular accessory pathway. *J. Cardiovasc. Electrophysiol.* 2004;15(1):118.

37 Tchou P, Lehmann MH, Jazayeri M, Akhtar M. Atriofascicular connection or a nodoventricular Mahaim fiber? Electrophysiologic elucidation of the pathway and associated re-entrant circuit. *Circulation.* 1988;77(4):837–848.

38 Sternick EB, Cruz FES, Timmermans C, et al. Electrocardiogram during tachycardia in patients with anterograde conduction over a Mahaim fiber: old criteria revisited. *Heart Rhythm.* 2004;1(4):406–413.

39 McClelland JH, Wang X, Beckman KJ, et al. Radiofrequency catheter ablation of right atriofascicular (Mahaim) accessory pathways guided by accessory pathway activation potentials. *Circulation.* 1994;89(6):2655–2666.

Answers to self-assessment questions

5.1 Atrial flutter

1 C
2 C
3 B
4 A
5 C
6 C
7 C

5.2 Atrial tachycardia

1 B
2 C
3 A

5.3 Atrial fibrillation

1 C
2 B
3 A
4 C
5 B
6 A
7 D
8 D

5.4 Automatic junctional tachycardia

1 A
2 C

5.5 AVNRT

1 B
2 C
3 B
4 A
5 C
6 A
7 C
8 D
9 C
10 A

5.6 AVRT

1 B
2 D
3 C
4 D
5 A
6 B
7 D
8 A
9 B

10 C
11 C
12 C
13 A
14 C
15 A
16 B
17 A
18 C
19 D
20 C

CHAPTER 6
Differential diagnosis of wide complex tachycardia

Self-assessment questions

1 A 52-year-old man, who suffered from uncomplicated inferior wall myocardial infarction 3 years ago, became aware of palpitations 4 months ago. Palpitations would last for several hours during which he had no other symptoms. During one such episode he came to the emergency room. Palpitations had persisted for 3 hours. BP was 106/70. Patient was alert and in no distress. ECG strip is shown.

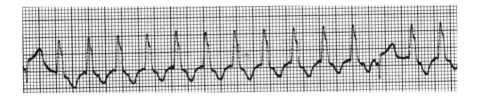

What will be the next step?
A IV adenosine.
B 200 mg of PO flecainide and continue maintenance dose.
C Cardioversion.
D Valsalva maneuver.

Essential Cardiac Electrophysiology: The Self-Assessment Approach, Second Edition. Zainul Abedin.
© 2013 Blackwell Publishing Ltd. Published 2013 by Blackwell Publishing Ltd.

2 A 67-year-old female whose baseline ECG shows prolong PR interval, RBBB
and old inferior MI presents to ER with palpitations. 12 lead ECG is shown
below. What is the likely diagnosis?

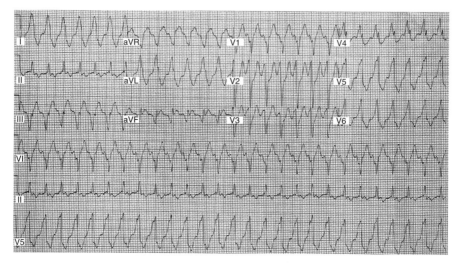

A SVT with aberrant conduction.
B VT.
C Pre-excited tachycardia.
D SVT bystander accessory pathway conduction.

6.1 Wide complex tachycardia (WCT)

Causes of WCT

1 Ventricular tachycardia: 80% of all WCT are due to ventricular tachycardia (VT).
2 Supraventricular tachycardia (SVT): in the presence of functional or persistent bundle branch block (BBB), electrolyte abnormalities and antiarrhythmic drugs.
3 Pre-excited tachycardia with positive concordant pattern in precordial leads.
4 Ventricular paced rhythm.

Differential diagnosis[1-6] (Table 6.1)

Clinical features

- WCT in the presence of previous myocardial infarction (MI) is likely to be due to VT.

Electrocardiographic features[7]

- Presence of atrioventricular (AV) dissociation, capture or fusion beats is highly suggestive of VT.
- In lead V1 triphasic complex with RBBB morphology and initial portion of the QRS similar to sinus rhythm is suggestive of SVT. Broad monophasic complexes are suggestive of VT.
- In lead V1 with LBB morphology the QRS demonstrates narrow (<30 ms) initial r and sharp smooth descent is likely to be due to SVT with aberrant conduction.
- Notching in the down slope of the QRS and an interval of 60 ms from the onset of the QRS to the nadir of the S wave is suggestive of VT.
- LBBB morphology with right axis deviation is invariably due to VT.
- RBBB morphology with normal axis is suggestive of SVT (uncommon in VT)
- Concordance pattern is uncommon in SVT. Positive concordance may be present in pre-excited tachycardia.
- Negative concordance in limb leads L1, L11, and L111 is suggestive of VT (northwest axis).
- Presence or preserved Q during WCT is suggestive of VT. Pseudo Q waves may be seen in AV nodal re-entry tachycardia (AVNRT).
- Absence of RS complex in precordial leads (concordant pattern) is suggestive of VT. If the RS pattern is present, the interval from onset of R wave to nadir of S wave of >100 ms is suggestive of VT.
- If the QRS duration during tachycardia is narrower than QRS duration during sinus rhythm, it is suggestive of VT[7].
- Occurrence of contralateral BBB during SR and WCT is highly suggestive of VT. If RBBB was present during sinus rhythm and LBBB developed during SVT, it will result in complete heart block (CHB) unless BBB pattern is due to peripheral conduction delay.

Table 6.1 Differential diagnosis of WCT[1].

Clinical features	SVT with AC	VT
H/O MI	Less likely	More likely
Cannon waves, variable S1		If present suggest AV dissociation
Carotid sinus pressure Valsalva, adenosine	Terminates tachycardia	Produces AV dissociation
ECG features		
QRS duration	<140 ms	>140 ms
QRS axis frontal plane	Normal	If right superior
RBBB morphology		
QRS in V1	Triphasic	Mono- or biphasic
QRS in V6	R/S ratio >1	R/S ratio <1
LBBB morphology		
QRS in V1	Narrow R, sharp descent	Notching, R to S >60 ms
QRS V6	RS	QR QS
LBBB RAD	Less likely	Likely to be VT
RBBB normal axis	Likely SVT	Less likely
Concordance pattern V lead	Uncommon	Common
Preserved Q during WCT	Unlikely	Common
AV dissociation, fusion, capture. number of V>A	Unlikely	Diagnostic of VT
RS pattern in V leads	Unlikely	Suggestive of VT
If RS pattern present in V Leads	RS less than 100 ms	RS >100 ms
QRS narrower during tachycardia than in SR	Unlikely	Likely
Contralateral BBB during WCT	Unlikely	Suggestive of VT
Change in axis from SR	<40 degrees	>40 degrees
QRS similar during SR and WCT	Suggestive of SVT	Uncommon
R in aVR	Unlikely	Suggestive of VT
Width of an initial R or Q wave >40 ms in aVR	Unlikely	Suggestive of VT
Ventricular activation–velocity ratio (Vi/Vt)	>1 mV	<1 mV

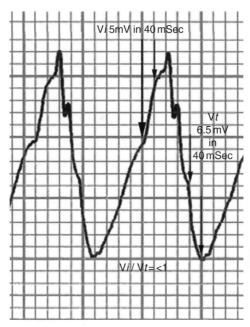

Figure 6.1 Assessment of V*i*/V*t* ratio.

- QRS alternans does not help in differentiating WCT.
- Some of the criteria may not be reliable in the presence of pre-existing BBB during sinus rhythm.
- In the presence of preexisting RBBB, AV dissociation, precordial concordance, right superior axis and monophasic R wave in V1 are highly suggestive of VT.
- If the WCT does not conform to any patterns of aberration it is likely to be due to VT.
- In lead aVR (1) presence of an initial R wave, (2) width of an initial R or Q wave >40 ms, (3) notching on the initial downstroke of a predominantly negative QRS complex, and (4) ventricular activation–velocity ratio (V*i*/V*t*), the vertical excursion (in millivolts) recorded during the initial (V*i*) and terminal (V*t*) 40 ms of the QRS complex, V*i*/V*t* >1 suggests SVT, and V*i*/V*t* ≤1 suggests VT (Figure 6.1).
- Presence of any criteria would suggest VT (Figures 6.2 and 6.3).

Exceptions to VT criteria
- Bundle branch re-entry tachycardia may mimic SVT with aberration of left bundle morphology. Presence of AV dissociation will help in making the correct diagnosis.
- VT can be irregular during first 30 seconds.
- Narrow complex VT is likely to originate from septum or the fascicle.

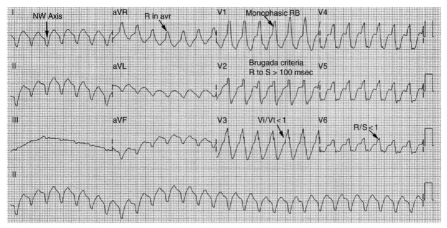

Figure 6.2 VT criteria.

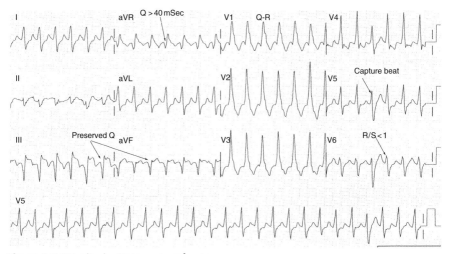

Figure 6.3 VT criteria. Note capture beats.

- Fusion complexes may occur with two ventricular ectopic foci.
- AV dissociation can be present in junctional tachycardia.

Differential diagnosis (Table 6.1)

References

1 Akhtar M, Shenasa M, Jazayeri M, Caceres J, Tchou PJ. Wide QRS complex tachycardia. Reappraisal of a common clinical problem. *Ann. Intern. Med.* 1988;109(11):905–912.
2 Olshansky B. Ventricular tachycardia masquerading as supraventricular tachycardia: a wolf in sheep's clothing. *J Electrocardiol.* 1988;21(4):377–384.

3 Wellens HJ, Bär FW, Lie KI. The value of the electrocardiogram in the differential diagnosis of a tachycardia with a widened QRS complex. *Am. J. Med.* 1978;64(1):27–33.

4 Wellens HJ. Electrophysiology: Ventricular tachycardia: diagnosis of broad QRS complex tachycardia. *Heart.* 2001;86(5):579–585.

5 Kindwall KE, Brown J, Josephson ME. Electrocardiographic criteria for ventricular tachycardia in wide complex left bundle branch block morphology tachycardias. *Am. J. Cardiol.* 1988;61(15):1279–1283.

6 Vereckei A, Duray G, Szénási G, Altemose GT, Miller JM. Application of a new algorithm in the differential diagnosis of wide QRS complex tachycardia. *Eur. Heart J.* 2007;28(5):589–600.

7 Arias MA, Domínguez-Pérez L, Pachón M, Rodríguez-Padial L. Wide QRS tachycardia complexes narrower than baseline: an uncommon electrocardiographic clue for ventricular tachycardia. *Europace.* 2008;10(11):1356.

Answers to self-assesement questions

1 C

2 B

CHAPTER 7

Ventricular tachycardia and ventricular fibrillation

Self-assessment questions

1 Which one of the following is not a risk factor for SCD?
   A Deafness
   B Left ventricular hypertrophy.
   C Na, Ca and K channel abnormalities.
   D Autonomic dysfunction such as increase in sympathetic and decrease in parasympathetic tone.

7.1 Ventricular arrhythmias in the presence of coronary artery disease

1 An 83-year-old man is brought to the emergency department because of palpitations that began four hours ago. He denies chest pain or dyspnea. He is alert and anxious. Blood pressure is 120/70 mmHg. He suffered from a myocardial infarction 7 years ago.
   Electrocardiogram is shown below.

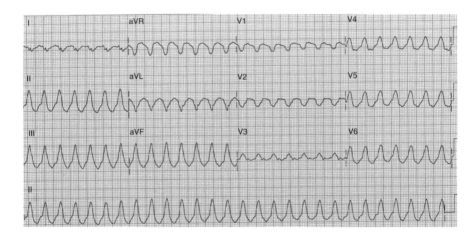

Essential Cardiac Electrophysiology: The Self-Assessment Approach, Second Edition. Zainul Abedin.
© 2013 Blackwell Publishing Ltd. Published 2013 by Blackwell Publishing Ltd.

Which of the following is the most likely diagnosis?

A Atrial flutter with 1:1 AV aberrant conduction

B Ventricular tachycardia

C AV reentrant tachycardia using an atriofascicular pathway

D Antidromic tachycardia utilizing right accessory pathway

2 Eight months ago, a 52-year-old man, who had a history of skipping of heart beats for several years, had an inferoposterior myocardial infarction. No clinical evidence of heart failure was noted during recovery.

Echocardiogram showed inferior akinesis and estimated left ventricular ejection fraction of 42%. Ambulatory electrocardiographic monitoring revealed frequent episodes of three-beat nonsustained monomorphic ventricular tachycardia.

The patient has no cardiovascular symptoms. His only medication is aspirin, 81 mg daily. Which of the following is most appropriate at this time?

A Electrophysiologic study.

B Amiodarone

C A β-adrenergic blocking agent

D An implantable cardioverter-defibrillator

3 A 56-year-old man, undergoing cardiac rehabilitation, complained of palpitations. He had a myocardial infarction 6 weeks ago. He has no history of angina pectoris, or syncope. Echocardiogram shows left ventricular ejection fraction of 30%.

Which of the following is the most appropriate next step?

A Observation

B 24-hour ambulatory electrocardiography

C An implantable cardioverter-defibrillator

D Electrophysiologic study

7.3 Ventricular arrhythmias in hypertrophic and dilated cardiomyopathy

1 Which one of the following is the risk factor for SCD in patients with IHSS?

A Age >50 years

B History of frequent PVCs

C Gene Mutation coding for troponin and tropomyosin

D LV wall thickness of >30 mm

2 You are asked to provide an opinion regarding a younger brother of a 28-year-old asymptomatic athlete who was found to have IHSS on an echocardiogram. This 21-year-old man is asymptomatic and his echocardiogram is normal. 12 lead ECG showed ST-T changes.

What will be your recommendations?

A This could be suggestive of carrier or preclinical state

B This is perhaps a juvenile pattern

C Patient should not be allowed to participate in competitive sports

D Coronary angiogram should be performed as these changes could be due to anomalous origin of the coronary arteries

3 In which of the following conditions echocardiographic findings suggestive of IHSS are unlikely to be present?

A Friedreich ataxia

B Noonan syndrome

C Amyloidosis

D Addison's disease

4 You are asked to evaluate a 17-year-old high school student who has been diagnosed to have IHSS. His main symptoms are palpitations and occasional non exertional chest pain; 24 hour ambulatory ECG monitoring revealed frequent PVCs and 3 to 4 beat nonsustain VT. There is no history of syncope or sustain VT. To further risk stratify what will be your recommendations?

A Electrophysiologic study

B Signal average ECG

C Stress test

D Cardiac catheterization and angiography

5 This patient expresses the desire to participate in high school football team. What will be your therapeutic recommendations?

A Start beta-blockers and allow him to participate in contact sports

B Start Disopyramide and allow him to participate in contact sports

C Start Digoxin and allow him to participate in contact sports

D Patient should refrain from participating in contact sports

6 In patients who have hypertrophic cardiomyopathy, which of the following findings is the strongest indicator of increased risk for sudden cardiac death?

A Mild exertional dyspnea

B Resting intraventricular pressure gradient

C Nonsustained ventricular tachycardia

D Mitral regurgitation on echocardiography

7.4 Bundle branch re-entry ventricular tachycardia

1 During electrophysiologic study a wide complex tachycardia is induced. Tracing is shown below.

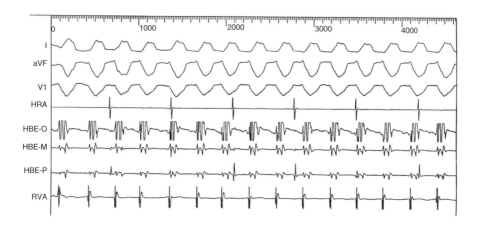

Which one of the following is likely to terminate and render tachycardia noninducible?

A AVN ablation

B Ablation of the focus in RVOT

C Ablation of the right bundle

D Ablation of the atriofascicular pathway.

2 Which one of the following conditions is unlikely to present with BBR-VT?

A Myotonic dystrophy

B Hypertrophic cardiomyopathy

C Ebstein anomaly

D Brugada syndrome

3 Which one of the following observation is unlikely to be present in BBR-VT?

A Short HV interval during VT when compared with HV in sinus rhythm as measured from the onset of surface QRS.

B Conduction abnormality of HPS during sinus rhythm

C VT with LB morphology.

D His electrogram precedes RB electrogram.

7.5 Channelopathies

Long QT syndrome and Torsade de pointes

1 A 22-year-old female, without deafness, presents with history of seizures. During EEG recording she has brief seizure. At that time fallowing rhythm strip is recorded. Serum potassium was 3.6 mEq/L. Echocardiogram was normal.

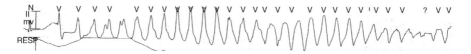

What will be your recommendation?
A Dilantin.
B Mexiletine.
C Keep serum potassium level >4.0 mEq/L.
D Implant ICD.

2 Which of the following channel/current activity will prolong the APD?
A Increase in I_{to}
B Block of I_{Na}
C Decrease in I_{Kr}
D Block of K_{ATP}

3 Which one of the following agents is least likely to prolong QT interval?
A Cefepime HCL
B Ketoconazole
C Haloperidol
D Trimethoprim-sulfa

4 A 46-year-old male was treated for hypertension with hydrochlorothiazide and felodipine and for diabetes with long-acting insulin. He developed low grade fever and cough. He was prescribed erythromycin and benadryl. Two days later he developed transient loss of consciousness lasting for 30 to 40 seconds, during which tonic and clonic movements were noted. Serum potassium was 3.7 mEq/L. Electrocardiogram done 3 weeks earlier was normal. Echocardiogram was normal.
What is the most likely cause this event?
A Hypoglycemia
B TDP
C Neurocardiogenic syncope
D Seizure disorder

5 You are asked to evaluate a 19-year-old woman who was found to have a QTc of 480 ms. Three months ago, her 25-year-old maternal aunt, who was recently diagnosed to have congenital long Q-T syndrome, died suddenly. The patient has no history of syncope or other cardiac symptoms. Her mother and 15-year-old brother are asymptomatic. There is no family history of deafness.
What will be your recommendations?
A Permanent pacemaker implant
B Initiate beta-blockers
C Implant ICD
D Observation

6 A 27-year-old female, on routine evaluation had ECG (shown below). She is asymptomatic. There is no family history of syncope, sudden cardiac death, deafness or prolong QT interval. Her echocardiogram is normal. Serum potassium is 4.0 mEq/L. She is not receiving any medications.

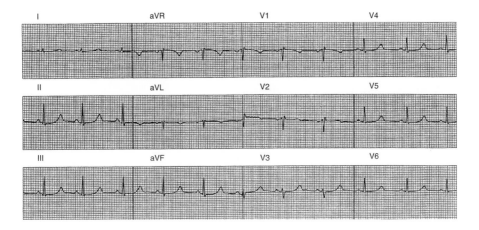

What will be your recommendation?
A Observation
B Beta-blockers
C Electrophysiologic study
D Permanent pacemaker implant

7 In a patient with long QT syndrome the risk of syncope, aborted cardiac arrest or sudden cardiac death is greatest during which of the following.
A First trimester
B Third trimester
C Immediate postpartum period
D First nine months postpartum

Arrhythmogenic right ventricular dysplasia/cardiomyopathy (ARVD/C)

1 A 17-year-old male presents to emergency room with a history of syncope. Cardiac monitoring reveals frequent PVCs but no ventricular tachycardia. Echocardiogram revealed mild RV dilatation. Cardiac MRI was inconclusive. Head up tilt test, RV angiogram and signal average ECG were normal.
What will be your recommendation?
A ICD implant
B Sotalol
C Amiodarone
D None of the above

2 A 40-year-old sales representative presents with progressively increasing dyspnea, fatigue and sever swelling around the ankles. Five years ago he had recurrent episodes of ventricular tachycardia. A diagnosis of ARVD/C was made. An ICD was implanted left pectoral region. At the time of initial implant R wave amplitude was 6 mV and pacing threshold was 0.6 V at 0.5 ms pulse width. On today's evaluation R wave amplitude was 1.5 mV and pacing

threshold was 2.5 V at 0.5 pulse width. In last 4 weeks four pleural taps were performed and each time 700 to 1000 mL of fluid was removed. Echocardiogram shows enlarged and hypokinetic RV.

Patient has not had ventricular arrhythmias in last 14 months. What will be your recommendation?

A Implant new ICD on the right side
B Start sotalol
C Consider cardiac transplant
D Surgically isolate RV

3 Which of the following findings is most likely to be present in arrhythmogenic right ventricular dysplasia?

A Areas of fatty infiltration without fibrosis in the myocardium
B Normal cardiac evaluations of family members
C Late potentials on signal-averaged electrocardiography
D No inducible arrhythmias on programmed electrical stimulation

Brugada syndrome

1 As a volunteer physician for Doctors without Borders you are posted in Cambodia. You are asked to evaluate a 17 year old male who had one episode of syncope. There is family history of sudden cardiac death. ECG shows type 1 Brugada pattern. What will be your recommendation?

A Flecainide
B Quinidine
C Beta-blockers
D Close observation No antiarrhythmics.

2 A 24-year-old asymptomatic subject presents with ECG diagnosis of Brugada syndrome. Family history is unremarkable. What will be your recommendation?

A ICD implant
B EPS
C Observation
D Beta-blockers

3 A 30-year-old man reported to the emergency room after an episode of syncope. While in the emergency room he had three episodes of ventricular fibrillation from which you were successfully resuscitated. Electrocardiogram is shown.

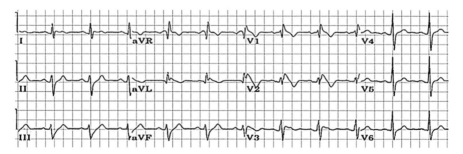

What will be your recommendations?
A Intravenous amiodarone
B Intravenous isoproterenol
C Oral metoprolol
D Intravenous magnesium

Catecholaminergic polymorphic ventricular tachycardia

1 A 21-year-old male presents to ER with exercise induced palpitations. Cardiac examination is normal. Echocardiogram is normal. ECG during stress test is shown.

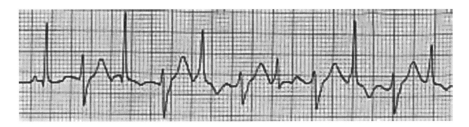

What is the likely diagnosis?
A Long QT syndrome
B Brugada syndrome
C CPVT
D BBRT-VT

2 A 16-year-old male presents to emergency department with abdominal pain. Diagnosis of acute appendicitis is made and surgery is recommended.
  There is no history of palpitations, syncope or seizures. His uncle had died suddenly at the age of 19.
  The patient's mother reported that the patient was found to be a carrier for RyR2 mutation. Her concern is that general anesthesia may induce malignant hyperthermia. Cardiac examination and echocardiogram are normal.
What will be your recommendations?
A Patient can safely under go surgery under general anesthesia
B ICD should be implanted prior to surgical intervention
C IV amiodarone should be started prior to surgery and should be continued after surgery
D Electrophysiologic study should be performed to assess the risk of inducible ventricular arrhythmias.

7.6 Ventricular tachycardia in structurally normal heart

1 A 50-year-old physician comes to the emergency department because of rapid palpitations that began 1 hour ago. He has had multiple episodes in the past year. Patient is in no distress. Pulse rate is 180 bpm, and blood pressure is 110/70 mmHg. Electrocardiogram is shown.

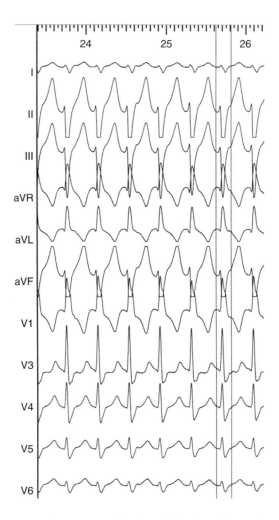

Adenosine, 6 mg intravenously, is administered, without any effect. Tachycardia terminates spontaneously 15 minutes later. Complete blood count, serum electrolytes and thyroid-stimulating hormone, chest radiograph, echocardiogram, cardiac magnetic resonance imaging scan are normal. Cardiac perfusion studies are normal.

Which of the following statements regarding this patient's tachycardia is most likely correct?

A It originates from the left ventricular outflow tract
B It originates from the right ventricular outflow tract
C It originates from the Purkinje system of the apical left ventricular septum
D It uses a left lateral AV accessory pathway

2 An 18-year-old woman is brought to emergency room for painful and swollen right knee that she suffered while playing tennis. In the ER following ECG was recorded. She denies any palpitations, chest pain or syncope. Physical

examination is normal. Serum electrolytes and blood count are within normal limit. Echocardiogram and cardiac MRI are normal.

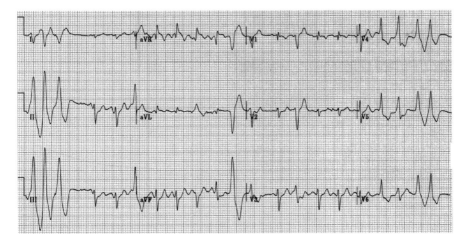

What will be your recommendations?

A Lidocaine 50 mg IV bolus and drip at 2 mg/min

B Begin oral flecainide

C Admit the patient and schedule for electrophysiologic study.

D Observation reassurance without further diagnostic and therapeutic intervention

3 A 36-year-old man seeks your advice regarding frequent palpitations. Last week he was in the emergency room with one such episode. Electrocardiogram recorded during that episode is shown.

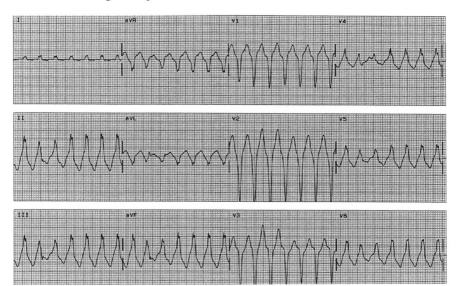

Ablation at which of the following sites is most likely to resolve the arrhythmias.
A Posterior free wall of the right ventricular outflow tract
B Left septal wall of the right ventricular outflow tract
C Lateral wall of the LV outflow tract
D Left ventricular basal-septum

4 A previously healthy 30-year-old man has sudden onset of palpitations and lightheadedness while playing soccer. Pulse rate was 190 bpm, and blood pressure is 100/58 mmHg. The arrhythmia terminates spontaneously, and he is brought to the hospital. Cardiac enzymes, electrocardiogram, echocardiogram, and treadmill exercise electrocardiogram are normal. Recordings obtained during electrophysiologic study are shown below.

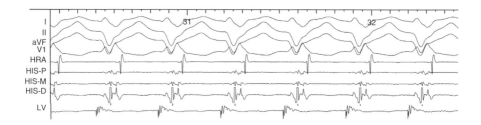

Which of the following statements is most likely correct regarding this condition?
A Intravenous administration of verapamil may result in hemodynamic collapse
B The tachycardia originates in the region of the left posterior fascicle
C Left lateral accessory pathway ablation will terminate the tachycardia
D An identical pace map is required for successful radiofrequency catheter ablation

7.7 Miscellaneous forms of ventricular arrhythmias

1 Which one of the following condition is least likely to present with bidirectional VT?
A Digitalis toxicity
B Herbal aconite poisoning
C Familial hypokalemic periodic paralysis
D Hypocalcemia

2 A 50-year-old man presents with frequent and symptomatic premature beats an occasional brief palpitations. He denies history of syncope. Other than premature beats on auscultation rest of the physical examination was unremarkable. Echocardiogram revealed ejection fraction of 40%. Electrocardiogram is shown. Radiofrequency catheter ablation is most likely to be successful if performed at which of the following sites?

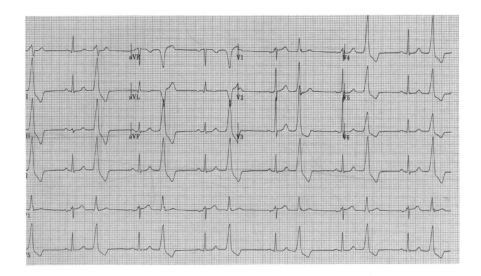

A Right ventricular outflow tract
B Noncoronary cusp of the aortic valve
C Left coronary cusp
D Lateral mitral annulus.

7.0 Ventricular arrhythmias

- Cardiovascular disease remains a major cause of sudden cardiac death (SCD).
- Fifty percent of all cardiac deaths are sudden. The majority of SCD are caused by ventricular arrhythmias. Its incidence increases with age.
- The high-risk subgroup includes patients with low ejection fraction, history of heart failure, resuscitated out of hospital cardiac arrest, previous myocardial infarction (MI).
- Ventricular arrhythmias generate high percentage of SCD but absolute numbers are low.
- In the general population the incidence of SCD is low, 0.1 to 0.2% but absolute numbers are high, 300 000 SCD per year.
- A large number of patients in general population will have to be treated to avoid small number of deaths.
- The risk of sudden death is highest in first 6–18 months after index event such as myocardial infarction or recent onset of heart failure. Risk of sudden death is proportionate to increasing number of coronary artery disease (CAD) risk factors.
- Structural abnormalities of the heart such as myocardial infarction, dilatation due to myopathy and left ventricular hypertrophy predispose to the genesis of ventricular life threatening arrhythmias. Use of these risk factors in identifying individual at risk of sudden cardiac death is limited.

- The incidence of ventricular arrhythmia induced SCD, as percentage of total mortality tends to be high in patients with congestive heart failure (CHF) in functional class II and III, however in patients with functional class IV bradyarrhythmias, asystole and pulseless electrical activity appears to be the cause of death.

Risk factors for SCD

1 Myocardial ischemia.
2 Left ventricular hypertrophy.
3 Na, Ca and K channel abnormalities.
4 Metabolic abnormalities such as hypokalemia, acidosis and stretch related modulations of ion channels.
5 Autonomic dysfunction such as increase in sympathetic and decrease in parasympathetic tone.
6 Drugs that could alter repolarization and cause Torsade de pointes.

In 80% of SCD victims no acute MI is found. Triggering mechanism appears to be ischemia.

Ventricular fibrillation (VF)[1]

- VF is a common arrhythmia noted in patients with out of hospital cardiac arrest.
- Slowing of VF rate after initial rapid onset may be due to ischemia and acid/base, electrolyte abnormality.
- Coronary artery disease is the most common substrate in patients with VF. Acute MI is found in 20% of patients with VF cardiac arrest and recurrence is less than 2% in 1 year in these patients. Recurrence is 30% if VF occurs in the absence of acute MI.
- Slowing of conduction may occur in the scar tissue of the healed MI predisposing to reentrant VT/VF.
- Twenty-five percent of patients with cardiomyopathy may develop VF cardiac arrest in first year.
- Identification of the high risk patients is difficult. In patients with hypertrophic cardiomyopathy, risk factors such as family history of sudden death, inducible VT during EPS may identify high risk group. Ejection fraction less than 35% remains a major risk factor for patients with ischemic or nonischemic cardiomyopathy although the sensitivity of these markers is low.
- During metabolic acidosis VF threshold is decreased and reverse is likely in metabolic alkalosis.
- Alkalization of the serum may retard class I antiarrhythmic related proarrhythmias.
- Prophylactic lidocaine should not be used in post MI patients.
- Defibrillator implant is the treatment of choice.
- Mortality remains 40% in 5 years irrespective of the treatment chosen.

7.1 Ventricular arrhythmias in the presence of coronary artery disease[2]

Ventricular tachycardia

- Occurrence of the arrhythmias is facilitated by the presence of substrate such as slowing of conduction (scar, anisotropy) dispersion of refractoriness, electrical triggers such as PVCs and physiologic modulating factors such as ischemia, electrolyte abnormalities, hypoxia and proarrhythmic drugs.
- Sustained monomorphic VT arises from the scar of healed myocardial infarction.
- Classification/definitions of the VT are outlined in Figure 7.1.

Definitions

On the basis of clinical characteristics

1 **Clinical ventricular tachycardia (VT)**: VT that has occurred spontaneously based on analysis of 12-lead ECG QRS morphology and rate. Haemodynamically unstable VT causes haemodynamic compromise requiring prompt termination.

2 **Idiopathic VT**: Occurs in the absence of clinically apparent structural heart disease. Idioventricular rhythm is three or more consecutive beats at a rate of <100/min that originate from the ventricles independent of atrial or atrioventricular (AV) nodal conduction.

3 **Incessant VT** is continuous sustained VT that recurs promptly despite repeated intervention for termination over several hours.

4 **Non-clinical VT** is induced by programmed ventricular stimulation that has not been documented previously. This term should be avoided. Induced VTs with a QRS morphology that has not been previously observed should be referred to as 'undocumented VT morphology'.

5 **Nonsustained VT** terminates spontaneously within 30 s.

6 **Presumptive clinical VT** is similar to a spontaneous VT based on rate and ECG or electrogram data available from implantable cardioverter-defibrillator

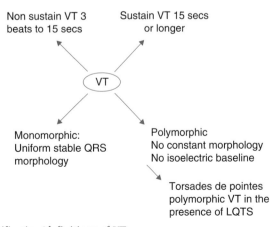

Non sustain VT 3 beats to 15 secs

Sustain VT 15 secs or longer

VT

Monomorphic: Uniform stable QRS morphology

Polymorphic No constant morphology No isoelectric baseline

Torsades de pointes polymorphic VT in the presence of LQTS

Figure 7.1 Classification/definitions of VT.

(ICD) interrogation, but without the 12-lead ECG documentation of either the induced or spontaneous VT.

7 Repetitive monomorphic VT: continuously repeating episodes of self-terminating non-sustained VT.

8 Sustained VT: continuous VT for ≥30s or that requires an intervention for termination (such as cardioversion).

9 Ventricular tachycardia: a tachycardia (rate >100/min) with three or more consecutive beats that originates from the ventricles independent of atrial or AV nodal conduction.

10 VT storm is considered three or more separate episodes of sustained VT within 24 h, each requiring termination by an intervention.

On the basis of electrocardiographic morphologies

1 Monomorphic VT has a similar QRS configuration from beat to beat Some variability in QRS morphology at initiation is not uncommon, followed by stabilization of the QRS morphology.

2 Multiple monomorphic VTs: refers to more than one morphologically distinct monomorphic VT, occurring as different episodes or induced at different times. Polymorphic VT has a continuously changing QRS configuration from beat to beat indicating a changing ventricular activation sequence.

3 Pleomorphic VT has more than one morphologically distinct QRS complex occurring during the same episode of VT, but the QRS is not continuously changing.

4 Right and left bundle branch block-like VT configurations: terms used to describe the dominant deflection in V1, with a dominant R-wave described as 'right bundle branch block-like' and a dominant S-wave as 'left bundle branch block-like' configurations. This terminology is potentially misleading as the VT may not show features characteristic of the same bundle branch block-like morphology in other leads.

5 Torsade de pointes (TDP) is a polymorphic VT associated with LQTS.

On the basis of mechanisms

1 Scar-related re-entry describes arrhythmias that have characteristics of reentry and originates from an area of myocardial scar identified from electrogram characteristics or myocardial imaging. Large reentry circuits that can be defined over several centimetres are commonly referred to as 'macrore-entry'.

2 Focal VT has a point source of earliest ventricular activation with a spread of activation away in all directions from that site. The mechanism can be automaticity, triggered activity, or microre-entry.

Factors associated with development of ventricular arrhythmias during MI:

1 Large MI
2 Septal involvement in MI
3 Left ventricular dysfunction

4 Hypotension during evolving MI

5 Ventricular fibrillation during early stages of MI

6 Conduction abnormalities.

- Patients with hemodynamically stable sustained ventricular tachycardia tend to have scars from MI, left ventricular aneurysm and left ventricular dysfunction when compared with patients whose first presentation is SCD.

Clinical manifestations during VT

- Heart rate during VT is a major determinant of homodynamic status.
- Other factors include systolic and diastolic dysfunction, ischemia, and degree of mitral insufficiency.

Electrocardiographic features for identifying the site of origin of VT

When attempting to localize the origin of the VT following points should be considered:

1 QRS width: QRS duration in septal VTs is less than the VTs originating from the free wall

2 QRS axis: Right superior-axis suggests that the VT is arising from apical septal or apical lateral region. QS pattern is seen in leads I, II, and III and QS or rS in V5 and V6.

Presence of QS complexes in inferior leads are due to spread of activation from inferior wall. QS pattern in precordial leads suggests activation moving away from the anterior wall.

VT with inferior-axis arises from the basal areas, right ventricular outflow tract, superior left ventricular septum, or basal lateral wall of the left ventricle. The inferior axis will point to left if VT is arising from the superior right free wall or superior left ventricular septum.

Left-axis deviation is present when in the presence of inferior infarction the VT exit site is near the septum. The axis moves to the right and superior as the site of the origin of the VT moves posterolaterally.

3 Bundle branch block (BBB) pattern: The BBB pattern is a result of the sequence of right and left ventricular activation. LBBB morphology is present in VTs arising from right ventricle or from LV side of septum.

4 Concordance: Positive concordance is present when the direction of the activation is anterior and apical and is generally present in VTs arising from the posterior basal area of the heart.

VT arising from the scar of inferior infarction, activation is from posterior to anterior resulting in R wave in precordial leads (V2 to V4). In the presence of RBBB this pattern may persist up to V6.

Negative concordance is seen in VTs arising from apical septum as a sequel of anteroapical MI.

5 Presence of QS or QR complexes: Presence of QS complexes in V4–V6 suggests apical origin of the VT.

- Frontal plane axis and QRS morphology may help localize the exit site and location of the VT circuit (Figure 7.2).

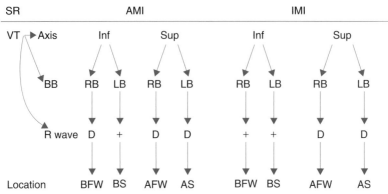

Figure 7.2 ECG algorithm for identifying the site of origin of VT. AFW = apex free wall. AMI = anterior MI. AS = apex septum. BB = bundle branch block. BFW = basal free wall. BS = basal septum. D = delayed R progression. IMI = inferior MI. LB = left bundle branch block morphology. RB= Right bundle branch block morphology. SR = sinus rhythm. += R wave present across precordial leads. − = R wave absent.

VT that manifest with left superior axis, include
1 VT arising from posteroseptal inferior myocardial infarction
2 Left posterior fascicular VT,
3 Interfascicular reentry,
4 Automatic fascicular VT,
5 Posterior papillary muscle VT,
6 Posterior mitral annular VT
- Posterior mitral annular VT has morphologic resemblance to VT from the crux

Mechanisms[3]
- Mechanism of the scar related VT is reentry, which can be initiated and terminated by programmed stimulation.
- The presence of mid-diastolic or presystolic potentials is suggestive of slow conduction facilitating reentry.
- The inverse relation between extra stimulus coupling interval and the interval to the first beat of VT suggest the presence of slow conduction.
- Majority of spontaneously occurring ventricular tachycardia are inducible.
- 20% of all VT are induced from RVOT when apical stimulation fails.
- Ventricular tachycardia, as in the setting of gene mutations for proarrhythmic drugs could be due to triggered activity.
- Ventricular tachycardia in this setting of a structurally normal heart could be due to focal mechanism.
- During programmed stimulation demonstration of resetting and concealed entrainment are suggestive of reentry.
- Reentrant VT can be terminated by overdrive.

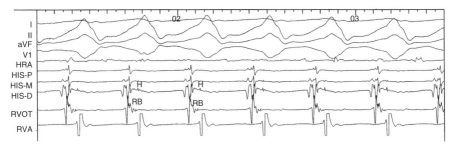

Figure 7.3 VT originating in the septum with retrograde activation of HPS. Right bundle precedes His electrograms. Underlying atrial rhythm is AF.

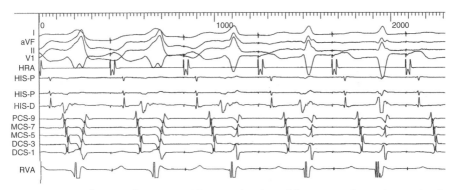

Figure 7.4 Atrial pacing during VT with normalization of the QRS as the VT is entrained.

Electrophysiologic features

- His bundle deflection preceding QRS complex is usually absent. If His electrogram is present the HV interval is shorter than the HV interval during sinus rhythm.
- Changing AH interval in the presence of constant but shorter HV interval indicates that the His is engaged retrogradly by VT.
- If His is retrogradly activated during VT, RB potential will precede His potential (Figure 7.3).
- If His is engaged by an antegrade impulse His electrogram will precede RB electrogram.
- Atrial pacing, if entrains the tachycardia with normal HV and QRS then it is highly suggestive of VT (Figure 7.4).
- The HV interval during VT should be compared with the HV interval during sinus rhythm. HV during VT may appear normal but will be shorter than the prolonged HV in sinus rhythm.
- The occurrence of HV interval that is shorter than the HV in sinus rhythm implies retrograde activation of the His with a conduction time to His being shorter than the antegrade conduction time to the rest of the ventricular myocardium. It also implies that the site of origin is in proximity of the Purkinje system.

- The Purkinje system may be part of the re-entrant circuit in patients with postinfarction monomorphic VT, resulting in a type of VT with a relatively narrow QRS complex that mimics fascicular VT.
- During BB re-entry tachycardia HV during VT may be same or longer than the HV during sinus rhythm (see Figures 7.15 and 7.16).
- In BB re-entry retrograde conduction occurs over the LB and antegrade conduction over the right bundle, the His electrogram precedes the RB electrogram.
- In BB re-entry tachycardia changes in V to V interval follow the changes in H to H interval. Right ventricular activation precedes left ventricular activation.
- Electrophysiologic study has low yield in patients who present with VF cardiac arrest due to ischemia.
- VT arise from surviving myocytes within the scar, conduction through these tissues is slow and inhomogeneous resulting in low amplitude ($<0.5\,mV$) and fractionated potentials (lasting for $>130\,ms$) that precedes the onset of the surface QRS.
- Substrate for VT after MI develops in the first 2 weeks but persists indefinitely.
- If a VT is induced 2 weeks after MI it remains reproducible 1 year later.
- Risk of developing VT is greatest (3–5%) in the first year after a MI but may occur 15–20 years later. Progression of coronary artery disease and worsening of left ventricular function may act as trigger.
- VT originating near the His bundle may have similar electrocardiographic and electrophysiological characteristics, regardless of whether the ablation site is in the right ventricle or aortic sinuses because of the close anatomical relationship of these structures and rapid transseptal conduction. When right ventricular mapping reveals an earliest ventricular activation in the HB region during VT, mapping in the right coronary cusp (RCC) and noncoronary cusp (NCC) should be added to accurately identify the site of origin.
- During wide complex tachycardia, ventricular tachycardia and antidromic reentrant tachycardia can be excluded if the H-V-A sequence is recorded while the surface QRS occurs after the His electrogram.
- Negative concordance could occur during a supraventricular tachycardia with functional LBBB.
- Precordial negative QRS concordance does not always mean that the wide QRS tachycardia is a VT.
- During tachycardia if there is AV dissociation and a His-bundle deflection is evident preceding each QRS two possibilities should be considered;
  1 Bundle branch re-entry VT
  2 VT with passive retrograde activation of the His bundle.
- These possibilities require assessment of coupling between the His and V and the sequence of activation.
  1 If oscillations in the H-H interval precede changes in the V-V interval and on termination there is no His following the last V passive retrograde activation from a ventricular tachycardia is unlikely.

2 During WCT with AV dissociation if the His bundle is activated from above possible diagnoses included.

   1 AV nodal reentrant tachycardia with upper common pathway block.

   2 Intrahisian reentry, splitting of the His potential.

   3 Focal junctional tachycardia.

   4 BBR VT.

- Differential diagnosis of narrow QRS VT should include ventricular tachycardia arising near the His Purkinje system especially in the postinfarction setting.
- There may be subtle differences in QRS morphology compared with during sinus rhythm.
- Programmed stimulation induces VT in over 90% of patients with a history of VT.
- Rate and QRS morphology of induced VT may differ from that observed during spontaneous tachycardia.
- Iinduction of VT signifies the presence of a fixed anatomic substrate associated with an increased likelihood of future spontaneous events.
- Episodes of sustained VT are a marker for increased mortality and reduce quality of life in patients who have implanted defibrillators.

Treatment[5,6]

- Hemodynamically unstable patients should be cardioverted.
- I.V. Procainamide appears to be superior to Lidocaine.
- Patients with incessant or recurrent VT may respond to IV Amiodarone. 30 day mortality remains high in this group (30 to 50%).
- Long-term treatment of choice is ICD.
- In AVID trial patients with hemodynamically stable VT and EF of greater than 40% were excluded from the trail but were fallowed in a registry. Mortality risks were found to be lower in this group.
- In patients with previous myocardial infarction, EF of 35%, spontaneous NSVT and inducible VT ICD implant improved survival by 20% in one year.
- Patients with low ejection fraction irrespective of nonsustain VT or inducibility during electrophysiologic study have been shown to derive survival benefit from prophylactic ICD implant.
- Antiarrhythmic medications can reduce the frequency of ICD therapies, but have low efficacy and side effects.
- Catheter ablation for VT should be considered early in the treatment of patients with recurrent VT.

Catheter ablation of VT is indicated for

- Symptomatic sustained monomorphic VT (SMVT), including VT terminated by an ICD, that recurs despite antiarrhythmic drug therapy or when antiarrhythmic drugs are not tolerated or not desired
- Control of incessant SMVT or VT storm that is not due to a transient reversible cause;
- Frequent PVCs, NSVTs, or VT that is presumed to cause ventricular dysfunction;
- Bundle branch reentrant or interfascicular VTs;

- Recurrent sustained polymorphic VT and VF that is refractory to antiarrhythmic therapy where each episode is triggered by PVC that Consistent electrophysiologic properties. Here the target of ablation is the triggering PVCs
- Haemodynamically tolerated SMVT due to prior MI preserved LV ejection fraction (>0.35) even if they have not failed antiarrhythmic drug therapy.
- Idiopathic VT.

VT catheter ablation is contra-indicated
- In the presence of a mobile ventricular thrombus (epicardial ablation may be considered);
- Asymptomatic PVCs and/or NSVT that are not suspected of causing or contributing to ventricular dysfunction;
- VT due to transient, reversible causes, such as acute ischaemia, hyperkalaemia, or drug-induced torsade de pointes.

Electrophysiologic criteria for selecting ablation site[2]
Electrogram recordings
- Activation entrainment and pace mapping are most useful
- Low-amplitude local potentials are easier to recognize with bipolar recordings.
- Rapid intrinsicoid deflection on the unipolar signal coincides with tall peak of the bipolar signal.
- Since ablation energy is delivered only through the tip electrode, it is imperative that the ablation target be located beneath the distal electrode, rather than the proximal electrode. Simultaneous recording of the unipolar electrograms from each electrode can allow this distinction.
- Relatively long-duration electrograms with multiple components are referred to as fractionated. It may represent depolarization and slow conduction of the adjascent myocytes
- Electrograms with a long isoelectric period (arbitrarily defined as >30–50 ms) between two spikes are said to be split potentials. Split potentials may represent block with activation around the site of block or two wavefronts moving in the same or opposite directions at different times.
- Bipolar recordings with 1 to 2 mm interelectrode distance and filtering at 10–400 Hz. should be considered
- Electrical activation sequence mapping during VT can be combined substrate mapping, entrainment mapping, and/or pace mapping.
- For focal VT, the earliest site of activation identifies the tachycardia origin that is targeted for ablation. The QRS provides a convenient fiducial point for mapping. Activation at the origin precedes the QRS onset.
- Unipolar signal (with high-pass filter setting <1 Hz) typically demonstrates a QS configuration consistent with the spread of activation away in all directions from the VT origin.
- In scar-related reentry, activation mapping is limited.
- Term 'site of origin' may be appropriate for focal VT, it is a misnomer in scar-related macroreentry. There is a continuous reentry path with no 'earliest point'.

- QRS onset occurs when the impulse reaches an exit along the border zone of the scar and propagates into the surrounding myocardium. Electrograms immediately preceding the QRS are recorded from the exit region.
- Electrograms recorded proximal to the exit site may appear between the QRS complexes as diastolic electrograms.
- Conduction abnormalities in areas of scar can cause bystander regions to depolarize during electrical diastole mimicking the timing of an isthmus site.
- Electrogram timing at an individual site may not be a reliable indicator that the site is a desirable ablation target, and entrainment methods are helpful for selecting ablation sites.
- Activation sequences combined with entrainment mapping and areas of pre-systolic activity and isolated potentials is used to guide ablation.

Activation time
- Endocardial activation time is defined as the interval from the local earliest fractionated ventricular electrogram, continuous or isolated potential, of the mapping catheter to the onset of the QRS complex. Activation time of >-70 ms suggests proximity of the mapping/ablation catheter to area of slow conduction. Resetting has the following characteristics
  1 Extra stimulus delivered during VT results in less than compensatory pause.
  2 First VT beat (return cycle) after the extrastimulus is morphologically identical to subsequent VT beats.
  3 The return cycle is measured from the extrastimulus to the onset of first VT beat is same as tachycardia cycle length.
- Resetting occurs in more than 85% of stable VT (CL more than 270).
- Scar related VT is due to reentry. Properly timed premature pacing stimulus can enter the reentrant circuit and reset the tachycardia.
- Extrastimulus encounters an excitable gap within VT circuit. It collides, retrogradely, with the previous tachycardia beat and continues antegradely, thus advancing the next tachycardia beat by the duration of its prematurity.
- The ability to demonstrate resetting does not prove re-entry, automatic and triggered activity can also be reset.
- Triggered rhythm show constant return cycle length, 100 to 110% of VT cycle length.
- Resetting with fusion is suggestive of re-entry. This phenomenon is not seen in triggered activity.
- Resetting does not help in identifying the site of successful ablation.

Post-pacing interval
- On termination of the pacing, that entrained the tachycardia, the interval from the last pacing stimulus to first spontaneous depolarization at pacing site is called the post-pacing interval (PPI). If the pacing site is within the reentrant circuit then the PPI will equal the tachycardia cycle length (TCL). Pacing from the bystander sites will result in PPI longer than TCL. PPI should not be the sole criteria for selecting the ablation target.

- For PPI to be identical to TCL one has to speculate that the pacing site is identical to the recording site, and the revolution of last pacing stimulus around the reentrant circuit is identical the to a spontaneous revolution during VT. It may be difficult to precisely determine local activation time in the presence of broad, fractionated electrograms.

Concealed entrainment

- Entrainment utilizes the same physiology as resetting when overdrive pacing is used during tachycardia.
- During entrainment first paced beat interacts with tachycardia circuit however subsequent paced beats interact with previously reset tachycardia circuit.
- Continuous resetting of the circuit by pacing at a rate faster than VT cycle length results in acceleration of the tachycardia to pacing cycle length and resumption of the tachycardia on terminating the pacing fulfills the criteria for entrainment.
- Entrainment without evidence of surface or intracardiac electrogram fusion is called concealed entrainment. This generally occurs when pacing is performed from the isthmus of a tachycardia circuit.
- During concealed entrainment stimulus to QRS interval will be short if the pacing site is close to the exit of the isthmus and longest at the proximal entry site.
- Concealed entrainment suggests that the pacing is being performed from the isthmus of the VT circuit. However the predictive value for identifying the site for successful ablation is approximately 50%.

Stimulus to QRS and electrogram to QRS interval

- At sites with concealed entrainment, less than 30 ms difference between stimulus-QRS and electrogram-QRS intervals identifies the most useful criterion for successful ablation. Identical stimulus-QRS and electrogram–QRS intervals suggest that the catheter is in contact with an area of slow conduction within the reentrant circuit.

Isolated potentials

- Low-frequency fragmented continuous or isolated electrograms are often recorded from the tip of the mapping catheter.
- Isolated potential that can not be dissociated from VT also identifies the area likely to be a successful site for ablation.

Termination of VT without global capture

- Termination of the VT by a pacing stimulus that does not produce QRS suggests that the pacing stimulus was delivered in the re-entrant circuit.
- Ablation at a site where ventricular pacing or extrastimulus results in termination of VT without global capture is likely to yield positive results. This phenomenon indicates that the extrastimulus collided with orthodromically conducting reentrant beat within the VT circuit and terminated the tachycardia.

- Concealed entrainment, stimulus to QRS interval same as electrogram (isolated diastolic potentials) to QRS and PPI same as VT cycle length increases the likelihood of successful VT ablation[4].
- Entrainment mapping is limited to hemodynamically tolerated VTs.
- Majority of post-infarction VTs are not hemodynamically tolerated. Different approaches have been used to map and ablate these VTs, including:
  1 Non-contact mapping
  2 Pace-mapping for identifying the VT exit site
  3 Substrate mapping and identification of channels within scar tissue
  4 VT mapping with hemodynamic support.
  5 Identification of non-excitable tissue.
  6 Targeting of post-infarction premature ventricular complexes (PVCs).

Pace mapping
- Pace mapping is performed from the site of earliest activation by recording 12-lead ECG during pacing. The site where the paced QRS morphology replicates that of the VT is likely to be near the origin for a focal VT or an exit region for scar-related reentry.
- The optimal site should exactly match the tachycardia QRS, including individual notches as well as major deflections.
- Pace mapping can be useful if the targeted arrhythmia is difficult to induce.
- For scar-related VTs, pace mapping at the exit region will match the VT QRS
- large reentry circuits and abnormal conduction may produce similar QRS morphology to VT while pacing from normal areas outside the exit
- Pace mapping can be combined with a voltage map during substrate mapping to define the potential exit.
- When pacing from regions of slow conduction the stimulus to QRS interval may exceeds 40 ms
- Entrainment mapping is useful for identifying reentry circuit sites and recognizing bystander sites in stable VT.
- Entrainment is performed by pacing faster than VT.
- During reentrant VT, a stable QRS morphology with resumption of tachycardia on termination of pacing indicates that each stimulated wavefront has reset the reentry circuit, entraining the tachycardia.
- Entrainment can be confirmed by the presence of constant fusion, progressive fusion, or evidence of conduction block terminating tachycardia.
- Pacing should be performed at a cycle length 10–30 ms shorter than the VT cycle length, and at pacing output that is just above threshold to avoid capture of remote myocardium.
- Post-pacing interval approximates the tachycardia cycle length when pacing in the reentry circuit.
- The post-pacing interval increases with increasing conduction time between the pacing site and circuit.
- If pacing slows conduction in the circuit, the post-pacing interval may prolong.

- If QRS complex during entrainment is the same as that during VT, called concealed entrainment, entrainment with concealed fusion, or exact entrainment, pacing site is likely to be in an isthmus.
- At these isthmus sites, the S-QRS interval, which indicates the conduction time from the pacing site to the exit, is the same as the electrogram to QRS interval.
- At bystander sites that are adjacent to the reentry circuit isthmus, entrainment may occur without QRS fusion, but the post-pacing interval (PPI) will exceed the VT cycle length and the S-QRS will exceed the electrogram to QRS interval.
- Sites with long S-QRS (>70% of the VT cycle length) with concealed fusion and a PPI=TCL indicating that the site is in the circuit may be proximal to the isthmus region (inner loops), with a lower likelihood of VT termination by RF ablation.
- Sites that are in an outer loop of the reentry circuit along the border of the scar may demonstrates post-pacing interval that approximates the VT cycle length, but with QRS fusion during entrainment.
- Some outer loop sites may be misidentified as exit sites or inner loop

Substrate-based approaches for selecting target sites for VT ablation[4]

- This approach reduces or eliminates the need for mapping during prolonged periods of hemodynamically unstable VT.
- Myocardial scar is identified by:
  1 Low-voltage regions on ventricular voltage maps,
  2 Areas with fractionated electrograms,
  3 Unexcitability during pace mapping,
  4 Evidence of scar on myocardial imaging,
  5 Area of known surgical incision.

Identification of scar

- Scar tissue can be identified by bipolar electrogram amplitude. Using a 4 mm tip electrode filtered at 10–400 Hz, normal LV endocardial electrograms have a peak-to-peak amplitude > 1.53–1.55 mV.
- Areas of low voltage (<0.5 mV or even less) are designated as 'dense scar', these regions can still contain viable myocytes and reentry circuit isthmuses.
- Signal amplitude between 0.5 and 1.5 mV is designated as intermediate low voltage found near the border zone of the scar.
- Radiofrequency lesions are generally confined within the low-voltage region to reduce the damage to functioning myocardium.
- Areas of electrically unexcitable scar can be defined and marked based on a high pacing threshold (> 10 mA at 2 ms during unipolar pacing.
- Causes of scar related VT
  1 Prior MI,
  2 Arrhythmogenic right ventricular cardiomyopathy (ARVC),
  3 Sarcoidosis,

4 Chagas' disease,

5 Dilated cardiomyopathy,

6 After cardiac surgery for congenital heart disease (particularly Tetralogy of Fallot) or valve replacement.

- The substrate supporting scar-related reentry is characterized by
  ○ Region of slow conduction,
  ○ Unidirectional conduction block
- Reentry occurs through surviving muscle bundles, commonly located in the subendocardium, but that can also occur in the mid-myocardium and epicardium
- Surviving muscle bundles commonly located in the subendocardium but also in the midmyocardium and epicardium, traverse the borders and penetrate the scar.
- Substrate mapping is is an attempt to identify areas likely to support reentry based on anatomy and electrophysiological characteristics during stable sinus or paced rhythm. This approach can facilitate ablation of multiple VTs, pleomorphic VTs, and VTs that are unmappable due to haemodynamic instability or that are not reliably inducible.
- In haemodynamically stable VTs, substrate mapping can be combined with activation sequence or entrainment mapping directed to a region of interest.
- Substrate mapping relies on identification of the scar, based on electrogram voltage in an electroanatomic map.
- Markers for reentry circuit exits, channels (isthmuses), and regions of slow conduction, identified based on pace mapping and electrogram properties, are then targeted for ablation.
- More extensive ablation over a relatively large area within the scar may be required.
- Cardiac fibrosis in the ventricles produces separation of ventricular myocyte bundles diminishind coupling and slow conduction.
- This promotes development of conduction block, and facilitates reentry in regions of ventricular scar resulting from infarction or cardiomyopathy.
- Fibrosis that separates conducting myocyte bundles also results in fractionated electrograms, potential targets for catheter ablation.
- Areas of ventricular fibrosis can be identified from the presence of low-amplitude bipolar electrograms, allowing the use of electroanatomic "voltage maps" to identify regions likely to contain ventricular reentrant circuits.
- In the left ventricle, the average bipolar electrogram amplitude is 4.8 mV (recorded with a bipolar interelectrode spacing of 2 mm and filtered at 10–400 Hz).9 A 60% reduction in electrogram amplitude to <1.55 mV accurately identifies regions of infarct scar.
- Large amounts of collagen and connective tissue may be present between the muscle bundles. These properties, rather than altered action potential characteristics, contribute to the formation of relatively insulated slow conduction channels through the scar.
- Scar detection has been defined as bipolar voltages <1.5 mV, with lower voltages (variously defined as 0.1–0.5 mV) indicative of more dense scar.

- The location of surviving muscle bundles within the scar can be identified by the detection of delayed low-voltage diastolic potentials, which occur after completion of the surface QRS.
- Most vulnerable component of the circuit appears to be the slow conduction channel insulated either anatomically (by fibrosis) or functionally (due to heterogeneous refractoriness, or direction-dependent and rate-dependent differences in conduction).
- Longer stimulus-to-QRS and electrogram-to-QRS intervals suggest a more proximal location in the slow conduction channel, whereas shorter times suggest a location near the exit to normal myocardium, coincident with onset of the surface QRS.
- Finding of late diastolic potentials, or SR pace-maps with exact reproduction of the VT morphology and long stimulus-to-QRS intervals, may enhance the probability that a slow conduction channel has been identified.
- SR pace-mapping is used to define the exit sites for all induced VTs, both stable and unstable.
- Linear lesions (3–4 cm) are placed parallel to the scar border centered on the exit site defined by pace-map matches. These lesions are placed 1 to 2 cm inside the 1.5-mV isopotential line.
- This approach may be effective in eliminating both stable and unstable VT in patients with advanced ischemic cardiomyopathy and frequent multidrug-resistant VT.
- Postinfarction PVCs usually arise from the infarct scar, and their site of origin often corresponds to the exit site of a reentrant VT. Therefore, catheter ablation of the PVCs may render VT noninducible.
- These bundles are characterized by decreased gap junction density, as well as alterations in distribution, composition, and function.

Electro-anatomical mapping[4]:
- Electroanatomic mapping (EAM) refers to point by point contact mapping combined with the ability to display the location of each mapping point in three-dimensional space.
- This records intracardiac electrical activation in relation to anatomical location in a cardiac chamber of interest.
- Electroanatomic mapping systems integrate three main functions:
  1 Non-fluoroscopic localization of the ablation catheter within the heart;
  2 Display of electrogram characteristics, most commonly activation time or voltage, in relation to anatomic position; and
  3 Integration of electroanatomic information with three-dimensional images of the heart obtained from point by point sampling, intracardiac ultrasound, computed tomography (CT), or magnetic resonance imaging (MRI).
- One system utilizes low-level electromagnetic fields emanating from three separate coils beneath the patient that are measured from a location sensor embedded in the tip of the mapping catheter.

- This allows a three-dimensional reconstruction of the chamber of interest and colour-coded display of various electrophysiological parameters for endocardial or epicardial mapping
- An alternative technology determines electrode position based on the measurement of a high-frequency current emitted by three pairs of orthogonally placed skin patches.
- Intracardiac echocardiography (ICE) has been incorporated into EAM. The ICE probe, equipped with a location sensor and tracked by the mapping system, allows reconstruction of a three-dimensional shell of the chambers of interest before mapping and may help define irregular anatomic features, such as papillary muscles.

Limitations of mapping systems
- Cardiac and respiratory motion reduce anatomic accuracy.
- Patient movement relative to the location signal or reference sources invalidates the anatomic maps
- Data are acquired point by point, such that a stable tachycardia or haemodynamic support is required for the definition of a complete activation sequence.
- Point by point mapping requires skills with catheter manipulation.
- Catheter induced mechanical trauma can terminate VT or induce ectopic beats.
- A non-contact mapping system consists of a catheter with MEA 64 (Microelectrode array) unipolar electrodes over an inflatable balloon.
- The potential for clots to form on the splines necessitates careful attention to anticoagulation during the procedure.
- Because accuracy decreases as the distance between the MEA and endocardium increases, it should be used with caution in large ventricles

RF ablation for ventricular tachycardia Table 7.1
- Permanent tissue injury occurs at temperatures exceeding 49°C.
- The RF electrode heats as a consequence of its contact with the tissue.
- Heating is limited by coagulation of proteins on the electrode that occurs at electrode temperatures exceeding 70°C.
- Power of 30–50 W is typically applied in the temperature control mode and titrated to an electrode temperature of 55–70°C or an impedance fall of 10–15 ohm.
- Careful attention to temperature, impedance, and power is important.
- Brisk heating at low power (e.g., <15 W) may indicate the location of the electrode in a low flow area and limited lesion creation, despite electrode heating.
- A brisk fall in impedance of >18 ohm may indicate substantial tissue heating and may warrant a reduction in power to avoid steam pops even though measured temperature is <60°C.
- Irrigation of the ablation electrode allows the delivery of more power before temperature increases to the point of coagulum formation, increasing the size of RF lesions.
- Two different types of electrode irrigation are available.

Table 7.1 Ventricular tachycardia likely to be considered for RF ablation.

Site of origin of VT	QRS Morphology
RVOT VT	LBBB Inferior axis
LV idiopathic VT	RBBB superior left or right axis
Bundle Branch reentry VT	LBBB occasionally RB
Scar related VT:	LBBB
RV dysplasia	LBBB
Fallot tetralogy	
Prior MI	
Sarcoidosis	
Chagas disease	

- An internal irrigation catheter circulates 5% dextrose solution at room temperature in a closed loop through the tip electrode.
- Open irrigation catheters infuse saline that emerges through pores in the ablation electrode, cooling the electrode and providing cooling of the tissue–electrode interface.
- There is low risk of coagulum formation with open irrigation.
- External irrigation result in intravascular saline administration which may aggravate congestive heart failure.
- Electrode irrigation increases the disparity between tissue temperatures and temperatures recorded from within the electrode. If tissue temperatures exceed 100°C, an explosion of steam within the tissue can occur with an audible 'pop'. These pops can cause perforation.
- A 3.5 mm electrode with external irrigation at 10–25 mL/min for power up to 30 W and 30 mL/min for power of >30 W is commonly used.
- For endocardial ablation, starting power of 30–35 W and increasing it to achieve an impedance fall of 10–15 ohm while maintaining electrode temperature <40–45°C is reasonable.
- Patients with structural heart disease undergoing left heart catheterization have a risk of stroke or thromboembolism of ~1%.

Anticoagulation during ablation
- Anticoagulation during the procedure may be considered, particularly for long procedures, when multiple venous catheters or when extensive ablation is required.
- Anticoagulation is warranted for patients with a history of prior venous thromboemboli, and/or who have known risk factors for thrombosis (e.g., Factor V Leiden) or have right to left intracardiac shunts that pose a risk of paradoxical embolism. Following the procedure, long-term anticoagulation is not required.

- During the procedure, systemic anticoagulation with intravenous heparin is recommended as for patients with structural heart disease. Ventricular tachycardia in these patients is usually ablated with a small number of focal lesions. After ablation, anticoagulation is not required.
- Imaging to assess the presence of a left ventricular thrombus is warranted prior to endocardial left ventricle mapping in patients with structural heart disease.
- A mobile left ventricular thrombus is a contraindication to left ventricle endocardial mapping and ablation. Evidence of laminated thrombus is not a contraindication to ablation.
- Anticoagulate with warfarin for 4–6 weeks prior to elective ablation may be considered when laminated thrombus is present.
- Some electrode arrays that may be thrombogenic require an ACT >300 s. Anticoagulation is not needed for epicardial mapping and ablation.
- During initial follow-up, anticoagulation is recommended with aspirin (75–325 mg daily) or warfarin for 6–12 weeks.

Anesthesia during ablation
- General anesthesia is usually required for ablation procedures in children. Adults are at risk for airway obstruction, other respiratory compromise and haemodynamic instability, or in high-risk patients with other major co-morbidities.
- A major disadvantage of general anesthesia is the potential for suppressing VT inducibility. Isofurane does not interfere with inducibility of supraventricular re-entrant arrhythmias.
- Halothane propofol may decrease and inducibility of VT.
- General anesthesia may cause vasodilation and impair reflex responses to hypotension during induced VT, although this can often be countered with volume administration and vasopressors.
- When ablating in the proximity of the phrenic nerve paralytic agents should be avoided as these may prevent identification of the phrenic nerve by high output pacing.
- Antiarrhythmic drugs (including beta-blockers) should be discontinued for 4–5 half-lives before the procedure.
- After ablation of idiopathic VT, most patients can be discharged without antiarrhythmic drugs, although it may be prudent to gradually taper beta-blockers.
- Following successful catheter ablation, amiodarone may be discontinued.
- Cardiac tamponade is reported in ~1% of procedures.
- No detrimental effect of ablation on LV function has been demonstrated.

Imaging prior to or during ablation
- When scar-related VT is suspected, imaging can be used to characterize the location/extent of the myocardial scar that is likely to contain the VT substrate.
- Magnetic resonance imaging using delayed Gd enhancement pulse sequences can be used to identify scar with good spatial resolution.

- Magnetic resonance imaging is limited in the VT population because many patients have implanted permanent pacemakers or defibrillators.
- imaging with a 1.5 T magnet in patients with pacemakers or defibrillators (after changing the pacing mode to either 'demand' only or 'asynchronous' for pacemaker-dependent patients, and disabling magnet response and tachy-arrhythmia functions) has been demonstrated.
- Intracardiac echocardiography is used to define three-dimensional ventricular chamber geometries and to observe contact between the catheter tip and underlying tissue that can be helpful during ablation on irregular structures such as papillary muscles.
- Intracardiac echocardiography has been used to visualize the proximity of the ablation catheter tip to an adjacent coronary artery when ablating in the left ventricular outflow tract (LVOT) or aortic valve cusps,
- Coronary angiography can be used to visualize the proximity of coronary arteries to ablation catheter.
- Post-procedural imaging is indicated when there is haemodynamic deterioration or instability.
- Transthoracic echocardiography is performed to assess the presence of pericardial effusion and tamponade, valve injury, or deterioration of ventricular function.

Assessment of coronary artery and peripheral vascular disease
- Evaluation for the presence of obstructive coronary artery disease prior to VT ablation, for scar-related VTs should be considered by coronary angiogram or exercise or pharmacological stress evaluation because
- Previous myocardial infarction is the commonest cause of scar related VT.
- Prolonged episode of VT required to allow activation and entrainment mapping during which there is a potential risk of hypotension and myocardial ischemia.
- Revascularization improves outcome. Recurrent SMVT is rarely due to acute myocardial ischaemia.
- Types and burden of sustained and nonsustained VT should be identified and quantified prior to performing catheter ablation. This information can be used to focus on the exit region suggested by the VT morphology.
- Assessment for peripheral vascular disease should be considered to anticipate any problem with vascular access or postprocedural vascular complications, if present transseptal approach to the left heart may be considered.

Transcoronary ethanol ablation
- Transcoronary ethanol ablation may be considered when both endocardial and epicardial ablation fail to control severely symptomatic, drug refractory VT.
- Alcohol ablation has several limitations. There is significant potential for extensive myocardial damage and complications including heart block, worsening heart failure, ventricular rupture, and death. A satisfactory target vessel cannot always be identified or cannulated.

Endpoints for ablation

- There are three endpoints for VT ablation:
  1 Non-inducibility of clinical VT
  2 Modification of induced VT cycle length (elimination of all VTs with cycle lengths equal to or longer than spontaneously documented or targeted VT)
  3 Non-inducibility of any VT (excluding ventricular flutter and fibrillation).
- Clinical VT is induced VTs with same 12-lead ECG QRS morphology and approximate cycle length as a spontaneous VT.
- Other VTs should be designated as presumptive clinical or as previously undocumented VT morphology
- Non-inducibility of clinical VT immediately post-procedure is associated with a lower risk of VT recurrence
- During follow-up, clinical success was defined as >75% reduction in VT episodes.
- In patients with recurrent episodes of PMVT or VF, ablation of a limited number of uniform premature ventricular complex (PVC) morphologies that were documented to trigger spontaneous episodes has been associated with a substantial reduction in recurrences during long-term follow-up.

Depressed ventricular function associated with frequent ventricular ectopy

- Frequent PVCs more than 20% of sinus beats in a 24-hour Holter monitor can result in a reversible form of cardiomyopathy
- The critical number of PVCs and the time course required to cause a cardiomyopathy are not known.
- Triggered activity and automaticity are probably the mechanisms of focal PVCs.
- Premature ventricular complexes in the setting of prior MI may originate from scar areas and may have similar QRS morphology as post-infarction VT, suggesting that reentry maybe the mechanism.
- Ablation is guided by activation mapping. Pace mapping can be used if PVCs are not frequent, but is less accurate.
- Site of origin of PVCs may include RVOT, LV, coronary cusps, and the pulmonary artery.
- Success is greater when only RVOT PVCs are present.
- Ventricular function improves following ablation.
- Antiarrhythmics could be used for a short duration to demonstrate if suppression of PVCs improves left ventricular function.
- Multiple morphologies of PVCs could reduce procedural success.
- Mechanism by which PVCs cause cardiomyopathy is not known. Possibilities include
- PVCs can cause relative bradycardia as the aortic valve may not open, leading to ineffective myocardial perfusion.
- Chronic ischemia due to increased demand and lack of supply may occur.
- Like right ventricular pacing, PVCs can alter activation, but the extent of dyssynchronous ventricular activation may be site dependent.

VT ablation in patients with implanted defibrillators

- When the indication for ablation is recurrent ICD shocks or antitachycardia pacing therapies, a 12-lead electrocardiogram of the VT may not be available.
- In such cases, stored intracardiac electrograms provide a measurement of the VT cycle length.
- RF ablation may affect myocardial VT substrate and the pacing and sensing functions of an ICD.
- Because programmed electrical stimulation and RF current are sensed by ICDs, these devices must be reprogrammed prior to the ablation procedure to prevent oversensing and unintended delivery of antitachycardia therapies.
- Tachycardia detection zones must be programmed 'off'.
- The ICD can still be used to deliver commanded shocks to terminate VT that is not interrupted by overdrive pacing.
- For patients who are pacemaker-dependent, the noise reversion response of the ICD should be programmed to an asynchronous mode before RF current is applied.
- For patients who are not pacemaker-dependent, the ICD is usually programmed to asynchronous noise reversion mode at a low pacing rate.
- Stimulation thresholds and intracardiac electrogram amplitudes should be measured before and after ablation to ensure appropriate pacing and sensing by the ICD.
- Following ablation tachycardia detection must be reprogrammed 'on'.
- Even when all VTs have been rendered non-inducible by ablation, the recurrence rate remains substantial so that secondary prophylaxis remains indicated

7.2 Electrocardiographic features of Epicardial VT

- Pseudo-delta wave ≥ 34 ms
- Precordial maximum deflection index ≥ 0.55
- Epicardial VTs from basal inferior LV are characterized by Q waves in lead II, III, or aVF.
- VTs arising from healed posteroseptal inferior myocardial infarction, have a left superior axis with a positive concordance from leads V2 to V6, with variable QRS wave patterns in lead V1.
- ECG morphology of this VT may be similar to maximally preexcited posteroseptal accessory pathways.
- ECG morphology can differentiate VT arising from the crux (left superior axis) from outflow tract VT (inferior axis).
- ECG features that predict an epicardial origin for LV-VTs include:
  1 Time to earliest rapid deflection in precordial leads (pseudodelta wave) ≥ 34 ms,
  2 Interval to peak of R wave in lead V2 (intrinsicoid deflection time) ≥ 85 ms,
  3 Time to earliest QRS nadir in precordial leads (shortest RS complex) ≥ 121 ms.
- Following characteristics may help differentiate epicardial VT from the crux from other VTs with similar morphology arising from the endocardium.

1 Deeply negative delta like waves in the inferior leads,
2 Prominent R wave in lead V2,
3 Maximum deflection index ≥ 0.55

Ablation Epicardial approach[6]

- Ablation from the epicardium may be required in non-ischaemic cardiomyopathy.
- Attempted epicardial access fails in ~10% of patients.
- Epicardial fat can limit lesion creation.
- Open or closed loop irrigation allows the delivery of energy at power settings (25–50 W). capable of creating deep lesions (up to 5 mm) that can be effective even in the presence of adipose tissue.
- Some degree of pericardial bleeding is recognized in ~30% of cases.
- Mild or modest bleeding usually resolves and can be carefully monitored with repeated aspiration of the pericardial space, as the procedure continues.
- Severe bleeding requiring surgical intervention can potentially occur.
- Radiofrequency injury to coronary arteries can cause acute thrombosis Based on available data and experience, a distance of > 5 mm between the ablation catheter and an epicardial artery is commonly accepted.
- The left phrenic nerve is potentially susceptible to injury along its course adjacent to the lateral left ventricle wall. Proximity to the nerve can be detected by pacing (typically at 10 Ma or greater stimulus strength) to detect diaphragmatic stimulation, allowing its course to be marked on a three-dimensional map.
- Detection by pacing is prevented by the use of paralytic agents during general anaesthesia. Catheter ablation should be avoided at sites adjacent to the phrenic nerve. Air in the pericardial space can increase the defibrillation threshold, requiring emergent evacuation if defibrillation is required.
- Symptoms of pericarditis are common after the procedure, occurring in ~30% of cases. Symptoms usually resolve within a few days with anti-inflammatory medications.
- In patients with coronary artery disease, epicardial ablation appears to be more frequently required for inferior wall infarct VTs than for those from anterior wall infarcts.
- Epicardial reentry circuits are frequent in Chagas' disease.

7.3 Ventricular arrhythmias in hypertrophic and dilated cardiomyopathy

Heart failure and hypertrophy

- Mortality is 40% in four years. Half of it is due to sudden death.
- Fibrosis, apoptosis, hypertrophy, dispersion of refractoriness, neuroendocrine activation, electrolytes abnormalities and drugs are the common factors that may precipitate arrhythmias.
- In left ventricular hypertrophy (LVH) action potential prolongation is due to decrease in I_{to}. This results in non-homogeneous repolarization and propensity for early after-depolarizations (EAD).

- Hypertrophied myocytes may produce delayed after-depolarizations (DAD) due to increase in Ca load.
- Abnormal pacemaker current (I_f) has been reported in LVH. Intensity of I_f current increases with β̃adrenergic stimulation.
- In LVH the density of I_{to} is reduced. The density of I_{CaL} and I_K is unchanged and density of I_f is increased.
- Hemodynamic overload may re-express fetal channel proteins such as T type calcium channel.
- I_{K1} (inward rectifier) is reduced by 40% in the failing heart. I_{K1} contributes to final phase of repolarization and sets resting membrane potential. Its reduction results in prolongation of the terminal phase of repolarization.

Stretch-activated ion channels (SAC)
- Stretch may activate chloride channel and I_{Ks}.
- Stretch decreases resting potential and induces premature depolarization by activating inward depolarizing sodium current.
- Sustain increase in preload causes shortening of action potential duration (APD) and refractoriness.
- SAC can be blocked by gadolinium, streptomycin, and spider venom peptides.
- Unlike intraventricular pressure which is equally distributed throughout the left ventricle, wall stress may differ according to regional differences in circumference, wall thickness and compliance. This could explain heterogeneous shortening of APD.
- Shortening of refractoriness and presence of slow conduction favors VF.
- Dilatation of the heart, which shortens refractoriness and hypokalemia, which decreases conduction velocity, when combined can cause serious arrhythmias.
- Ventricular dilatation causes shortening of refractoriness at rapid heart rate and not at slow heart rates. Shortening of refractoriness may predispose to arrhythmia.
- Beneficial effects of the beta blockers in CHF may be due to slowing of the heart rate and restoring the refractoriness.
- I_{Ks} is increased by mechanical stretch. This may cause abbreviation of APD in a rate dependent manner and decrease refractoriness.
- Dilatation may result in increase defibrillation threshold.
- Renin–angiotensin system (RAS), where the angiotensin-converting enzyme (ACE) plays a central role, are the kallikrein–kininogen and angiotensin-converting enzyme 2 (ACE2) pathways.
- Higher renin levels are associated with increased risk of cardiovascular disease mortality. Blocking these pathways with ACE inhibitors, angiotensin receptor blockers, or aldosterone inhibitors decreases risk of SCA.

Tachycardia-induced myocardial changes
- Changes in effective refractory period (ERP) and calcium loading occurs earlier then autonomic changes, which may take several weeks.
- Tachycardia-induced low intracellular magnesium in ventricular myocytes may contribute to abnormal repolarization in congestive heart failure.
- Tachycardia also reduces repolarizing potassium currents.

- Heterogeneity of sympathetic stimulation of the myocardium due to reduction of β-receptors may result in arrhythmias.
- Short-term tachycardia results in activation of $I_{K,ATP}$ channel, which may contribute to shortening of APD after tachycardia.
- Rapid pacing decreases I_{to}.
- Prolonged increase or decrease in cytosolic calcium increases or decreases sodium current respectively.

Ventricular arrhythmias in patients with heart failure

- Incidence of CHF increases with the patient's age. Mortality approaches 50% in patients with class IV CHF. With increasing severity of heart failure the mechanism of death shifts from tachyarrhythmias to bradyarrhythmias.
- Mechanisms that increase the vulnerability of failing heart to ventricular arrhythmias include:
  - Ischemia produces shortening of action potential and slowing conduction in ischemic zone and predisposes to reentry.
  - Left ventricular hypertrophy results in increase of APD.
  - Changes in Ion channels and currents may occur.
  - In CHF increase in APD is due to reduced I_{to} and I_K. I_f current is increased resulting in increased automaticity.
  - The activity of Na/K ATPases is decreased, thus increasing the susceptibility to digoxin induced arrhythmias.
  - In CHF there is alteration in gap junction and decrease in density of connexi-43, which results in slowing of conduction.
  - Increased sympathetic activation promotes automatic and reentrant arrhythmias.
  - Elevated norepinephrine levels correlate with poor prognosis.
  - Electrolyte abnormalities such as hypokalemia and hypomagnesemia may induce DAD.
- The piperazine derivative ranolazine, used for the treatment of chronic angina, is an anti-ischemic agent that has been shown to selectively inhibit the late sodium current ($I_{Na,late}$) in cardiac myocytes.
- In the failing heart, the late sodium current ($I_{Na,late}$) is increased leading to an Na$^+$ accumulation in cardiac myocytes
- Increased Na$^+$ concentration reverses the mode direction of the Na$^+$/Ca^{2+}-exchanger, contributing to a Ca^{2+} overload in the cell.
- Increased diastolic Ca^{2+} impairs relaxation leading to diastolic dysfunction. By inhibiting the $I_{Na,late}$, ranolazine is expected to prevent (or reduce) sodium accumulation in the myocyte. This should improve calcium extrusion through the Na$^+$/Ca^{2+}-exchanger and thereby improve relaxation of the myocardium and decrease diastolic dysfunction.

Ventricular arrhythmias in hypertrophic cardiomyopathy (HCM)[7–10]

- Hypertrophic cardiomyopathy is caused by gene mutation of either β myosin heavy chain or α tropomyosin or cardiac troponin T and I or cardiac myosin binding protein C or regulatory myosin light chain (Table 7.2).

Table 7.2 Chromosome location of the genes for cardiac proteins.

Chromosomes	Encoding proteins
1q32	Troponin T
19p13	Troponin I
15q22	α-tropomyosin
11p11	Myosin-binding protein C
3p21 and 12q23–p21	Myosin light chains
15q14	Actin

- Thirty-five to 50% of HCM patients have a mutation in the cardiac major histocompatibility complex gene, 15 to 25% due to mutations of myosin-binding protein C, 15 to 20% due to mutations of the cardiac troponin T gene, less than 5% due to mutations of the tropomyosin gene.
- Unexplained abnormalities of the electrocardiogram in first-degree relatives of patients with HCM may be suggestive of a carrier or preclinical state.
- Mutations of the troponin T gene results in mild to moderate hypertrophy, however it is associated with poor prognosis and a high risk of sudden death.
- These mutations express in autosomal dominant fashion. Penetrance and expression may be variable and age related.
- Mutations result in abnormal force generation that causes hypertrophic response.
- Prevalence of HCM is low, about 0.2% in the general population.
- Hypertrophy usually occurs during adolescence and period of rapid somatic growth. It has been noted to occur in elderly.
- Myocardial hypertrophy is out of proportion to the hemodynamic load.
- Occurrence of sustain VT is uncommon however non-sustained VT is frequent.
- The cardinal histologic feature of HCM is myofibrillar disarray occupying 20% or more of at least one pathologic tissue block.
- The annual mortality rates from HCM are approximately 6% in patients diagnosed while children and approximately 3% in patients diagnosed as adults

Classification of the HCM based on imaging
1 Asymmetric septal hypertrophy (ASH): predominantly affects the septum.
2 Apical hypertrophy: Affects the apex of the left ventricle (Japanese type). It demonstrates narrow apex during angiographic study, giant negative T waves in the precordial ECG leads, there is no intraventricular pressure gradient, symptoms are mild. It has benign course with low mortality. Atrial fibrillation may occur.
3 Idiopathic subaortic stenosis (IHSS): septal hypertrophy resulting in obstruction.
4 Hypertrophy and obstruction localized to mid segment of the left ventricle.
- Although the diagnosis of HCM is made on the basis of echocardiographic findings, a single normal echocardiogram does not exclude HCM in a child or adolescent.

Cardiac hypertrophy suggestive of HCM may be seen in

1 Amyloid, glycogen storage disease, or tumor involvement of the septum.
2 Friedreich ataxia.
3 Generalized lipodystrophy.
4 Hyperparathyroidism.
5 Infants of diabetic mothers.
6 Lentiginosis.
7 Neurofibromatosis.
8 Noonan syndrome.
9 Pheochromocytoma.

Risk factors for sustained ventricular arrhythmia and sudden death (Box 7.1)

- The incidence of sudden death in patients with HCM is approximately 2 to 4%.
- Nonsustained VT is associated with increased risk of sudden cardiac death. Presence of nonsustained VT has low positive predictive value and high negative predictive value. Absence of nonsustain ventricular tachycardia indicates relatively good prognosis. Presence of nonsustained VT indicates possible high risk group that may require further risk stratification.
- Family history of sudden cardiac death, nonsustained VT, marked hypertrophy, marked left atrial dilation, and abnormal blood pressure response to exercise, identifies a high-risk group.
- The commonest cause of SCD in HCM is VT.
- The mechanism of ventricular arrhythmia may be reentry due to (1) disarray of hypertrophied myocytes and fibrosis, (2) ischemia.
- The major causes of ischemia are as follows:
  1 Impaired vasodilator reserve due to thickness and narrowing of the intramural coronary arteries.
  2 Increased oxygen demand due to hypertrophy and outflow obstruction.
  3 Elevated filling pressures with resultant subendocardial ischemia.
- A higher incidence of accessory pathways has been reported.
- Adolescence is a vulnerable period for sudden death especially in male.

Box 7.1 Risk factors for SCD in HCM

- Syncope
- Age < 30 years
- History of sustain ventricular arrhythmias
- Family history of SCD
- Abnormal blood pressure response to exercise
- LV wall thickness > 30 mm
- Gene Mutation coding for troponin and tropomyosin
- Nonsustained VT

- 25% of HCM have abnormal blood pressure response during exercise. This may be due to inappropriate vasodilatation during exercise. These patients tend to have small left ventricle cavities. Left ventricle cavity C fiber or baroreceptor stimulation may contribute to inappropriate vasodilatation. Abnormal blood pressure response is associated with increase risk of sudden death.
- 40% of SCD occur during or immediately after exercise.
- Patients with left ventricle wall thickness of more than 30 mm are at increased risk of SCD.
- Family history of SCD is an important risk factor. This may be due to more malignant mutation in certain families.
- Exertion-related syncope is ominous symptom in young patients with HCM.
- The presence of non-sustained VT may increase the risk of sudden death but the positive predictive value is low.
- A short PR interval is commonly seen in patients with HCM may reflect enhanced AV node conduction. This may facilitate rapid conduction during atrial arrhythmia.
- Conduction system disease and AV block may occur in HCM.
- QT dispersion, signal average ECG, heart rate variability and programmed stimulation are not helpful in risk stratification because of low positive predictive value.
- History of sudden cardiac death and sustained VT are important risk factors.
- Low risk patients are characterized by lack of symptoms, absence of family history of SCD, normal blood pressure response to exercise and no ventricular arrhythmias.
- Electrophysiologic study with programmed stimulation, as a means of identifying high risk patients has low yield.
- Prognosis correlates with the degree of hypertrophy, in patients with sever hypertrophy (>30 mm) there is 2% per year risk of sudden death.
- Three age peaks of presentation have been proposed: adolescence, the early 40s, and the early 60s.
- The clinical presentation of HCM (syncope, sudden cardiac death, severe effort-related chest discomfort, or dyspnea) tends to be more common when HCM presents in adolescence.
- HCM is inherited in an autosomal-dominant pattern in 50 to 75% of cases. Its prevalence is thought to be 1 per 500 in the general US population and higher in African American individuals.
- In HCM, long-term survival up to 30 years may follow after successful resuscitation from cardiac arrest.
- Arrhythmogenic events do not portend other adverse clinical outcomes such as occurrence of heart failure or need for surgical myectomy, or septal ablation.
- Abnormal blood pressure response to exercise may occur in up to a third of HCM cases and is associated with an increased risk of death, particularly in the young. It has 15% positive predictive value for SCD in HCM.
- Blood pressure response to exercise differs among carriers of the R92W mutation in the cardiac troponin T gene (*TNNT2*), which has been associated

with an increased risk of sudden cardiac death in young males; and carriers of mutations in the cardiac β-myosin heavy chain gene (*MYH7*); and their noncarrier relatives.

- Blood pressure response to exercise is influenced by genotype and gender in patients with HCM.
- Common mutations in HCM are the genes encoding beta cardiac myosin heavy chain (*MYH7*), cardiac troponin T (*TNNT2*), and myosin binding protein C.
- Phenotypes resulting from these genetic defects vary greatly, mutations in TNNT2 have frequently resulted in an increased susceptibility to SCD, often in the presence of mild or absent cardiac hypertrophy.
- Failure of blood pressure to increase appropriately in response to exercise has been recorded in 8%–33% of ungenotyped patients with HCM.
- Abnormal blood pressure responses were defined as either:
  ○ An initial increase in SBP with a subsequent fall of >20 mmHg compared with the blood pressure value at peak exercise or a continuous decrease in SBP throughout the exercise test of >20 mmHg compared with resting blood pressure (termed hypotensive responses); or
  ○ An increase of <20 mmHg in SBP from resting state to peak exercise (termed a flat response).
1 Markedly abnormal ECGs in young athletes may represent the initial expression of underlying cardiomyopathies that may not manifest until many years later and be associated with adverse outcomes. Athletes with such ECG patterns merit continued clinical surveillance.
2 Presence or absence of LV outflow tract obstruction may not be associated with prognosis.

Atrial arrhythmias in HCM
- SVT and AF may occur in up to 30% of the patients and may be due to left atrial enlargement.
- Left atrial enlargement may be due to LV diastolic dysfunction, mitral regurgitation or atrial muscle fibrosis.
- Patients with persistent or paroxysmal atrial fibrillation should be anticoagulated.
- Amiodarone or Sotalol can be used to maintain sinus rhythm. If that fails Ca channel blockers or beta-blockers can achieve rate control.

Treatment[11-13]
- Strenuous physical activity should be prohibited in all patients with HCM even in the absence of symptoms.
- Unsuspected HCM is the most common finding at autopsy in young competitive athletes who die suddenly.
- Cardiovascular screening before participation in competitive sports may identify asymptomatic patients with silent HCM and may prevent unexpected sudden death.
- Digitalis should be avoided.
- The majority of patients with HCM require only medical management.

- Beta-blockers exert negative chronotropic response and decrease myocardial oxygen consumption thus alleviate ischemia.
- Verapamil by depressing myocardial contractility may decrease left ventricle outflow gradient and improve diastolic filling.
- Disopyramide, an antiarrhythmic drug that alters calcium kinetics reduces contractility, may produce symptomatic improvement by reducing pressure gradient.
- Prophylactic use of amiodarone in high-risk patients may decrease the occurrence of SCD.
- Amiodarone is effective in the treatment of both supraventricular and ventricular tachyarrhythmias.
- Insertion of a dual-chamber DDD pacemaker may be useful in some patients especially elderly with an outflow gradient and severe symptoms.
- Pacing for the treatment of medically refractory HCM is currently a class IIb indication by the ACC/AHA guidelines.
- When pacing is applied in the patient with HCM, AVI has to be short enough to result in ventricular depolarization by the paced event. However, the shortest AVI may not provide optimum hemodynamics. AV node ablation has been recommended to ensure paced ventricular depolarization.
- It may help 10% of HCM patients. Symptoms are improved and the gradient may be reduced by 20 to 25%.
- Surgical or chemical septal ablation could be considered in symptomatic patients with significant gradient.
- Complications of the percutaneous technique include, (1) development of RBBB, (2) complete heart block.
- ICD is the treatment of choice in high-risk patients[12,13].
- Five percent of the patients in high risk group, who receive ICD for primary prevention of SCD, may experience appropriate discharge per year.
- Time to first appropriate shock, after the initial ICD implant may be quite variable and may extend to 10 years.
- Likelihood of appropriate discharge was similar in patients with 1, 2, or 3 or more risk markers.
- A single marker of high risk for sudden death may be sufficient to justify consideration for prophylactic defibrillator implantation in selected patients with HCM.

Dilated cardiomyopathy[14]

- Ventricular arrhythmias are common in dilated cardiomyopathy (DCM) irrespective of etiology.
- The causes of dilated cardiomyopathy include CAD, valvular or hypertensive heart disease, pregnancy, infections or alcohol.
- Thirty-five percent of patients with DCM may have autosomal dominant familial disease.
- X-linked form of inheritance is seen in infants and children. It may be due to mutation in the Lamin A/C gene. It is associated with conduction defects, variable skeletal muscle involvement, and reduced survival to adulthood. Female carriers may have mild form of DCM.

- The gene responsible for this disorder codes for dystrophin, a cytoskeletal protein responsible for structural support to myocytes by producing a mesh of sarcolemma.
- Subendocardial scarring provides substrate and hypokalemia, hypomagnesemia and circulating catecholamines may be the modulating factors for arrhythmias.
- Ejection fraction of less than 35% is the single most predictor of mortality.
- Other markers of mortality include low serum sodium, elevated plasma norepinephrine, renin and BNP.
- The presence of LBBB and AV blocks are the markers of poor outcome.
- Ventricular arrhythmias are common but have low positive predictive value.
- Programmed electrical stimulation is not a reliable predictor of SCD in DCM.
- Frequent PVCs may result in tachycardia induced cardiomyopathy.

Genetics
- DCM occurs as a hereditary disease in up to one third of patients with "idiopathic" DCM.
- Mutations in the Lamin A/C gene are associated with familial DCM and AV conduction disease
- Phospholamban (PLN) is a crucial regulator of myocardial Ca^{2+} transients and of cardiac contractility Heterozygous deletion of arginine 14 in the gene encoding phospholamban (*PLN-R14Del*) may cause familial dilated cardiomyopathy
- Attenuated R amplitudes have been identified as an early ECG phenotype in familial dilated cardiomyopathy due to the *PLN-R14Del* mutation.

Calcium, heart failure, and arrhythmias
- Arrhythmias may result from a wide pathophysiologic spectrum including scar, neuronal, hormonal, and metabolic sequelae of heart failure, systolic dysfunction.
- Abnormal calcium handling is central to both contractile dysfunction and arrhythmogenesis.
- In systole, calcium release from the sarcoplasmic reticulum initiates excitation–contraction coupling, whereas in diastole, calcium is extruded by the sodium–calcium exchanger and undergoes reuptake via sarcoplasmic reticulum calcium adenosine triphosphatase (SERCA2a).
- With systolic dysfunction, diastolic calcium concentration increases because of reduced expression of SERCA2a and altered expression of the sodium–calcium exchanger.
- In heart failure and atrial fibrillation, CaMKII expression and, late INa activity are increased.
- CaMKII may increase late I_{Na}.
- Increased late INa contributes to ventricular as well as atrial arrhythmias,
- Inhibition of CaMKII and late I_{Na} produce antiarrhythmic effects.
- Ranolazine (a specific late I_{Na} inhibitor) reduces late I_{Na}
- Diastolic dysfunction and spontaneous PVCs induced by Na-dependent Ca overload are ameliorated by ranolazine.
- Increased late I_{Na} may also play a role in diastolic dysfunction.

Box 7.2 Causes of mortality in DCM

EF <35%
NYHA classification
Third heart sound
Syncope
Low serum sodium
Increased plasma norepinephrine
Increased plasma rennin
Elevated levels of natriuretic peptide
Presence of LBBB, first and second-degree AV block, AF
Frequent PVCs, non-sustained VT
Subsequent pregnancy in patients with documented peripartum
   cardiomyopathy

Causes of mortality in DCM (Box 7.2)
- Fifty percent of all deaths in DCM are sudden and majority of those may be due to VT.
- In majority of patients with advanced heart failure the cause of sudden death may be bradyarrhythmias and pulseless cardiac electrical activity, rather then tachyarrhythmias.
- Ischemia and MI may also be responsible for mortality in patients with DCM.

Predictors of mortality[15]
- The incidence of nonsustained VT increases with worsening CHF.
- The role of programmed stimulation in risk stratification of patients with DCM is poorly defined. Even in patients who present with ventricular tachycardia or SCD programmed stimulation may fail to induce index arrhythmia. Polymorphic VT could be induced. It has no prognostic significance.
- Patients with DCM who present with decreased left ventricular ejection fraction (LVEF) and syncope should be considered for prophylactic ICD insertion even if the electrophysiologic study is negative.
- Signal average electrocardiogram, heart rate variability, QT dispersion and T wave alternans are not helpful in predicting outcome in patients with DCM.
- It is accompanied by elevation of plasma levels of tumor necrosis factor-alpha.

Treatment
- The optimum pharmacologic treatment for CHF includes ACE inhibitors, adrenergic receptor blocking agents, digitalis, diuretics and aldosterone antagonists.
- The use of ace inhibitors and beta-blockers may decrease the mortality by 30%.
- Identification and treatment of ischemia, electrolyte abnormalities should be considered.
- The use of phosphodiesterase inhibitors, as an inotropic agent, increases mortality.

- Amiodarone may be effective in controlling symptomatic ventricular arrhythmias and decreasing SCD in patients with DCM. Efficacy and tolerance of amiodarone decreases with decreasing EF and duration of the treatment.
- Biventricular pacing, by resynchronizing ventricular contraction and improving conduction, reduces diastolic mitral regurgitation, improves symptoms of LVF and may improve survival.
- Current indication for ICD in patients with DCM include cardiac arrest survivors, syncopal VT or spontaneous sustain VT and/or EF <35.
- Sustained monomorphic VT (SMVT) is not common in nonischaemic-dilated cardiomyopathies, but 80% of those that occur are due to scar-related re-entry, with the remainder due to bundle branch re-entry or a focal origin.
- Scars are probably due to progressive fibrosis.
- Compared with post-infarction VT, areas of scar are smaller, but patients who present with SMVT typically have multiple morphologies of inducible VT.
- Magnetic resonance imaging with delayed Gd enhancement and voltage mapping demonstrates that scars are often adjacent to a valve annulus.
- Transmural scar is rare and intramural scars are common. These features likely account for the general perception that ablation of VT is more difficult when compared with that in the post-MI population.
- When endocardial ablation fails, epicardial mapping usually shows that more extensive scar is present in the epicardium.
- Catheter ablation employs the approaches for scar-related VT after exclusion of bundle branch reentry.

7.4 Bundle branch re-entry ventricular tachycardia[16]

- Tachycardia may present with LBBB or RBBB morphology depending on the antegrade conduction over RB or LB respectively. LBBB morphology is common.
- It is a macroreentrant tachycardia incorporating the His bundle, RBB, LBB, and transseptal myocardial conduction as critical components.
- The re-entry wavefront circulates retrogradely up one bundle branch (most commonly the left bundle) and down the other (most commonly the RB), giving rise to VT that usually has a typical LBBB configuration that can be the same as the QRS configuration during sinus rhythm.
- Introduction of RV premature beat at short coupling interval results in retrograde block in RB. Transeptal delay and shorter refractory period of the LB allows the impulse to proceed over LB. If the RB recovers from its refractoriness, the impulse may conduct antegradely over RB and initiate re-entrant tachycardia (Figure 7.5).
- The VT can usually be induced by programmed right ventricle stimulation; induction may occur with left ventricle stimulation, short–long–short extrastimuli sequences, isoproterenol infusion, sodium channel blockade, atrial stimulation, or an irregular rhythm from atrial fibrillation or flutter.
- During entrainment from the right ventricle apex, the post-pacing interval–VT cycle length difference is typically 30 ms or less.

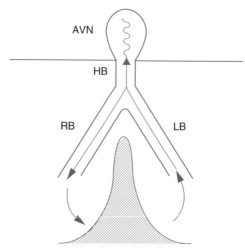

Figure 7.5 Schematic of BBR-VT, antegrade conduction through RB and retrograde conduction through LB.

- An inverse relationship exists between retrograde conduction delay in LB and recovery of the antegrade conduction over RB.
- Recording and analysis of His bundle and bundle branch activation sequence during tachycardia is essential for the diagnosis of BB VT.
- Introduction of the premature beats with short to long cycle length changes the refractoriness of the HPS allowing the reentry to occur.
- BBRT commonly presents with LB morphology. Reverse re-entry loop may occur if the LB refractoriness exceeds that of RB.
- LV pacing or extastimuli do not facilitate RB type BBRT.
- In patients with structurally normal heart BBR tends to be self limiting because of the spontaneous blocks in retrograde limb (LB).
- The presence of conduction abnormalities in HPS facilitates BBR.
- BBRT commonly occurs in the presence of structural heart disease such as dilated cardiomyopathy with severe left ventricle dysfunction and conduction abnormalities in the HPS.
- RBBB configuration tachycardias occur when the LB is used anterogradely, or are due to interfascicular reentry tachycardia involving both fascicles of the left-sided Purkinje system that may coexist with bundle branch reentry.
- In interfascicular re-entry right axis deviation indicates antegrade activation over left anterior fascicle and retrogrades over the left posterior fascicle; and left axis deviation occurs when the circuit revolves in the opposite direction. The tachycardia cycle length is usually <300 ms; near syncope, syncope, or cardiac arrest are common presentations.

Clinical manifestations
- BBR-VT may result in presyncope, syncope and sudden death.
- It is commonly associated with structural heart disease and low ejection fraction.

- This mechanism should be considered in VTs occurring in the presence of dilated cardiomyopathy.
- BBR VT may also be seen in:
  1 Myotonic dystrophy
  2 Hypertrophic cardiomyopathy
  3 Ebstein anomaly
  4 Fallowing valvular surgery
  5 Proarrhythmia due to Na channel blockers.

Electrophysiologic features (Boxes 7.3 and 7.4)

- The baseline electrocardiogram shows either sinus rhythm or AF. Nonspecific IVCD of LBB type and prolonged PR interval are common findings.
- During tachycardia right or left bundle branch block pattern and AV dissociation is present (Figure 7.6).
- Intracardiac electrograms reveal prolonged HV interval (average 80 ms).
- Six percent of all inducible ventricular tachycardias have bundle branch re-entry as their mechanism.
- Tachycardia is induced by RV programmed stimulation. It may require introduction of short to long cycle length premature beats.
- Isoproterenol infusion may facilitate induction of the tachycardia.
- Infusion of procainamide may facilitate induction of tachycardia by increasing conduction delay in HPS.

Box 7.3 Electrophysiologic features of BBR-VT

- During tachycardia QRS morphology is commonly LBBB type.
- AV dissociation.
- His electrograms precedes each V
- HV interval during tachycardia > HV in baseline.
- Changes in V-V interval fallow the changes in H-H.
- Delay in HPS conduction facilitates induction.
- Block in bundle branches or HPS will terminate the tachycardia.
- Ablation of RB renders tachycardia noninducible.

Box 7.4 Observations suggestive of BBR-VT.

- Idiopathic dilated cardiomyopathy.
- Conduction abnormality of HPS during sinus rhythm.
- VT with LB morphology.
- HV interval during VT same or longer than HV in sinus rhythm when measured from H to onset of QRS.
- H electrogram precedes RB electrogram.
- If entrained by A pacing, the QRS morphology is similar to QRS morphology during VT.

- The HV interval during LBB morphology tachycardia tends to be similar or longer than HV interval during sinus rhythm. During tachycardia HV interval depends on the conduction characteristics of contralateral bundle (Figures 7.7 and 7.8)
- The sequence of activation of His and bundle branch is essential in diagnosing the type of VT. During tachycardia with LBB morphology LB activation is followed by His and then RB activation. The sequence of activation is reversed in RBB morphology VT.
- Tachycardia terminates with a block in His Purkinje tissue (no LB or His electrogram following last QRS).

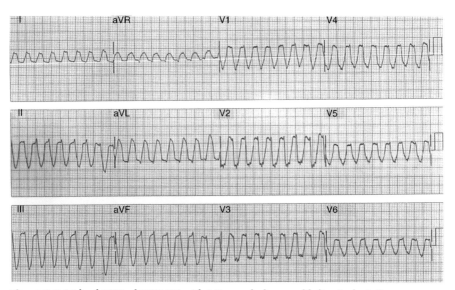

Figure 7.6 12 lead ECG of BBR-VT with LB morphology and left axis deviation.

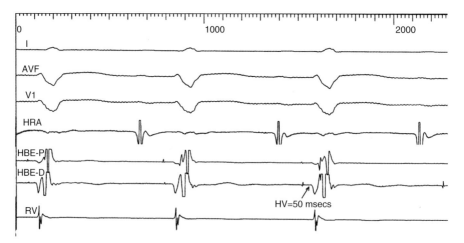

Figure 7.7 Intracardiac electrograms during sinus rhythm. LB morphology.

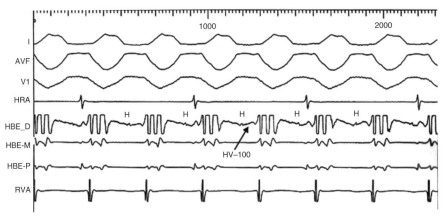

Figure 7.8 BBR-VT. H precedes each QRS. HV longer than HV in sinus rhythm.

- During tachycardia changes in H to H interval precede the changes in V to V interval. This helps differentiates BBR-VT from myocardial origin VT with incidental HPS activation.
- Introduction of premature impulses during the tachycardia may reverse the circuit.
- The QRS morphology during entrainment by atrial pacing is identical to that of BBR VT. However during right ventricle pacing the QRS morphology is different.
- Difference between PPI and tachycardia cycle length tends to be less than 30 ms.

Differential diagnosis of BBR-VT
- VT of myocardial origin may present with incidental HPS activation preceding QRS however V to V cycle length variation dictates H to H variation. Often H can not be discerned during this type of tachycardia
- Supraventricular tachycardia with aberrancy may be mistaken for BBR-VT, especially if there is 1:1 retrograde conduction is present. His and BB activation is antegrade in SVT and resembles the activation during sinus.
- Atriofascicular reentry tachycardia presents with LBB morphology. However RBB activation precedes His activation in this tachycardia and excludes BBR VT with LBB morphology. There is 1:1 AV relation and atrial premature beats preexcite the right ventricle.
- Variation in the V-V cycle length is preceded by variation in the His-His interval, which suggests bundle branch re-entry as the mechanism
- SVT including atriofascicular AV re-entrant tachycardia can be ruled out by the observation of atrial dissociation during tachycardia and the long AV block cycle length.
- Antidromic nodofascicular tachycardia can be excluded by the long VH time,
- Junctional tachycardia can be excluded by the observation of a short PPI during entrainment from the right ventricle apex.
- During bundle branch re-entry with a RBBB configuration, the LB is activated anterogradely and the RB is activated in the retrograde direction

Treatment
- Treatment of choice for BBR VT is ablation of the RB[17].
- The right bundle branch is the preferred ablation target. Even in patients with baseline LBBB, right bundle ablation does not usually produce heart block, but back-up bradycardia pacing is required in ~30% of patients.
- Ablation of the left bundle branch may be considered when LBBB is present during sinus rhythm, but is more difficult and has risks of left heart catheterization.
- There is concern that LBBB may be more likely to adversely affect ventricular function than RBBB. Long-term outcome depends on the underlying cardiac disease.
- A permanent pacemaker should be implanted if post ablation HV interval is 100 msec or longer.
- ICD implant should be considered if myocardial VT occur spontaneously or are inducible or if EF less than 35%.
- Despite successful BBRT ablation, many patients remain at risk of sudden death due to concomitant scar-related VTs and/or LV dysfunction.

7.5 Ventricular arrhythmias in the presence of channelopathies

Cardiac action potential
- APs constitute changes in the membrane potential of cardiomyocytes.
- The membrane potential is established by an unequal distribution of electrically charged ions across the sarcolemma (electrochemical gradient) and the presence of conducting ion channels in the sarcolemma.
- Opening and closing (gating) of ion channels produces transmembrane ion currents resulting in AP formation.
- Ion channels consist of pore-forming α-subunits and accessory β-subunits.
- α- and β-subunits are made of large protein families that possess comparable amino acid sequences.
- This is reflected in the names of the subunits and their genes. For example, the gene encoding the α-subunit of the cardiac Na+ channel is called SCN5A: sodium channel, type 5, α-subunit. The α-subunit channel is termed Nav1.5: Na+ channel family, subfamily 1, member 5; the subscript "V" means that channel gating is regulated by transmembrane voltage changes (voltage dependent). The current it produces is termed as INa (Table 7.3).
- The direction of ion currents (into the cell [inward] or out of the cell [outward]) is determined by the electrochemical gradient of the corresponding ions.
- The current amplitude (I) depends on the membrane potential (V) and the conductivity (G) of the responsible ion channels.
- This relation is expressed in equation form as $I = V \times G$ (as resistance [R] is the reverse of conductivity: $I = V/R$ [Ohm's law]), implying that the current amplitude reacts linearly ("ohmically") in response to membrane potential changes.

Table 7.3 Genetic and molecular basis of cardiac ion currents.

Current	β-Subunit	Gene	β-subunit(s)/ accessory proteins	Gene	Blocking agent
I_{Na}	Nav1.5	SCN5A	β1 β2 β3 β4	SCN1B SCN2B SCN3B SCN4B	Tetrodotoxin
I_{to},fast	Kv4.3	KCND3	MiRP1 MiRP2 KChIPs DPP6	KCNE2 KCNE3 Multiple genes DPP6	4-aminopyridine *Heteropoda* spider toxins
I_{to},slow	Kv1.4	KCNA4	Kvβ1 Kvβ2 Kvβ3 Kvβ4	KCNB1 KCNB2 KCNB3 KCNB4	4-aminopyridine
$I_{Ca,L}$	Cav1.2	CACNA1C	Cavβ2 Cavα2δ1	CACNB2 CACNA2D1	Cations (Mg^{2+}, Ni^{2+}, Zn^{2+}) Dihydropyridine Phenylalkylamines Benzothiazepines
$I_{Ca,T}$	Cav3.1 Cav3.2	CACNA1G CACNA1H			Similar as $I_{Ca,L}$ (potency may differ)
I_{Kur}	Kv1.5	KCNA5	Kvβ1 Kvβ2	KCNAB1 KCNAB2	4-aminopyridine
I_{Kr}	Kv11.1	KCNH2	MiRP1	KCNE2	E-4031
I_{Ks}	Kv7.1	KCNQ1	minK	KCNE1	Chromanol-293B
I_{K1}	Kir2.1	KCNJ2			Ba^{2+}
I_f (pacemaker current)	HCN1-4	HCN1-4			Cs^+

- Some currents do not act ohmically (so-called rectifying currents). The conductivity of channels carrying such currents is not constant but alters at different membrane potentials.
- Rectifying currents in the heart are the inward rectifying current (I_{K1}) and the outward rectifying currents.
- Channels carrying outward rectifying currents preferentially conduct K^+ ions during depolarization (potentials positive to K^+ equilibrium potential [approximately $-90\,mV$]) when the currents are outwardly directed.

- Channels carrying I_{K1} preferentially conduct K$^+$ ions at potentials negative to K$^+$ equilibrium potential when the currents are inwardly directed.
- I_{K1} channels also conduct a substantial outward current at membrane potentials between -40 and -90 mV. Within this voltage range, outward I_{K1} is larger at more negative potentials. Because membrane potentials negative to the K$^+$ equilibrium potential are not reached in cardiomyocytes, only the outward I_{K1} plays a role in AP formation.
- Resting potential of atrial and ventricular myocytes during AP phase 4 (resting phase) is stable and negative (approximately -85 mV) due to the high conductance for K$^+$ of the I_{K1} channels.
- Upon excitation by electrical impulses from adjacent cells, Na$^+$ channels activate (open) and permit an inward Na$^+$ current (I_{Na}), which gives rise to phase 0 depolarization (initial upstroke).
- Phase 0 is followed by phase 1 (early repolarization), accomplished by the transient outward K$^+$ current (I_{to}).
- Phase 2 (plateau) represents a balance between the depolarizing L-type inward Ca^{2+} current ($I_{Ca,L}$) and the repolarizing ultra-rapidly (I_{Kur}), rapidly (I_{Kr}), and slowly (I_{Ks}) activating delayed outward rectifying currents.
- Phase 3 (repolarization) reflects the predominance of the delayed outward rectifying currents after inactivation (closing) of the L-type Ca^{2+} channels. Final repolarization during phase 3 is due to K$^+$ efflux through the I_{K1} channels.
- In contrast to atrial and ventricular myocytes, SAN and AVN myocytes demonstrate slow depolarization of the resting potential during phase 4.
- Absence of I_{K1} allows inward currents (e.g., pacemaker current [I_f]) to depolarize the membrane potential.
- Slow depolarization during phase 4 inactivates most Na$^+$ channels and decreases their availability for phase 0.
- In SAN and AVN myocytes, AP depolarization is mainly achieved by $I_{Ca,L}$ and the T-type Ca^{2+} current.
- I_{Na} determines cardiac excitability and electrical conduction velocity by enabling phase 0 depolarization in atrial, ventricular, and Purkinje APs.
- α-subunit of cardiac Na$^+$ channels (Nav1.5, encoded by *SCN5A*) encompasses four serially linked homologous domains (DI–DIV), which fold around an ion-conducting pore.
- Each domain contains six transmembrane segments (S1–S6). S4 segments are responsible for voltage-dependent activation.
- At the end of phase 0, most channels are inactivated and can be reactivated only after recovery from inactivation during phase 4.
- Some channels remain open or reopen during phases 2 and 3, and they carry a small late Na$^+$ current (I_{NaL}).
- Na$^+$ channel dysfunction is linked to several inherited arrhythmia syndromes (Table 7.4),
- Long QT syndrome (LQTS) is a repolarization disorder with QT interval prolongation and increased risk for Torsades de Pointes ventricular tachycardia and ventricular fibrillation.

Table 7.4 Genetic basis of inherited cardiac diseases.

Type	Occurrence (or % of genotyped)	Gene	Protein	Protein function	Affected current
Long QT syndrome					
1	42–54%	KCNQ1	Kv7.1	α-subunit I_{Ks} channel	I_{Ks} decrease
2	35–45%	KCNH2	Kv11.1	α-subunit I_{Kr} channel	I_{Kr} decrease
3	1.7–8%	SCN5A	Nav1.5	α-subunit Na$^+$ channel	I_{NaL} increase
4	<1%	ANK2	Ankyrin-B	Adaptor protein	None
5	<1%	KCNE1	minK	β-subunit I_{Ks} channel	I_{Ks} decrease
6	<1%	KCNE2	MiRP1	β-subunit I_{Kr} channel	I_{Kr} decrease
7	Rare	KCNJ2	Kir2.1	α-subunit I_{K1} channel	I_{K1} decrease
8	Rare	CACNA1C	Cav1.2	α-subunit Ca^{2+} channel	$I_{Ca,L}$ increase
9	Rare (1.9% in one study)	CAV3	Caveolin-3	Component of caveolae (co-localizes with Nav1.5 at sarcolemma)	I_{NaL} increase
10	<0.1%	SCN4B	β4	β-subunit Na$^+$ channel	I_{NaL} increase
11	Rare (2% in one study)	AKAP9	Yotiao	Mediates I_{Ks} channel phosphorylation	Inadequate I_{Ks} increase during β-adrenergic stimulation
12	Rare (2% in one study)	SNTA1	α1-syntrophin	Regulates Na$^+$ channel function	I_{NaL} increase
Short QT syndrome					
1	Three families	KCNH2	Kv11.1	α-subunit I_{Kr} channel	I_{Kr} increase
2	Two case reports	KCNQ1	Kv7.1	α-subunit I_{Ks} channel	I_{Ks} increase
3	One family (two members)	KCNJ2	Kir2.1	α-subunit I_{K1} channel	I_{K1} increase
Brugada syndrome					
–	10–30%	SCN5A	Nav1.5	Na$^+$ channel (I_{Na})	I_{Na} decrease
–	Rare (one family)	GPD1-L	GPD1-L	Regulates intracellular Nav1.5 trafficking	I_{Na} decrease

(Continued)

Table 7.4 (*Continued*)

Type	Occurrence (or % of genotyped)	Gene	Protein	Protein function	Affected current
–	<1%	SCN1B	β1	β-subunit Na⁺ channel	I_{Na} decrease
–	<1%	SCN3B	β3	β-subunit Na⁺ channel	I_{Na} decrease
–	<1%	KCNE3	MiRP2	β-subunit I_{to},fast channel	I_{to},fast increase
–	<8.5%	CACNA1C	Cav1.2	α-subunit Ca²⁺ channel	$I_{Ca,L}$ decrease
–	<8.5%	CACNB2	Cavβ2	β-subunit Ca²⁺ channel	$I_{Ca,L}$ decrease
Familial atrial fibrillation					
–	One (small) family	KCNE3	MiRP2	β-subunit I_{to},fast channel	I_{to},fast increase
–	Three families	KCNA5	Kv1.5	α-subunit I_{Kur} channel	I_{Kur} increase
–	One family	KCNH2	Kv11.1	α-subunit I_{Kr} channel	I_{Kr} increase
–	Two families	KCNE2	MiRP1	β-subunit I_{Kr} channel (may modulate I_{Ks} channel)	I_{Ks} increase
–	One family	KCNQ1	Kv7.1	α-subunit I_{Ks} channel	I_{Ks} increase
–	One family	KCNJ2	Kir2.1	α-subunit I_{K1} channel	I_{K1} increase

- LQTS type 3 (LQT3), mutations in *SCN5A* delay repolarization, mostly by enhancing I_{NaL}.
- Delayed repolarization may trigger early after-depolarizations (EADs are abnormal depolarizations during phase 2 or 3 due to reactivation of L-type Ca²⁺ channels).
- EADs are believed to initiate Torsades de Pointes.
- Drugs that block I_{NaL} (e.g., ranolazine, mexiletine) may effectively shorten repolarization in LQT3 patients.
- Mutations in genes encoding Na⁺ channel regulatory proteins may cause of LQTS.

Long QT syndrome[18–20]

- Despite the designation of LQTS as "congenital," the average age at LQTS diagnosis is 30 years.

- Diagnosis in the first year of life is made is made in approximately 4% of cases; neonatal LQTS is due to mutations in the three ion channels commonly associated with LQTS but has severe morbidity and mortality compared with LQTS in older patients.
- LQTS patients with cardiac symptoms in the first year of life represent an extremely high risk group.
- Twenty percent of LQTS remains genetically undetermined.
- Approximately 75% of clinically definite LQTS are caused by mutations in three genes: *KCNQ1* (LQT1), *KCNH2* (LQT2), and *SCN5A* (LQT3), which encode the major pore-forming alpha subunit of the macromolecular channel complexes Kv7.1 (I_{Ks}), Kv11.1 (I_{Kr}), and Nav1.5 (I_{Na}), respectively.
- LQTS type 1 and type 2 mutations are located in the α-subunits (*KCNQ1* or *KCNH2*) underlying cardiac delayed rectifier ion currents and may lead to loss of function by modifications of biophysical properties and deficient trafficking of α-subunits to the cell membrane.
- Clinically these differ in ECG T-wave patterns, clinical course, triggers of cardiac events, response to sympathetic stimulation, and effectiveness and limitations of beta-blocker therapy.
- The incidence of congenital LQTS has been estimated to be 1:5000.
- ECG-guided molecular screening provides a higher prevalence of LQTS, at least 1:2000.
- Incidence of Jervell and Lange–Nielsen syndrome is estimated to be 1:500 in congenitally deaf individuals.
- It is more severe with 90% of patients experiencing syncope, cardiac arrest, or sudden death by age 18 years, and mortality exceeds 25% even with medical therapy.
- Without treatment, 13% of patients and following a syncope 36% of patients with LQTS will suffer cardiac arrest or sudden death before age 40 years;
- Ninety percent of the mutation-positive cases may have single genotypes, remaining have more than one mutation.
- Genetic screening for the high-risk family member may help to diagnose and treat the LQT carrier.
- Mutation carrying relatives of LQTS proband can be prophylactically treated with medication.
- Beta-blockers may help prevent life-threatening arrhythmias in LQTS.
- The QT interval is the body surface representation of the interval from the beginning of ventricular depolarization to the end of ventricular repolarization.
- Any deviation or dispersion of either depolarization (e.g., BBB) or repolarization (e.g., enhanced action potential duration [APD] or its dispersion) prolongs the QT interval.

Measurement of QT interval

- QT interval is measured in LII or using the lead that shows the largest QT interval, which generally is lead V3 or V4.
- Various formulas are available for the measurement of QT interval (Box 7.5).

Box 7.5 Formulae for measuring QT interval

Bazett $QTc = QT / (RR / 1000)^{1/2}$

Fridericia $QTc = QT / (RR / 1000)^{1/3}$

Framingham $QTc = QT + 0.154 \times (1000 - RR)$

Hodges $QTc = QT + 1.75 \times (60000 / RR - 60)$

- Bazett and Fridericia correction formulas may overestimate the change in QT interval with change in the heart rate.
- For adult population, normal QTc values for males are 350 to 450 ms and for females are 360 to 460 ms, Boundaries of the normal QT determined by genetic studies are not different from those derived from population studies.
- Progesterone shortens action potential duration. This may be due to enhancement of the slow delayed rectifier K^+ current (I_{Ks}) under basal conditions and inhibition of L-type Ca^{2+} currents ($I_{Ca,L}$) under cAMP-stimulated conditions.
- The effects of progesterone were mediated by nitric oxide released via nongenomic activation of endothelial nitric oxide synthase.
- There is considerable overlap of QTc intervals between mutation-carriers and noncarriers.
- No single QTc value separates all LQTS patients from healthy controls, males with QTc ≥470 ms and females with QTc ≥480 ms should be considered to have LQTS even if they are asymptomatic and have a negative family history.
- Bazett formula, is used for calculating QTc (i.e., to correct QT for heart rate) which undercorrects at fast heart rates and overcorrects at slow heart rates.
- The Fridericia formula ($QT_F = QT/RR^{1/3}$) does not use the square root function.
- Although QTc values >470 ms are not seen among healthy individuals when their heart rate is 60 to 70 bpm, 2% of healthy adults (and more children) have QTc ≥480 ms when their heart rate is greater than 90 bpm.
- Whenever a "long QTc" is found during sinus tachycardia, ECG should be repeated when the heart rate slows down.
- Defining QTc may be difficult in the presence of physiologic sinus arrhythmia because the QT shortening in response to heart rate changes is not immediate leading to little change in the uncorrected QT interval as the R-R interval shortens and lengthens with respiration but leading to "long" QTc during sinus rate acceleration and normal QTc during deceleration.
- U waves are not often seen in leads I, aVR, and aVL, so determinations of QT in those leads could be performed.
- QTc ≥460 ms during the shortest R-R interval, or marked variability (>40 ms) of the uncorrected QT during sinus arrhythmia, may favors the diagnosis of LQTS.
- The majority of the general population QTc is between 400 and 450 ms.

- LQTS still is possible within this range, and whenever the clinical history requires exclusion of LQTS, additional tests are indicated.
- The first step is to periodically repeat a resting ECG because of the considerable day-to-day variability in QTc of patients with LQTS.
- Forty percent of patients with LQTS will have QTc >500 ms at least once during long-term follow-up, but only 25% will have that degree of QT prolongation during their initial evaluation.
- The second step is to review the ECGs of all family members because LQTS has dominant inheritance, and some family members may have obvious QT prolongation.
- Attention should be given to the T-wave morphology, which differs according to the LQTS genotype.
- Holter recordings only rarely will show spontaneous arrhythmias but may reveal characteristic T-waves changes during sleep or following postextrasystolic pauses.
- 24-h Holter recordings allow dynamic evaluation of QT interval including the effect of sinus pauses.
- A challenge test with either intravenous epinephrine or adenosine may provide additional information.
- The epinephrine challenge test is useful for identifying patients with LQT1.
- LQT1 is the more common genotype and is commonly missed. Other LQTS genotypes may present with abnormal T waves, LQT1 demonstrate broad T waves, which can be interpreted as normal.
- The duration of the QTc carries important prognostic information.

Epinephrine QT stress test[21,22]

- Normal response of healthy individuals to epinephrine infusion is an appearance of prominent U wave without increase in the QTC interval.
- 30-ms or greater increment of the uncorrected QT during low-dose epinephrine infusion and appearance of notched T waves (with T2 > T1) can be considered diagnostic of LQT1 and LQT2, respectively.
- In LQT1 there is paradoxical increase in the uncorrected QT interval during infusion of low-dose epinephrine.
- Epinephrine QT stress test involves a 25-minute infusion protocol (0.025–0.3 µg/kg/min). The paradoxical QT response is defined as a ≥30-ms increase in QT during infusion of ≤0.1 µg/kg/min epinephrine.
- The median change in QT interval during low-dose epinephrine infusion may range from −23 ms in the gene-negative group, 78 ms in LQT1, −4 ms in LQT2, and −58 ms in LQT3.
- Overall, the paradoxical QT response has sensitivity of 92.5%, specificity 86%, positive predictive value 76%, and negative predictive value 96% for LQT1.
- The epinephrine QT stress test can unmask concealed LQT1 with a high level of accuracy.
- Injection of adenosine during sinus rhythm invariably causes sudden short-lasting bradycardia, followed by sinus tachycardia. These rapid changes in heart rate are accompanied by marked QT changes.

- Adenosine injection is a useful test for diagnosing LQT2, its value in patients with borderline QT prolongation remains to be defined.
- Disturbances of repolarization that may result in arrhythmias include:
- Reverse use dependence, agents like sotalol causing prolongation of the QT interval during slower heart rate.
- Proarrhythmia is not limited to disturbances of repolarization; disturbances of conduction velocity, refractory period and automaticity also cause proarrhythmia.
- The combination of slow conduction velocity (CV) with short ERP is detrimental, leading to shortening of the cardiac wavelength ($\lambda = CV \times ERP$), which facilitates re-entry.
- Mutation carriers with rate-corrected QT intervals in the lowest quartile (<446 ms) had a 40-year event rate under 20%, compared with an event rate of almost 80% in the highest quartile (>499 ms).
- QT prolongation could be a predictor of subsequent mortality in patients recovering from acute myocardial infarction, diabetes, advancing age, chronic heart failure, autonomic dysfunction, hypertrophic cardiomyopathy and muscular dystrophy.
- More than 600 mutations in at least 11 genes have been identified in LQTS patients
- Most of these genes encode for proteins composing cardiac ion channels, and, of these, more than 90% of mutations are found in five genes (*KCNQ1, KCNH2, SCN5A, KCNE1,* and *KCNE2*).
- There are a total of 12 LQTS-susceptibility genes.
- LQT4-12 accounts for less than 5% of LQTS cases.
- *CAV3* (LQT9), *SCN4B* (LQT10), and *SNTA1* (LQT12), encode proteins that function in part as sodium-channel interacting proteins (ChIPs).
- When coexpressed with an otherwise intact sodium-channel alpha subunit, mutant caveolin-3, mutant sodium channel beta 4 subunit, or mutant alpha syntrophin convert the NaV1.5 sodium channel complex into late sodium current.
- Similarly, mutations in *AKAP9* disrupt the I_{Ks} ChIP, yotiao, causing an LQT1-like loss of function.
- LQTS mutation carriers, who lack a prolonged QT interval and, therefore, escape clinical diagnosis, have a 10% risk of a major cardiac event by age 40 years if left untreated.
- LQTS shows both autosomal recessive and autosomal dominant patterns of inheritance: A rare autosomal recessive disease associated with deafness (Jervell and Lange–Nielsen), caused by mutation in two genes that encode for the slowly activating delayed rectifier potassium channel (*KCNQ1* and *KCNE1*).
- A common autosomal dominant form known as the Romano–Ward syndrome is caused by mutations in 10 different genes.
- Six of the 10 genes encode for cardiac potassium channels.
- Acquired LQTS refers to a syndrome similar to the congenital form but caused by Exposure to drugs that prolong the duration of the ventricular action potential

- QT prolongation secondary to cardiomyopathies including dilated or hypertrophic cardiomyopathy,
- Abnormal QT prolongation can be associated with bradycardia or electrolyte imbalance.
- The acquired form of the disease is far more prevalent than the congenital form, and may have a genetic predisposition.
- Multiple concomitant risk factors such as hypokalemia, left ventricular hypertrophy and I_{Kr} blockade and genetically determined reduced activity of the cytochrome P450 enzymes CYP2D6 and CYP3A may be involved in prolongation of the QT interval.

M cells

- In LQTS, preferential prolongation of the APD in M-cell leads to an increase in the QT interval as well as an increase in TDR, which contributes to the development of spontaneous as well as stimulation-induced TdP.
- M cell action potential prolongs more than that of epicardium or endocardium in response to a slowing of rate or in response to agents that prolong APD.
- M cells with the longest APD typically are found in the deep subendocardium to midmyocardium in the anterior wall.
- M cells also have been identified in the deep layers of papillary muscles, trabeculae, and interventricular septum.
- The prolonged APD of the M cell appears to be due to a weak slowly activating delayed rectifier current I_{Ks} and a stronger late I_{Na} and sodium/calcium exchange current compared with epicardial and endocardial cells.
- These ionic characteristics leave M cells susceptible to an action from variety of pharmacologic agents.
- Agents that block the rapidly activating delayed rectifier current I_{Kr} or I_{Ks} or that increase calcium channel current I_{Ca} or late I_{Na} generally produce much greater prolongation of the APD of the M cell than of epicardial or endocardial cells.
- Differences in the time course of repolarization of the three predominant myocardial cell types contribute to the inscription of the T wave of the ECG.
- Voltage gradients developing as a result of the different time course of repolarization of phases 2 and 3 in the three cell types give rise to opposing voltage gradients on either side of the M region, which are in part responsible for the inscription of the T wave.
- In the case of an upright T wave, the epicardial response is the earliest to repolarize and the M cell action potential is the last.
- Full repolarization of the epicardial action potential coincides with the peak of the T wave, and repolarization of the M cells is coincident with the end of the T wave.
- The duration of the M-cell action potential therefore determines the QT interval, whereas the duration of the epicardial action potential determines the QT peak interval.

- The interval between the peak and end of the T wave (T_{peak}–T_{end} interval) in precordial ECG leads has been suggested to provide an index of TDR.
- TDR, rather QT prolongation, underlies the principal substrate for the development of TdP.
- Agents that reduce net repolarizing current via a reduction in IKr or IKs or augmentation of I_{Ca} or late I_{Na} increase TDR.
- Reduction in I_{Kr} or augmentation of late INa produce a preferential prolongation of the M-cell action potential leading to prolong QT interval and increase in TDR, predisposing to development of EAD.
- Not all agents that prolong the QT interval increase TDR. Chronic administration of amiodarone produces a greater prolongation of APD in epicardium and endocardium but less of an increase in the M region, thereby reducing TDR.
- Sodium pentobarbital is another agent that prolongs the QT interval but reduces TDR. Pentobarbital has been shown to produce a dose-dependent prolongation of the QT interval, accompanied by a reduction in TDR.
- TdP is not observed under these conditions, nor can it be induced with programmed electrical stimulation.
- Amiodarone and pentobarbital have in common the ability to block I_{Ks}, I_{Kr}, and late I_{Na}. This combination produces a preferential prolongation of the APD of epicardium and endocardium so that the QT interval is prolonged, but TDR. is actually reduced and TdP does not develop.
- Cisapride blocks both inward and outward currents.
- Chromanol 293B induced block of I_{Ks} increases QT without augmenting TDR. It prolongs APD of the three cell types homogeneously without increasing TDR.
- TdP does not occur.
- β-adrenergic agonists such as isoproterenol abbreviate the APD of epicardial and endocardial cells but not that of the M cell, resulting in a marked accentuation of TDR and the development of TdP.
- This may explain why patients with LQTS, particularly LQT1, are so sensitive to sympathetic stimulation and support the hypothesis that the risks associated with LQTS are not due to prolongation of the QT interval but rather to the increase in spatial dispersion of repolarization that usually, but not always, accompanies prolongation of the QT interval.

Tp–Te interval
- QT interval is an accepted measure of ventricular repolarization, the interval from the peak of the T wave to the end of the T wave (Tpe) is considered a more sensitive index of abnormal repolarization and may reflect dispersion of repolarization.
- Beta-adrenergic stimulation with exercise or epinephrine is helpful in identifying subjects with occult LQT1.
- Epinephrine bolus (but not steady state epinephrine) increased Tpe in LQT2 patients.
- One possible explanation for phenotype/genotype discordance observed in LQTS is the repolarization reserve hypothesis, which implies that multiple

challenges to cellular repolarization are required to produce clinical QT prolongation. For example, a subject exposed to an I_{Kr}-blocking drug may show QT prolongation only if there is coexistence of hypokalemia or an underlying genetic abnormality in repolarization

- Erythromycin causes concentration-dependent prolongation of repolarization, competitively blocking I_{Kr} receptors.
- Normal Tpe interval is <100 ms. a Tpe of over 100 ms in the baseline state is uncommon in control subjects
- Tpe interval has been suggested as a noninvasive surrogate for transmural dispersion of repolarization.
- Role of the Tpe interval as a measure of transmural dispersion remains controversial, it is accepted as a measure of abnormal, heterogeneous repolarization.

Classification of long QT syndrome[18,23,24]

- There are 12 forms of inherited LQTS have been identified and are associated with mutations in the genes encoding ion channels or their associated proteins.
- Mutations have been identified in genes encoding the α subunits of voltage-gated K^+, Na^+, and Ca^{2+} channels (LQT1, LQT2, LQT3, LQT7, LQT8), in genes encoding auxiliary subunits of K^+ and Na^+ channels (LQT5, LQT6, LQT10), and in the gene encoding the cytoskeletal membrane adaptor protein ankyrin-B (LQT4), *AKAP9* (LQT11) and the scaffolding protein caveolin-3 (LQT9) cytoskeletal protein syntrophin (LQT12).
- Prolongation of repolarization results from reduction of outward repolarizing (potassium) currents (loss-of-function mutations) or from a persistent or late influx of depolarizing (sodium or calcium) ions (gain-of-function mutations) during an action potential.
- LQTS is associated with SCD caused by torsade de pointes (TdP) triggered by EAD.
- The Na^+/Ca^{2+} exchanger (NCX) has a stoichiometry of 3 Na^+ 1 Ca^{2+} and generates an inward depolarizing current in the forward mode as calcium is extruded from the cell. NCX may play a role in maintaining the action potential plateau.
- LQTS identified primary mutations in genes coding for pore-forming subunits (*KCNQ1*, *KCNH2*, *SCN5A*, *KCNJ2*, *CACNA1C*) or beta subunits (*KCNE1*, *KCNE2*, *SCN4B*) of ion channels critical for the cardiac action potential, thus defining LQTS as a cardiac channelopathy.
- In 20% to 30% of cases, genetic analysis of all ion channel subunits fails to identify the gene responsible for the LQTS phenotypes in affected patients.
- Genetic defects have been uncovered in genes coding for scaffolding (*CAV3*), adapter (*ANK2*, *AKAP9*), and cytoskeletal proteins (*SNTA1*), which act as channel interacting proteins (ChIPs) with an effect on ion channel trafficking, posttranslational modification, and kinetics.
- A-kinase anchoring proteins (AKAPs) recruit signaling molecules and present them to downstream targets to achieve efficient spatial and temporal control of their phosphorylation state.

- In the heart, sympathetic nervous system (SNS) regulation of cardiac action potential duration (APD), mediated by β-adrenergic receptor (βAR) activation, requires assembly of AKAP9 (Yotiao) with the I_{Ks} potassium channel α subunit (KCNQ1).
- *KCNQ1* mutations that disrupt this complex cause type 1 long-QT syndrome (LQT1).
- Mutation of a channel may result in either gain of function or loss of function. For an example SQTS 1 and LQTS 2, caused by gain and loss of function of I_{Kr}; SQTS2 and LQTS1, caused by gain and loss of function of I_{Ks}; SQTS3 and Andersen–Tawil syndrome (LTQS7), caused by gain and loss of function of I_{K1}; and Timothy syndrome (LQTS8) and SQTS and Brugada syndrome, caused by a gain and loss of function of L-type calcium channel.
- C-terminally located missense mutations tend to be clinically benign phenotype compared with those located in the pore region.
- *KCNH2* and *KCNQ1* mutations exerting a dominant-negative effect (i.e., mutations that cause >50% reduction in channel function) may lead to a more malignant outcome than nonpore mutations, which tend to cause haploinsufficiency (i.e., mutations that cause ≤50% reduction in channel function).
- LQT1 patients who are carriers of *KCNQ1* mutations located in the transmembrane portion of the KCNQ1 protein tend to have worst outcome.
- Family members may carry the same mutation but manifest the disease with variable clinical symptoms.
- This may be due to polymorphisms located on LQTS genes which may profoundly impact cardiac repolarization and the effect of the primary mutation. Five to 7% of LQTS probands carry more than one mutation. This may affect the severity of clinical manifestations among family members.
- Some of these inherited channelopathies appear to be mirror images of each other:
  - SQTS1 and LQTS2, caused by gain and loss of function of I_{Kr}
  - SQTS2 and LQTS1, caused by gain and loss of function of I_{Ks}
  - SQTS 3 and Andersen–Tawil syndrome (LTQS7), caused by gain and loss of function of I_{K1}
  - Timothy syndrome (LQTS8) and the new clinical entity comprised of SQTS and Brugada syndrome, caused by a gain and loss of function of L-type calcium channel.

Micro RNA
- MicroRNAs are small RNA fragments of 22 and 61 nucleotides.
- 34 different miRs are specific to the heart
- Activity of the miRs can regulate ion channels by decreasing RNA availability for the transcription of the ion channel subunits. Loss of these subunits would lead to a rapid loss of functional channels, giving a mechanism for molecular changes under physiological or pathological stress.
- There are two miR-1 targets: Kir2.1, a channel responsible for the inward rectifier K+ current (I_{K1}), and connexin-43 (Cx43), the primary gap junction

protein in the ventricle. These channels, which maintenance conduction velocity in the heart, were decreased in ventricular tissue in the presence of increased miR-1, resulting in slowing of conduction and a propensity for arrhythmias.

- In AF as compared with ventricular arrhythmias miR-1 is decreased with reciprocal increase in Kir2.1.
- Contraction duration in symptomatic LQTS mutation carriers tends to be longer in the subendocardium than in the midmyocardium, indicating transmural mechanical dispersion, which is not present in asymptomatic and healthy individuals.
- The *NOS1AP* (nitric oxide) gene influences cardiac repolarization within the normal physiological range.

T wave and U wave

- Multiple structural, metabolic, genetic, autonomic, psychological, and pharmacologic factors affect T-wave appearance.
- Similar T-wave patterns can be caused by diverse conditions and often are difficult to distinguish.
- Some relatively specific T-wave patterns (e.g., those corresponding to genetic forms of long QT syndrome or proximal left anterior descending artery occlusion) have been identified, most of the less prominent T-wave changes are bundled under the term nonspecific.
- The T wave reflects ventricular repolarization.
- Termination of the T wave is usually coincident with the closure of the aortic valve and termination of mechanical systole.
- The U wave follows the T wave as a separate wave under physiological conditions and begins with the second heart sound at the beginning of ventricular relaxation.
- The U wave is usually monophasic positive, best visible within a heart rate range of 50 to 100 bpm and the amplitude seldom exceeds 0.2 mV.
- Unlike the QT interval, the interval from the end of the T wave to the apex of the U waves is nearly rate independent.
- After a sudden increase of the cycle length during atrial fibrillation or after premature beats, the timing of the U wave does not change but it leads to an encroachment of the T wave by the U wave.
- The U wave is often difficult to differentiate from the T wave under pathophysiological conditions such as long QT syndrome.
- The origin of the U wave remains controversial possibilities include electrical or a mechanoelectrical phenomenon.
- The three major hypotheses for the origin of the U wave are that it is caused by:
  1 Repolarization of the His Purkinje system, unlikely because tissue mass is too small to register on the surface ECG. Moreover, the interval between the end of the T wave and the apex of the U wave is constant at different heart rates, whereas the difference between Purkinje action potential duration and that of ventricular muscle increases as heart rate slows and decreases at faster rates.

2 Repolarization of papillary muscle or M cells, Unlikely because M cells are responsible for a second component of the T wave, often confused as an accentuated or inverted U wave. Terms T1 and T2 are used to describe the two contiguous repolarization waves or bifurcated T wave, which is distinct from the U wave. The T wave and U wave are separate deflections, as could be shown in patients with acute myocardial ischemia, in which the monophasic transformed ventricular complex is independent of the shape and timing of the U wave.

3 Stretch-induced DAD caused by distension of the ventricular wall during diastole, a mechanoelectrical effect. It suggests the origin of the U wave as afterpotential that is caused by stretching of the circular muscle layers of the left ventricle. U wave coincides with ventricular relaxation.

- The end of the T wave coincides with the second heart sound.
- Mechanical function is unaltered in SQTS patients despite a dramatic acceleration of repolarization. Ejection times, isovolumic contraction, and relaxation were not significantly different in SQTS and control groups.
- These results suggest that the marked abbreviation of the ventricular action potential has little effect on the time course of the calcium transient, cell shortening, or mechanical contraction of the ventricles.
- Such independence of mechanical systole from changes in repolarization forces is also evident in patients with a long QT syndrome, in which the time course of mechanical systole is similar to that of control subjects.
- In patients with SQTS, the U wave is separated from the T wave by >100 ms,
- The timing of aortic valve closure and the start of isovolumic relaxation coincided with the beginning of the U wave.
- The U wave is the only component of the ventricular complex on the electrocardiogram (ECG) that cannot be derived from the ventricular action potential.
- The maximal amplitude of the U wave (usually in leads V2–V3) ranges from 3 to 24% of the T wave and seldom exceeds 0.2 mV, even when ventricular relaxation accelerates during sympathetic stimulation.
- Negative U-wave in lead where it should be positive is a marker of cardiac pathology.

LQT1

- It is due to mutation of gene *KCNQ1* located on chromosome 11. It is the most common form of mutation.
- Loss-of-function mutations in the gene *KCNQ1* encoding the Kv7.1 K$^+$ channel cause long QT syndrome type 1 (LQT1).
- KCNQ1 channels (Q1) co-assemble with KCNE1 β-subunits (E1), forming a channel that generates the slowly activating delayed rectifier K+ current IKs.
- In LQT1 T waves are broad based (Figure 7.9).
- Alleles for the long QT syndrome are more often transmitted to daughters than to sons.
- Mutation in *KCNQ1* and *KCNE1* results in Jervell and Lange–Nielsen (JLN) syndrome. It is accompanied by deafness. QT prolongation in this syndrome

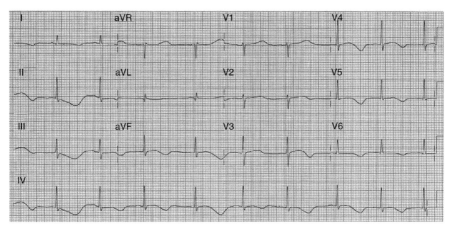

Figure 7.9 Broad T waves. T wave alternance in LQT1.

is autosomal dominant and deafness is transmitted as autosomal recessive disorder.

- Romano Ward syndrome presents as QT prolongation without deafness.
- JLN phenotype occurs when an offspring inherits mutant *KCNQ1* gene from both parents and is therefore homozygous. This results in deafness. Parents are heterozygous and are not deaf.
- It is due to single residue substitution such as replacement of alanine by valine or glutamic acid. This results in amino acid change and loss of function.
- In patients with LQT1 sympathetic stimulation prolongs QT interval and causes torsades de pointes. Sympathetic stimulation abbreviates APD in epicardium and endocardium but not in M cells resulting in transmural dispersion.
- Different response of the three cell types to adrenergic stimulation is related to level of augmentation of I_{Ks}, which is strong in epicardium and endocardium and weak in M cells.
- Augmented I_{Ks} in epicardium and endocardium abbreviates APD and causes dispersion of repolarization and broad base T waves.
- Potassium channel openers shorten the QT interval in LQT1.
- Beta-blockers may be useful for the treatment of patients with LQT1, because it inhibits isoproterenol induced transmural dispersion of repolarization. Beta-blockers may help LQT2 but not LQT3 patients (Table 7.4).
- Kv7.1, encoded by *KCNQ1*, is the α-subunit of the channel responsible for I_{Ks}.
- Co-expression of KCNQ1 with minK-encoding *KCNE1* yields currents that resemble I_{Ks}.
- I_{Ks} is markedly enhanced by β-adrenergic stimulation through channel phosphorylation by protein kinase A (requiring A-kinase anchoring proteins [AKAPs]) and protein kinase C (requiring minK).
- I_{Ks} contributes to repolarization, especially when β-adrenergic stimulation is present.
- I_{Ks} block prolongs AP duration minimally under baseline conditions but markedly under β-adrenergic stimulation

- The KCNE family includes KCNE2 to KCNE5, also known as minK-related peptides or MiRP1–MiRP4)
- In heterologous expression KCNQ1 can associate with each of the KCNE2–KCNE5 subunits.
- Missense mutation annotated as p.Arg231Cys (R231C-Q1) has been reported in LQT1, *KCNQ1-A341V* mutation is a malignant mutation.
- The I_{Ks} current is a major contributor to cardiac action potential repolarization.
- Loss of function of this channel may result in prolongation of action potential duration and QT interval causing long QT syndrome types 1 and 5.
- Gain-of-function mutation in I_{Ks}, which shortens APD, will result in shortening of the QT interval in the ventricle and in the atria.
- In a familial form of AF due to a serine to glycine substitution at amino acid 140 (S140G) in *KCNQ1* results in a gain of function in the I_{Ks} current.
- Affected family members may paradoxically exhibit a prolonged long QT interval.
- IKs is essential for cardiac action potential repolarization, especially when β-adrenergic tone is high or when the rapid delayed rectifier (I_{Kr}) current is suppressed.

LQT2[25–27]

- It is due to mutation of the gene *KCNH2* located on chromosome 7. It is responsible for expression of the protein HERG and codes for α subunit of the I_{Kr} channel, a rapidly activating delayed rectifier potassium current.
- LQT2 is characterized by low amplitude notched T waves (Figure 7.10).
- d-Sotalol, an I_{Kr} blocker, mimics LQT2 and acquired LQTS. It causes greater prolongation of APD in M cells and slows phase-3 repolarization in all the cell layers. This results in prolongation of QT interval and low amplitude T waves.
- Hypokalemia and I_{Kr} block results in marked slowing of repolarization and low amplitude notched T waves.
- The start of the T wave corresponds to the onset of epicardial AP plateau. Final repolarization of epicardium causes peak of second component of T wave. Final repolarization of M cells defines end of T wave.
- Exogenous administration of potassium may correct repolarization abnormality in LQT2 and in acquired LQTS.
- Nicorandil, a potassium channel opener, abbreviates long QT interval and reduces transmural dispersion in LQT1 and LQT2 that are secondary to reduced I_{Ks} and I_{Kr} respectively.
- LQTS-related cardiac events, during a 40-week postpartum interval, may occur in women harboring mutations in *KCNH2* (LQT-2).
- Members of the ether-a-go-go (ERG) K[+] channel family are expressed in endocrine cells and in the nervous system. Anterior pituitary cells express ERG channels, and blockade of these channels by the class III antiarrhythmic agent E-4031 leads to cell membrane depolarization and increased excitability, which, in turn, may perturb prolactin secretion by these cells[16].

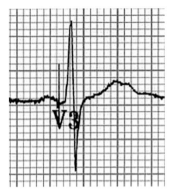

Figure 7.10 Notched T wave in LQT2.

- Symptomatic triggers in congenital LQT are gene specific:
- In LQT1 often after continuous physical exercise (swimming)
- Startled auditory stimuli in LQT2.
- α1 adrenergic stimulation may result in prolongation of action potential duration of his Purkinje fibers in long QT syndrome. Patients with LQT2 who do not respond to beta-blockers may respond to α1- and beta-blockers (e.g., labetalol).
- Patients with drug-induced LQTS have underlying subclinical genetic mutations that become clinically manifest when treated by QT-prolonging medications.
- All patients with LQTS, including those with suspected but unconfirmed diagnosis should avoid QT-prolonging medications.
- Newly developed drugs undergo for their "torsadogenic potential," limited data are collected for the "Brugadogenic potential" of these drugs.
- Methadone has been used to treat opiate addiction for almost 50 years. It is an I_{Kr} channel blocker that can provoke torsades de pointes.
- Drugs that either block the I_{Kr} channel or, use the same metabolic pathway (CYP3A4) may increase the serum level of the parent compound and result in QT prolongation.

LQT3

- Ten per cent of genotype-positive LQTS subjects carry mutations in *SCN5A* encoding the major cardiac voltage gated sodium channel NaV1.5 resulting in LQT3 disease subtype.
- LQTS-associated *SCN5A* mutations confer a gain-of-function characterized by impaired inactivation and increased persistent sodium current.
- Mutation of *CAV3*, *SCN4B* and *SNTA1* that encode proteins that interact with NaV1.5 may result in increased persistent sodium current and prolongation of QT interval.
- The mutant *CAV3* results in a two- to threefold increase in late sodium current similar to the increased late sodium current associated with LQT3-associated *SCN5A* mutations.

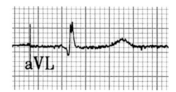

Figure 7.11 Stretched out ST and normal appearing T LQT3.

- The mutation is in cardiac sodium channel gene, *SCN5A* located on chromosome 3. This mutation results in sustained inward current during repolarization resulting in gain of function and prolongation of APD in M cells, increase in QT interval and late appearing T waves (Figure 7.11). M cells exhibit a large late sodium current.
- Mutation in same sodium channel without gain of function causes Brugada syndrome.
- Single amino acid substitution of *SCN5A* at residue 1623 causes LQT3, however similar mutation at position 1620 causes Brugada syndrome.
- Mexiletine causes I_{Na} block in M cells resulting in abbreviation of APD and QT interval in LQT3. This effect may be of value in treatment of LQT1, LQT2, and LQT3.
- Increase heart rate, spontaneous or pacing induced, will abbreviate the slow kinetic of late Na current and shorten the QT interval in LQT3.
- Bradycardia either spontaneous (during sleep) or drug induced (beta-blockers) will prolong APD and QT interval in LQT3 patients.
- Mexiletine and other sodium channel blocking drugs suppress persistent sodium current and may correct the QT interval in subjects with LQT3.
- Ranolazine, a blocker of physiologic plateau sodium current, has been demonstrated to suppress persistent Na current for certain LQT3 mutations.
- Blocking sodium channels in the setting of LQT3 may sometimes evoke ECG changes of Brugada syndrome.
- *SCN5A* mutation resulting in gain of function may play a role in atrial fibrillation. Flecainide may be useful in the treatment of both conditions.
- β-adrenergic receptor antagonists, are less efficacious in LQT3.
- LQT3 patients seem to have less frequent arrhythmic events but a greater propensity to die despite beta-blocker therapy.
- Sudden death may be the first symptom.
- Beta-blockers may be less effective rather than contraindicated in LQT3 patients.
- A *SCN5A* mutation does not automatically imply that it is disease-causing.
- Thus, asymptomatic LQT3 subjects have a good prognosis as is the case in Brugada syndrome.
- ICD therapy should not be recommended for all LQT3 patients but may be considered in asymptomatic LQT3 subjects with excessive QT prolongation and/or other possible markers for cardiac events, such as T-wave alternans, prolonged sinus pauses, strong family history of sudden cardiac death, and/or a functionally significant *SCN5A* mutation.

- LQT3 genotype carriers who are older than 40 years may have higher cumulative lethal event rate compared with LQT1, or LQT2.
- Sodium channel blocker mexiletine may shorten the QT interval by an average of 90 ms.
- Response to mexiletine may not be consistent and may be mutation specific. Similar results have been reported for flecainide.
- Ranolazine, which reduces late sodium channel current, shorten QTc interval in patients with LQT3-ΔKPQ mutation.
- ECG response may not correlate with clinical efficacy.

LQT4[28]
- LQT4 has been linked to mutations in *ANK2*, which encodes the structural protein ankyrin-B that, when mutated, results in altered localization and expression of ion channels.
- Patients with *ANK2* mutations do not uniformly have prolonged QT intervals.
- Mutations in *ANK2* represent a nonchannel form of LQTS.
- Mutations in *CAV3* also represent a nonchannel form of long QT syndrome.
- LQT4 may present with "sick sinus syndrome associated with bradycardia."

LQT5
- It is caused by mutation of gene *KCNE1* located on chromosome 21. This gene is responsible for expression of the protein MinK which co assembles with protein KvLQT1 to form I_{Ks}.
- A mutation in *KCNE1*, the 129 amino acid single membrane-spanning peptide β-subunit that associates with the voltage-gated KCNQ1, results in loss of function of slow delayed rectifier current (I_{Ks}), which causes the long QT syndrome type 5 (LQT5).
- This mutation, Y81C, is located in the post-transmembrane domain region of the KCNE1 (minK) channel in close proximity to three other LQT5 mutations (S74L, D76N, and W87R).

LQTS6
- It is due to mutation of the gene *KCNE2* located on chromosome 21. It is responsible for the expression of the protein MiRP1. It codes for the β subunit of the I_{Kr} channel. Defect results in faster deactivation of the current.

Andersen–Tawil syndrome (ATS) LQTS7[29,30]
- ATS (LQT7) is autosomal-dominant characterized by skeletal muscle periodic paralysis, distinctive facial, frequent ectopy, but relatively rare episodes of TdP, secondary to loss of function (dominant-negative) mutations in *KCNJ2*, which encodes Kir2.1, the channel conducting the inward rectifier current I_{K1}.
- Thirty percent of ATS patients do not have an identifiable mutation in *KCNJ2*.
- There are no obvious phenotypic differences that distinguish individuals with and those without a mutation in *KCNJ2*.

- It is not clear if patients with *KCNJ2* mutations are at greater, lower, or similar risk of life-threatening arrhythmias compared with those who are *KCNJ2*-mutation negative.
- ATS is notable for its variable penetrance (not all subjects manifest all three phenotypes) and variable expressivity (the severity of the expressed phenotype varies considerably). The neuromuscular manifestations of ATS consist of intermittent weakness, often in the setting of progressive interictal weakness.
- The distinctive physical characteristics include low-set ears, micrognathia, syndactyly, clinodactyly, short stature, and scoliosis.
- Cardiac manifestations of ATS include QT and QU interval prolongation, prominent U waves, frequent premature ventricular contractions (PVCs), polymorphic VT, and bidirectional VT.
- Burden of ventricular ectopy is often high, degeneration into life-threatening arrhythmias is relatively uncommon
- Distinguishing individuals with stable but frequent ventricular ectopy and those at risk of sudden cardiac death remains a challenge.
- It results in disorder of both cardiac and skeletal muscle excitability. ATS is unique among ion channelopathies, implying a defect in an ion channel expressed in both tissues.
- Variable expressivity is typical of ATS with individual *KCNJ2* mutation carriers manifesting any or none of the classic triad features
- Symptoms such as syncope and sudden cardiac death are rare.
- Despite frequent episodes of polymorphic and bidirectional VT, ATS patients are often asymptomatic and unaware of their underlying rhythm disturbance.
- Pharmacological therapy is not effective at reducing the frequency of ventricular ectopy.
- Many ATS patients are asymptomatic in the face of a large tachycardia burden some are at risk for life-threatening events. These patients may benefit from ICD implant.
- Reduced Kir2.1 current contributes to the development of DAD and ventricular arrhythmias in Andersen syndrome.
- U-wave is modulated by either an I_{K1} decrease or an I_{K1} increase with a corresponding increase or decrease of its amplitude.
- The terminal part of the action potential is predominantly regulated by the inward rectifier repolarizing current I_{K1}.

Timothy syndrome (LQT8)[31]

- Timothy syndrome, also referred to as LQT8, is a rare congenital disorder characterized by multiorgan dysfunction, including prolongation of the QT interval, lethal arrhythmias, webbing of fingers and toes, congenital heart disease, immune deficiency, intermittent hypoglycemia, cognitive abnormalities, and autism.
- Timothy syndrome has been linked to loss of voltage-dependent inactivation due to mutations in *CACNA1C*, the gene that encodes CaV1.2, the α-subunit of the calcium channel.

- Mutations in *CACNA1C* encoding the L-type calcium channel cause a "gain of function" of I_{Ca} due to slowed inactivation, which directly prolongs the QT interval similar to the other forms of LQTS.

LQT9

- Genes *CAV3*, which encodes caveolin-3, and *SCN4B*, which encodes NavB4, an auxiliary subunit of the cardiac sodium channel.
- Caveolin-3 spans the plasma membrane twice, forming a hairpin structure on the surface, and is the main constituent of caveolae, which are small invaginations in the plasma membrane.
- Mutations in *CAV3* and *SCNB4* both produce a gain of function in late I_{Na}, causing an LQT3-like phenotype.
- *SCN5A*-encoded cardiac sodium channel localized in caveolae, whose major component in the striated muscle is caveolin-3 (CAV3).
- Mutations in *CAV3* may result in LQTS.
- There are four mutations in *CAV3*-encoded caveolin-3. The mutant *CAV3* results in a two- to threefold increase in late sodium current compared with wild-type *CAV3*.
- It is similar to the increased late sodium current due to *SCN5A* mutations associated with LQT3.
- Caveolins has been incriminated in the pathogenesis of cancer, atherosclerosis and vasculoproliferative diseases, cardiac hypertrophy and heart failure, muscular dystrophies, and diabetes mellitus.

Clinical presentation[32]

- One in 3000–5000 persons is a carrier of LQTS gene. Sixty percent of gene carriers may present with syncope in early teen years. Three to four thousand children and young adults may succumb to sudden death each year[15].
- Recurrent syncope and resuscitated cardiac arrest are the hallmark of high risk patient. Sudden death may be the first manifestation of the LQTS.
- During follow up, 30% of cardiac arrest survivors may have recurrence and 19% of patients who present with syncope may continue to have symptoms inspite of beta-blockers[15].
- Some gene carriers may have normal QTc yet may suffer from syncope or cardiac arrest.
- Ten percent of family members of LQTS patients who have QT interval of less than 440 may present with cardiac arrest
- Patients may present with syncope or cardiac arrest due to Tdp. There is usually a family history of syncope, long QT or sudden death. Thirty percent of LQTS cases are sporadic without family history.
- Sudden infant death (SID) could be due to LQTS.
- In patients with LQTS1, SCD may occur during increased sympathetic activity such as fright, anger, sudden awakening or physical activity such as exercise or emotional stress however in patients with LQTS3 it may occur during sleep.

- Symptoms may be caused or aggravated by QT prolonging drugs and hypokalemia.
- Occurrence of cardiac events at rest or during sleep is commonly seen in LQT2 and LQT3.
- LQTS1 and LQTS2 are likely to be symptomatic. LQTS3 is more likely to be lethal. LQT4 patients may have PAF.
- Homozygous *KVLQT1* and *KCNE1* mutations are associated with congenital deafness (Jarvell and Lange–Nielsen syndrome).
- Compared to the background prevalence of 0.1%, early-onset AF may occur in almost 2% of patients with genetically proven LQTS.
- The average age at diagnosis of AF is 25 years (range 4–46 years).
- Early-onset AF (age <50 years) is more common in patients with LQTS.

Electrocardiographic features[33]

- Electrocardiographic changes consist of prolongation of QT interval corrected for the heart rate and measured in LII.
- In patients with LQTS1 T waves tend to be smooth and broad (Figure 7.10), however it tends to be low amplitude and notched in LQTS2. Late onset but normal appearing T waves are seen in LQTS3.
- The QT interval, corrected for the heart rate, of 440 ms in male and 460 ms in females is considered as abnormal. QT interval becomes longer after puberty in females.
- The extent of QT prolongation does not correlate with symptoms. Marked prolongation of the QT interval (more than 600 ms) may be associated with Tdp.
- T wave abnormalities are more noticeable in precordial leads.
- The appearance of notched T wave during recovery phase of exercise is seen in LQTS patients but not in control subjects.
- QT dispersion is common in patients with LQTS.
- Dispersion of repolarization improves after anti-adrenergic therapy.
- The persistence of QT dispersion after beta-blocker therapy identifies high-risk patients.
- T wave alternans is a marker of electrical instability. It is generally seen during emotional or physical stress in patients with LQTS. It identifies high-risk patients.
- Patients with LQTS may have sinus pauses and bradycardia. These changes may precede occurrence of Tdp.
- Echocardiogram may show increase rate of thickening in early phase of systole and slowing of thickening and plateau in late phase.
- Verapamil may normalize contraction, may be due to decrease in intracellular calcium and EAD.
- Paradoxical prolongation of the QT interval by >30 ms, on infusion of the epinephrine at a rate of 0.025–0.3 µg/kg/min for 5 minutes may identify patients who otherwise have borderline QT prolongation. Sensitivity and negative predictive value is high[19].

Molecular genetics and risk stratification[34]

- Screening for gene mutation should be limited to patients and family members in whom the clinical diagnosis of LQTS is clear or suspected[5].
- Abnormal gene test confirms the diagnosis; however, a negative test does not exclude LQTS.
- Screening of asymptomatic carriers may help in counseling about use of certain drugs, anesthesia or prenatal planning[4].
- Mexiletine, a sodium channel blocker, may shorten QT interval in LQT3 and to a lesser extent in LQT1 and LQT2.
- Three percent of LQT1 patients and 61% of the patients with LQT3 had cardiac event during sleep.
- Ninety-seven percent of patients with LQT1 had a cardiac event during physical or emotional stress while 33% with LQT3 had such events.
- Patients with LQT2 behave more like LQT3. Both these groups have normal I_{Ks}.
- Among LQTS gene carriers only 14 to 33% may have phenotype expression.
- Silent carriers may have ventricular arrhythmias on exposure to certain triggers such as QT prolonging drugs or hypokalemia.
- The probability of successfully identifying genotype by molecular method is 30–50% because of the lack of knowledge about all the possible genes involved in LQTS.
- Molecular diagnosis is 100% sensitive and specific for affected family members of a genotype proband.
- An asymptomatic gene carrier may need counseling about the reproductive risks and the risk of exposure to certain drugs.
- Syncope or cardiac arrest is the presenting symptom in majority of the probands.
- LQTS is common among females.
- Nitric oxide synthase 1 adaptor protein (NiOS1AP) gene may be associated with QT-interval variation.
- C-terminally located missense mutations result in clinically more benign phenotype compared with those located in the pore region.
- Mutations in the pore region of the *KCNH2* gene are at increased risk for arrhythmia-related cardiac events compared to patients with nonpore mutations.
- LQT1 patients who are carriers of *KCNQ1* mutations located in the transmembrane portion of the protein have a poor prognosis.
- Five to 7% of LQTS probands carry more than one mutation and poor outcome,
- *KCNH2* and *KCNQ1* mutations exerting a dominant-negative effect (i.e., mutations that cause >50% reduction in channel function) may lead to a more malignant outcome than nonpore mutations, which tend to cause haploinsufficiency (i.e., mutations that cause ≤50% reduction in channel function).
- Family members may carry same mutation but manifest variable clinical manifestations.

Risk factors for sudden cardiac death in long QT syndrome[35]

1 Personal history of aborted sudden cardiac death.
2 T-wave alternans.
3 Prolonged sinus pauses.

4 QTc exceeding 550 to 600 ms.
5 Syncope.
6 Female gender.
7 More than one mutation in the same patient.
8 Age: occurrence of events in the first year of life.
9 History of death of a sibling is associated with an increased risk of syncope. It is not associated with an increased risk of aborted cardiac arrest or death.
10 QTc ≥ 0.53 is strongly associated with an increased risk of any cardiac event, including aborted cardiac arrest and death.
11 Personal history of syncope is associated with aborted cardiac arrest or death, particularly if the syncope was recent.
   • Beta-blockade is associated with a reduction in the risk of aborted cardiac arrest or death. Iindividual expression of the LQTS trait, not the penetrance of the gene mutation within a family, is important for risk assessment.
   • Each family member with a suspected or confirmed inherited channelo-pathy must be evaluated clinically for risk without regard for severity of symptoms among siblings.

Therapeutic options in LQTS[36,37]

Gene-specific therapy for LQTS (Table 7.4)[38]
• Potassium channel openers shortens QT interval in LQT1.
• Beta-blockers reduce incidence of syncope and sudden cardiac death in patients with congenital LQTS1 by inhibiting adrenergic induced transmural dispersion of repolarization[7].
• LQT1 events occur during exercise and emotion, beta-blockers are likely to be effective in this group.
• Exogenous administration of potassium and increase in extracellular potassium may correct repolarization abnormality in LQT2 and acquired LQTS.
• Beta-blockers may be useful in treating patients with LQTS2
• Nicorandil, a potassium channel opener, abbreviates long QT interval and reduces transmural dispersion in LQT1 and LQT2 which are secondary to reduced I_{Ks} and I_{Kr} respectively.
• There is no need to limit physical activity if QT shortens during exercise test.
• Na channel blocker Mexiletine, which suppresses the late reopening of sodium channel shortens QT interval in LQT3.
• Niflumic acid, an I_{Ks} activator, has been shown to shorten QT in LQT1 and LQT5.
• M cells have a large late I_{Na}. Mexiletine causes I_{Na} block in M cells resulting in abbreviation of APD. This effect may be of value in treatment of LQT1, LQT2 and LQT3.
• Pacemaker are likely to be effective in LQT3, as faster heart rate will abbreviate the slow kinetic of late Na current and shortens QT interval. Permanent pace-maker may be helpful in preventing bradycardia during rest and sleep.
• These patients may be at a lesser risk of syncope during exercise. Beta- blockers are likely to be less effective or even contraindicated in LQT3.
• Mortality in untreated patients is 20% in the first year and 50% in 5 years. Those patients who were treated with beta-blockers had yearly mortality of 0.9%.

- Incidence of sudden cardiac death as a first event is 7%.
- Propranolol, 2–3 mg/kg, remains initial choice of therapy in symptomatic patients.
- Nadolol, because of its longer half-life, could also be used effectively in LQTS patients.
- Patients with spontaneous (LQTS3) or drug-induced bradycardia may benefit from pacemaker insertion.
- In patients who present with cardiac arrest there may be 13% reoccurrence in spite of treatment with beta blockers. These patients may benefit from ICD.
- Patients who have reoccurrence of syncope in spite of β Blockers should be considered for ICD.
- A pacemaker should be considered in patients with bradycardia; however it should never be considered as a sole therapy for LQTS and must be used in conjunction with beta-blockers.
- Patients with LQT3 who have bradycardia at rest may benefit from a pacemaker.
- Twenty percent of patients with LQTS may need a pacemaker.
- ICD should be programmed with a long detection interval to avoid recurrent shocks for self-terminating TDP. Rate smoothing feature may prevent pauses[3].
- Post shock pacing should be programmed at a faster rate to avoid pauses and bradycardia that might reinduce TDP.
- Patients with long QT syndrome, type 1 (LQT1) experience most cardiac events during exercise; only 3% of arrhythmic episodes occur during rest or sleep.
- Beta-blockers are effective in this group of patients.
- Ninety percent of LQT1 patients treated with beta-blockers may remain free of arrhythmic recurrences.
- Cardiac events in LQT3 patients occur at rest or during sleep (65%) and occasionally occur during exercise (4%). In this group of patients, beta-blockers are less effective; more than 32% of patients experience symptoms despite therapy.
- Beta-blockers are extremely effective in LQTS1.
- Beta-blockers noncompliance and use of QT-prolonging drug are responsible for almost all life-threatening "BB failures."
- Beta-blockers are appropriate therapy for asymptomatic patients and those without his trio cardiac arrest.
- Routine implantation of cardiac defibrillators in such patients does not appear justified.
- Diabetes mellitus and QTc-affecting drugs determined QTc prolongation and may be predictors of SCD in coronary artery disease.
- Idiopathic abnormal QTc prolongation may result in fivefold increased odds of SCD.
- High risk patients presenting with T-wave alternans or the appearance of prolonged sinus pauses or a QTc exceeding 550 to 600 ms, syncope should be considered for prophylactic ICD implant and or left cardiac sympathetic denervation (LCSD).
- If the patient presents with cardiac arrest, consider implant an ICD, initiate or continue with β-blockers, and then perform LCSD to minimize the probability of shocks.

Table 7.5 Treatment options in LQTS.

Electrocardiogram	Symptoms	Family history	Treatment
Prolong QTc	None	None	None
Prolong QTc	None	SCD, syncope due to LQTS	Beta-blockers
Prolong QTc	Syncope	SCD, syncope due to LQTS	Beta-blockers, ICD
Prolong QTc	SCD		Beta-blockers, ICD

Management of asymptomatic patients with LQTS (Table 7.5)

- Sudden death may be the first manifestation in 7 to 9% of patients with LQTS. This risk tends to be higher in LQT3 than LQT1.
- All the patients with LQTS should be treated with β blockers
- Beta-blockers should be strongly considered in patients with LQTS and congenital deafness, neonate and infants in first year, history of sudden death in a sibling, T wave alternans, QTc greater than 600 ms and a request from family members.
- Family members should be educated about CPR.
- Patient should be provided with a list of drugs that could prolong QT interval.
- All symptomatic patients and asymptomatic children with LQTS1 and LQTS2 should be treated with beta blockers but not those with LQTS3.
- Raising serum potassium level may shorten the QT interval in LQTS2.
- Patients with LQTS3 may benefit from the Na channel blocker mexiletine.

Left cardiac sympathetic denervation

LCSD could be considered in patients with:

- Syncope only despite beta-blocker therapy. Surgical antiadrenergic therapy effectively complements pharmacologic therapy and becomes sufficient for most patients.
- Patients already implanted with an ICD who receive multiple appropriate shocks.
- To reduce the frequency of shocks lengthen the ventricular tachycardia detection time, thus allowing brief self-terminating episodes of torsades de pointes to end spontaneously and program post shock pacing at a higher rate and for a longer duration to avoid pauses.
- Unilateral.
- Stellate ganglion ablation (right or left) results in:
  - 70% increase in threshold for ventricular fibrillation,
  - Lack of ensuing postdenervation supersensitivity.
- Thus, after LCSD it is more difficult to fibrillate and the effect is permanent because following preganglionic denervation there is no reinnervation.
- Lower half of the left stellate ganglion is removed together with the first four thoracic ganglia. The upper half of the stellate ganglion should remain intact in order to avoid Horner syndrome.

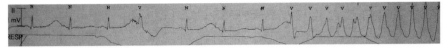

Figure 7.12 This ECG strip demonstrates prolong QT interval, T wave alternans and pause dependent TDP.

Table 7.6 Drugs causing LQT and TDP.[23]

Antiarrhythmics	Disopyramide, procainamide, quinidine, amiodarone, bretylium, sotalol
Antimicrobial	Erythromycin, trimethoprim-sulfa
Antihistamine	Astemizole, terfenadine
Antifungal	Fluconazole, itraconazole, ketoconazole.
Antiprotozoal	Chloroquine, pentamidine, quinine, mefloquine, halofantrine
Psychotropic	Chloral hydrate, haloperidol, lithium, phenothiazines, pimozide, tricyclic antidepressants
GI prokinetic	Cisapride.
Other	Indapamide, probucol, amantadine, tacrolimus, vasopressin
HypoK Hypo Mg induced by	Diuretics, steroids, cathartics, liquid protein diet.

Torsade de Pointes (TDP)[39]

- First described by Dessertenne as twisting of the QRS morphology around a imaginary axis. Dessertenne described torsade de pointes (TdP) as a ventricular arrhythmia having *"tantôt la pointe en haut et tantôt la pointe en bas,"* which in electrocardiographic terms means a twisting of the QRS complexes.
- Torsade de Pointes (TDP) is a polymorphic VT associated with LQTS (Figure 7.12).
- Quinidine and hypokalemia produce EAD and triggered activity resulting in TDP (Table 7.6).
- The initial event in TDP is EAD induced triggered activity.
- TDP often occurs fallowing a short long short cycle length.
- The term TDP should be reserved for polymorphic VT associated with LQTS.
- In the absence of LQTS, the term polymorphic VT should be used.
- In addition to twisting of the QRS complexes there may be change in the amplitude.
- LQTS is due to abnormality of potassium and sodium currents. This results in prolongation and dispersion of repolarization, which leads to EAD-induced triggered activity in HPS.
- The balance between inward (Na, Ca and Na/Ca exchange) and outward (K) currents determines duration of repolarization.

Table 7.7 Drugs interfering with cytochrome P-450 enzyme.

Antifungal	Fluconazole, itraconazole, ketoconazole, metronidazole
Serotonin reuptake inhibitors.	Fluoxetine, fluvoxamine, sertraline
HIV protease inhibitors.	Indinavir, ritonavir, saquinavir
Dihydropyridine	Felodipine, nicardipine, nifedipine
Antimicrobial	Erythromycin
Others	Grapefruit juice. Hepatic dysfunction

Table 7.8 Short QT syndrome.

Type	Function	Chromosome	Current	Affected Gene/Channel
SQT1	Gain of Function	7q35	I_{Kr}	KCNH2
SQT2	Gain of Function	11p15	I_{Ks}	KCNQ1
SQT3	Gain of function	17q23.1–24.2	I_{K1}	KCNJ2, Kir2.1
SQT4	Loss of function	12p13.3	I_{Ca}	CACNA1C, CaV1.2
SQT5	Loss of Function	10p12.33	I_{Ca}	CACNB2b, CaVβ2b

- Acquired LQTS can be due to the following mechanisms[21] (Tables 7.7 and 7.8):
  - I_{Ks} or I_{Kr} channel block by quinidine, procainamide, sotalol, cesium and bretylium. These actions can be reversed by potassium channel openers such as pinacidil and cromakalin.
  - Suppression of I_{to} channel in M cells.
  - Increase in I_{Ca} activity.
  - Continuous activation of I_{Na} during repolarization will also result in prolongation of the QT interval. This can be blocked by lidocaine.
- More then one mechanism may be responsible for prolongation of the QT interval.
- Bradycardia and low serum potassium have synergistic effect on prolonging repolarization and inducing TDP.
- High plasma levels of the drugs either due to high dose or lack of clearance may increase the risk of initiating TDP. Reduced clearance may be due to inhibition of the cytochrome P-450 enzyme.
- Bradycardia, short–long cycle length, T wave alternans and hypertrophy results in dispersion of refractoriness and thus may predispose to TDP.
- Neither the ventricular rate nor the QRS width at the time of bradyarrhythmia predicts the risk of TdP. Corrected QT (QTc), and T(peak)–T(end) intervals correlates with the risk of TdP. T(peak)–T(end) interval of >120 ms may indicate high risk for TDP.
- LQT2-like "notched T waves" may occur in patients with TDP

Polymorphic VT and normal QT interval

- It occurs in the presence of structural heart disease and ischemia and normal QT interval.
- Polymorphic VT may occur in the absence of structural heart disease such as in Brugada syndrome which is characterized by RBB pattern, ST segment elevation in V1–V3, normal QT interval.
- Genetic abnormality includes mutation in Na channel *SCN5A* resulting in rapid recovery of sodium channel function form inactivation (opposite of LQT3) or in a nonfunctional sodium channel.

Acquired LQTS

- Bradycardia, hypokalemia and QT prolonging drugs may precipitate TDP.
- The initiating event in TDP is EAD in the presence of dispersion of repolarization.
- IV Magnesium sulfate, increase heart rate by pharmacological agents or by pacing suppresses polymorphic VT.

Short QT syndrome (SQTS)[40,41]

- A diagnosis of SQTS should be considered when patients with QTc <360 ms present with cardiac arrest, malignant syncope, or atrial fibrillation at a young age.
- The cutoff values for short QT intervals were defined as 320 ms (very short) and 340 ms (short).
- The prevalence of QT interval <320 ms is 0.08%, and the prevalence of QT interval <340 ms is 0.3%.
- QTc <330 ms is rare.
- To clarify the diagnosis of "short QT" ECGs should be repeated at different heart rates to assess QT duration and T-wave morphology.
- Patients with SQTS have a flat QTc/R-R relationship. These patients have QTc intervals in the low–normal range at heart rates greater than 80 bpm that fail to prolong adequately at slower heart rates.
- Repeated resting ECGs showing different QT intervals at different heart rates may help distinguish patient with innocent QTc shortening during brady-cardia from the rare SQTS patient with a flat QTc/R-R relationship.
- Healthy males have taller T waves and shorter ST segments than do healthy females, and T-wave amplitude increases as heart rate decreases such characteristics are more striking in SQTS.
- Patients with symptomatic SQTS have tall peaked T waves with a very short J-point to T-wave-peak interval and no flat ST segment (Figure 7.13).
- J_{point}–T_{peak} interval, uncorrected for heart rate, tends to be shorter in SQTS patients.
- An augmented T_{peak}–T_{end} interval may be due to increased TDR.
- An increase in outward repolarizing current can preferentially abbreviate endocardial/M-cell action potential, thus increasing TDR and creating the substrate for reentry.
- Polymorphic VT can be induced with programmed electrical stimulation.

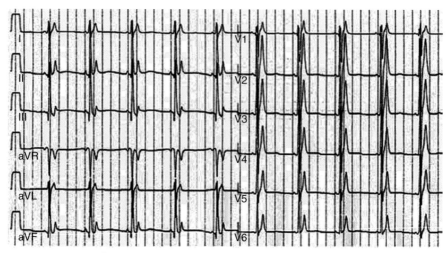

Figure 7.13 Short QT.

- The increase in TDR is accentuated by isoproterenol, leading to easier induction and more persistent VT/VF.
- There is clear separation of the T wave and U wave in patients with SQTS.
- In patients with SQTS, the U wave is separated from the T wave by >100 ms.
- Normal T_{peak}–T_{end}/QT ratio is 0.13 to 0.21. Increase in ratio is associated increased vulnerability to ventricular tachyarrhythmias.
- High T_{peak}–T_{end}/QT ratio on standard 12-lead ECG reflects increased transmural dispersion of repolarization and increased vulnerability to ventricular tachyarrhythmias.
- Subjects with short QT interval without shortened early repolarization and with normal T_{peak}–T_{end}/QT ratio do not seem to be at risk for serious arrhythmias.
- The same relationship has been observed in long QT syndrome, where the threshold value of the T_{peak}–T_{end}/QT ratio of 0.28 differentiated symptomatic from asymptomatic patients
- Normal J_{point}–T_{peak} interval is >150 ms.
- Mechanical function is unaltered in SQTS patients despite a dramatic acceleration of repolarization. Ejection times, isovolumic contraction, and relaxation were not significantly different in SQTS and control groups.
- Short QT syndrome is an inherited syndrome characterized by QTc ≤360 ms and a high incidence of VT/VF in infants, children, and young adults.

Classification of SQTS (Table 7.8)
- SQTS1 is a result of gain of function mutation in *KCNH2* resulting in enhanced I_{Kr}.
- SQTS2 is aresult of missense mutation in *KCNQ1* causing gain of function in I_{Ks}.

- SQT3 is caused by mutations in *KCNJ2* and results in overexpression of IKir2.1 and enhanced I_{K1}. It is associated with QTc intervals <330 ms, not quite as short as SQT1, and SQT2.IK1 suppression results in QT-interval prolongation enhanced Kir2.1 expression is associated with familial atrial fibrillation
- SQT4 is caused by loss of function mutations in the gene *α1-CACNA1C* encoding for Cav1.2 calcium channel.
- SQTS5 is a result of mutation in *β-CACNB2b*.
- Mutations in the α- and β-subunits of the calcium channel may also lead to ST-segment elevation, creating a combined Brugada/SQTS.
- In SQT1, SQT2, and SQT3, the ECG commonly displays tall peaked symmetric T waves due to acceleration of phase 3 repolarization.
- SQTS is more common in men. Males tend to have lower heart rate and shorter QTc than females.
- Patients with idiopathic VF have normal QT intervals that fail to prolong during sinus bradycardia.
- All-cause or cardiovascular mortality does not differ between subjects with a very short or short QT interval and those with normal QT intervals (360 to 450 ms).
- There were no sudden cardiac deaths, aborted sudden cardiac deaths, or documented ventricular tachyarrhythmias among subjects with a QTfc <340 ms.
- Short QT interval does not appear to indicate an increased risk for all-cause or cardiovascular mortality in middle-aged individuals.

Arrhythmogenic right ventricular dysplasia/cardiomyopathy[42–44]

- Arrhythmogenic right ventricular cardiomyopathy (ARVC) is an autosomal dominant disease characterized by progressive fibrofatty replacement of the right ventricular myocardium and ventricular arrhythmias heart failure, and sudden cardiac death.
- It affects males disproportionately and carries an increased risk for sudden death, particularly during exercise.

Incidence and prevalence

- The prevalence of the disease in the general population is estimated at 0.02–0.1% or 1 in 5000. Male/female ratio is 2.7/1.0.
- In Italy (Padua, Venice) and Greece (Island of Naxos), prevalence of 0.4–0.8% has been reported.
- Occurrence of ARVD/C in Veneto region of Italy, in some clusters of families, has earned the term Venetian cardiomyopathy.
- ARVD/C is linked to mutations in proteins of the cardiac desmosome, a component of the intercalated disc essential for the mechanical coupling between cardiac cells.
- Disruption of cardiac gap junction integrity caused by recessive mutation of plakoglobin protein forming part of the scaffold of the desmosomes occurs in patients with Naxos disease.
- Naxos disease is characterized by palmoplantar keratosis and woolly hair and has been mapped on chromosome 17q21 which controls plakoglobin

Table 7.9 Type of ARVD and its chromosome location.

ARVD Type	ARVD1	ARVD2	ARVD3	ARVD4	ARVD5	ARVD6	ARVD7	ARVD8
Chromosome location	14q23–q24	1q42–q43	14q12–q22	2q32	3p23	10p12–14	10q22, 6p24	12p11

- Carvajal syndrome is caused by a recessive mutation of the gene leading to truncation of desmoplakin, a protein that is part of the scaffold in the desmosomes, fascia adherens junctions.
- Desmosomes are linked to the intermediate filament system of the cytoskeleton and maintains mechanical continuity of the architecture of heart tissue.
- Molecular change in both Carvajal and Naxos disease consists of a significant decrease of Cx43, a major protein in the gap junction channel that ensures low-resistance coupling between cardiac cells

Genetics/classification of ARVD/C[44]

- Transmission is autosomal dominant (Table 7.9).
- Fifty percent of the ARVD/C families do not show any linkage with the identified chromosomal loci
- There are three major types of myofilaments in heart and skeletal muscle: thick filaments, thin filaments, and intermediate filaments.
- The thick filaments consist of myosin, thin filaments are composed of actin. Intermediate filaments are made up of desmin.
- Intermediate filament links the Z-discs to each other, to the desmosomes and adherens junctions at the cell surface, and to the nuclear membrane.
- As force is generated by thick and thin filaments in the sarcomere, it is transmitted by the intermediate filaments to result in muscle contraction.
- Desmosomes provide a rigid link between neighboring cells, which allows them to withstand mechanical strain.
- In these structures, the extracellular portions of desmosomal cadherins mediate cell adhesion across the cell borders, while their intracellular modules bind to the plaque proteins plakoglobin (PG) and plakophilin, which in turn bind desmoplakin (DSP).
- DSP is associated with intermediate filaments, which establish a mechanical continuum across cells.
- Mutations in desmosomal genes can result in cardiac disease, including arrhythmogenic right ventricular cardiomyopathy (ARVC), cutaneous disorders (palmoplantar keratoderma), and multitissue syndromes (e.g., Naxos disease).
- Desmosomal adhesion is a prerequisite for proper gap junction formation and maintenance at cell–cell contact sites.
- Cx43 is the major ventricular gap junction protein, which ensures electrical coupling of neighboring cardiomyocytes. Changes in Cx43 have been demonstrated in ARVC patients bearing PKP2 mutations.
- The disease is clinically heterogeneous, with interfamilial and intrafamilial variability, ranging from benign to malignant forms with a high risk of sudden

cardiac death. The mode of inheritance is mostly autosomal dominant with incomplete penetrance.
- Mutations have been documented in eight different genes encoding desmosomal proteins:
  - Desmoplakin (DSP, ARVD8),
  - Plakophilin-2 (PKP2, ARVD9),
  - Desmoglein-2 (DSG2, ARVD10),
  - Desmocollin-2 (DSC2, ARVD11),
  - Plakoglobin (JUP, ARVD12)
  - TGFβ3 (ARVD1)
  - TMEM43 (ARVD5)
  - RyR2 (ARVD2)
    1 Mutations of JUP and DSP have been shown to cause recessively inherited ARVC manifesting with palmoplantar keratoderma and woolly hair, named Naxos and Carvajal syndrome, respectively.
    2 The cardiac ryanodine receptor gene RyR2 causes a distinct clinical entity, characterized by juvenile sudden cardiac death and effort-induced polymorphic VT. Whether this is a variant of ARVC/D remains controversial.
- The DES gene encodes desmin, which is a major intermediate filament protein of skeletal and cardiac muscle that provides structural and functional integrity by coordinating mechanical stress transmission, organelle positioning, organization and assembly of sarcomeres, signal transduction, and apoptosis.
- Mutations in the DES gene are associated with a variable clinical phenotype referred to as desmin-related myopathy
- The clinical phenotype encompasses "isolated" myopathies, pure cardiac phenotypes (including dilated cardiomyopathy [DCM] and restrictive cardiomyopathy [RCM]), cardiac conduction disease, and combinations of these disorders.
- Cardiologic and neurologic features may occur; cardiologic features can precede, occur simultaneously with, or follow manifestation of generalized neuromuscular disease.
- More than 40 DES mutations have been identified
- The majority of mutations are located in the α-helical rod domains of the gene.
- Mutations in the 2B segment of desmin are involved in skeletal muscle disease, whereas mutations in the 1B and tail domain cause cardiac disease.
- Inherited forms of both cardiomyopathy and muscular dystrophy are notable for marked genetic heterogeneity.
- Mutations in DES p.S13F may result in a range of phenotypes, from isolated cardiac disease to isolated skeletal muscle disease and various combinations of heart and skeletal muscle involvement.
- Different DES mutations have been reported to result in DCM, HCM, or restrictive cardiomyopathy (RCM), arrhythmogenic right ventricular dysplasia/cardiomyopathy (ARVD/C), but not left ventricular hypertrabeculation.
- All of these structural cardiomyopathies were identified among individuals with the identical DES p.S13F mutation.
- More rapid cardiac than skeletal muscle dysfunction may be due desmin's greater abundance in heart (2%) than skeletal muscle (0.35%), desmin may play a

more prominent role in the right ventricle than in the left. This may help to explain the occurrence of ARVD/C among carriers of the p.S13F DES mutation.

- Fifty percent of individuals with this disorder have a mutation in a component of the cardiac desmosome.
- DES mutations in ARVD/C patients extends this association for ARVD/C from the desmosome to the intermediate filaments,
- In patients with desmin mutation, arrhythmic manifestations are common.
- Conduction block may be present in all mutation carriers with progressive, age-dependent severity. RBBB may be the initial manifestation. SCD may occur.
- Majority of mutation carriers died, had cardiac transplantation, or had appropriate implantable cardioverter-defibrillator firing at young age.
- Severity of heart failure surpasses ARVD/C, and is quite similar to findings of increased cardiac mortality among those with a mutation in LMNA.
- Purkinje fibers contain abundant intermediate filaments composed of desmin which may explain common occurrence of heart block and arrhythmia.
- Lower extremity weakness is commonly seen with desmin mutations.

Pathological features[45,46]

- There is patchy loss of right ventricular myocytes with replacement by fibrofatty tissue and persistence of normal myocardial tissue in between. This may result in area of slow conduction that initiates reentrant ventricular arrhythmias.
- There is thinning of the right ventricular wall.
- Fibrosis contributes to slowing of conduction and provides substrate for arrhythmias.
- Fibrofatty replacement begins in the subepicardium or midmural layers and progresses to the subendocardium. It involves right ventricular outflow tract, apex, and infundibulum.
- It might also affect interventricular septum and posteroseptal and posterolateral wall of the left ventricle.
- Rarely, left ventricular involvement may appear first.
- Inflammatory changes with lymphocyte infiltration may be noted.
- Reduced Cx43 expression, possibly explaining the myocardial conduction delay that is typical of ARVC.
- Cardiac conduction velocity is determined in part by the presence of functional gap junctions. A nonuniform distribution of connexins can promote heterogeneities in conduction velocity that facilitate reentrant electrical activation and contribute to cardiac arrhythmogenesis.

Diagnosis[47]

- The diagnosis of ARVD is based on the presence of major and minor diagnostic criteria as suggested by international task force.
- The diagnosis is established by the presence of two major criteria or one major and two minor criteria or four minor criteria.
- Definite diagnosis of ARVD is made when all the four criteria are met. Diagnosis of probable ARVD is made when fewer criteria are present such as one major and one minor or three minor criterions (Table 7.10).

Table 7.10 Task force criteria for diagnosis of arrhythmogenic right ventricular dysplasia.

Major	Minor
Severe RV dilation, reduction of RV ejection fraction, localized RV aneurysms	Mild RV dilatation and/or reduced ejection fraction
Fibrofatty replacement of myocardium as proven by biopsy	T-wave inversion in leads V1–V3 or beyond (see Figure 7.1)
Epsilon waves or localized QRS prolongation (>110 ms) in leads V1–V3	Late potentials on signal-averaged ECG
Familial disease confirmed at necropsy or surgery	LBBB-type VT (sustained and nonsustained) or frequent PVCs (>1000/24 hours)
	Familial history of premature sudden death (<35 years) or clinical diagnosis based on present criteria

RV = right ventricle.

- Task force recommendations do not incorporate the findings of imaging such as MRI, angiography and echocardiogram nor does it specify which imaging technique should be preferred to examine and grade right ventricular morphology and function.

Electrocardiogram[48,49]
- ECG shows a regular sinus rhythm.
- QRS-duration is >110 ms in lead V1, a terminal deflection within or at the end of the QRS complex called epsilon wave may be present in lead V1–V3 in 30% of patients.
- QRS duration may be longer over right precordial leads (V1–V3) compared with lead V6.
- T-wave inversion in the right precordial leads is noted in 50% of patients (Figure 7.14).
- Signal average EKG tends to be abnormal.
- Holter monitor may show frequent PVCs and nonsustained VT.
- During stress test there may be ST segment changes over right precordial leads.
- During electrophysiologic study VT may be inducible by programmed stimulation.
- Idiopathic right ventricular outflow tract (RVOT) VT is important differential diagnosis of ARVD/C, and MRI, have been used for differentiating the two conditions.
- Twenty percent of patients with RVOT VT may have subtle structural abnormalities on MRI that preclude definitive diagnosis.

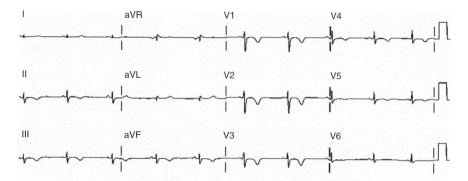

Figure 7.14 Low voltage ECG T wave inversion across precordial leads.

- Interpretation of imaging results (including MRI) is operator dependent Re-evaluation of patients initially diagnosed as having ARVD/C by MRI revealed that only 27% of these patients actually met the task force criteria, and the major cause of "misdiagnosis" was the presence of intramyocardial fat or wall thinning on MRI.
- ECG features in the original task force criteria included inverted T waves in the right precordial leads V2 and V3, epsilon waves, and localized prolongation (>110 ms) of the QRS complex in the right precordial leads V1–V3.
- Epsilon waves, a marker of delayed activation of the right ventricle, are a hallmark feature of ARVD/C and are considered a major criterion.
- Highly specific they lack sensitivity and are seen in only 25–33% of ARVD/C patients when evaluated by standard ECG.
- Use of highly amplified (20 mV) precordial leads and modified limb leads, can increase the detection of epsilon potentials to 75%.
- Other ECG features have been reported as markers of ARVD/C:
  ○ Ratio of QRS duration in V1+V2+V3/V4+V5+V6 ≥1.2,
  ○ Parietal block defined as QRS duration in leads V1–V3 that exceeds the QRS duration in lead V6 by 25 ms.
  ○ S-wave upstroke ≥55 ms in leads V1–V3.
  ○ Prolonged terminal activation duration, defined as the longest value in leads V1–V3 from the nadir of the S wave to the end of all depolarization deflections ≥55 ms.
  ○ QRS fragmentation.
- QRS fragmentation is an indicator of altered electrical activation in the myocardium as a result of structural derangements.
- QRS fragmentation can be used for the diagnosis of ARVD/C along with T-wave inversion if coronary artery disease can be excluded, localized QRS prolongation in right precordial leads and epsilon potentials.

Myocardial biopsy
- It lacks sensitivity as the tissue is obtained from interventricular septum, whereas pathological changes are more noticeable in the free wall of the right ventricle.

RV angiogram
- It shows dyskinetic bulging, localized in outflow tract, apex, and infundibulum the anatomic triangle of dysplasia, and the presence of hypertrophic trabeculae in other areas.

Echocardiography
- It shows right ventricular dilatation, enlargement of the right atrium, isolated dilatation of the right ventricular outflow tract, increased reflectivity of the moderator band, localized aneurysms, and decreased fractional shortening of the right ventricle. There is dyskinesis of the inferior wall and the right ventricular apex.
- In obese patients and in patients with pulmonary emphysema, transesophageal echocardiography is the preferred approach to visualize the right ventricle.
- Radionuclide angiography may demonstrate abnormal right ventricular function, but it is not an optimum imaging technique for ARVD/C.

Computed tomography
- It may demonstrate a dilated hypokinetic right ventricle, abundant epicardial fat, intramyocardial fat deposits and conspicuous trabeculation with low attenuation.
- Multislice computed tomography may be helpful in serial evaluation of ARVD/C patients with an implantable cardioverter defibrillator.

Cardiovascular MRI[50,51]
- It demonstrates intramyocardial fat deposits characterized by high-signal intensity areas indicating the substitution of myocardium by fat, focal wall thinning and wall hypertrophy, trabecular disarray, right ventricular outflow tract enlargement and ectasia, right ventricular aneurysms characterized dyskinetic bulges, diminished right ventricular function and enlargement of the right atrium.
- Sole reliance on fatty infiltrate may result in inappropriate over diagnosis of ARVD/C/C.
- Fibrosis may be more specific than intramyocardial fat deposit. Contrast enhanced signal acquisition is capable of demonstrating fibrosis.
- Cardiovascular MRI remains normal in idiopathic RVOT tachycardia.
- If fatty infiltration is demonstrated, the diagnosis of ARVD/C should be confirmed by demonstrating other right ventricular morphological and functional abnormalities. These findings should be confirmed by other imaging techniques such as echocardiography or angiography.
- Diagnosis of ARVD/C and therapeutic decisions must be made on the basis of Task Force criteria and not on structural abnormalities alone.
- Echocardiography should be the initial diagnostic approach.

SAEKG[52]
- All three components of the SAECG are associated with the diagnosis of ARVC/D. They include
- Filtered QRS duration (normal less than 120 ms)

- Low-amplitude signal duration (normal less than 20 ms)
- Root mean square amplitude of the last 40 ms of the QRS (normal more than 40 μV)
  1 The sensitivity of using SAEKG for diagnosis of ARVC/D is from 50 to 70% and specificity of 95%.
  2 SAEKG abnormalities does not vary with clinical presentation or reliably predict spontaneous or inducible VT and has limited correlation with ECG findings.

Immunohistochemical analysis
- Immunohistochemical analysis of heart biopsies showed nonspecific reduction of immunostaining for Cx43 reduced staining for junction plakoglobin (gamma-catenin) and it correlated well with ARVD/C, sensitive (91%), and specific (82%)

Differential diagnosis[53]
- Uhl's disease is characterized by a paper thin right ventricle. There is loss of myocardial muscle fibers due to apoptotic process.
- In Uhl's disease there is no gender difference (male/female ratio 1.3) or family history of SCD. It presents in early childhood, usually with congestive heart failure as the first symptom.
- Myocarditis and idiopathic cardiomyopathy should also be considered in differential diagnosis.
- VT with LB morphology and inferior axis may occur in ARVD/C and may be mistaken for idiopathic RVOT-VT, Sarcoidosis and congenital heart disease.
- In contrast with RVOT-VT, VT in ARVD/C demonstrates reentry multiple morphologies, and fragmented potentials
- Cardiac sarcoidosis with right ventricle involvement can mimic ARVD/C.
- Non-ischaemic cardiomyopathy and MI also cause right ventricle scar-related VTs.

High risk group[54]
- Patients with the following characteristics are considered at high risk for ventricular arrhythmias and SCD.
  1 Definite ARVD/C as defined by task force criteria.
  2 Sever structural right ventricular disease, diffuse right ventricular involvement.
  3 Increased QRS duration and T-wave inversion in leads V1–V3)
  4 Nonsustained or sustained VT.
  5 Syncope.
  6 Inducible sustained ventricular arrhythmia during electrophysiologic study.
  7 Desmoplakin mutation.
  8 Abnormal SAECG parameters or rapid progression of SAECG abnormalities.
  9 Resuscitated sudden cardiac arrest.
  10 Left ventricular dysfunction.
  11 Family history is not currently an identified risk factor because of variable penetrance.

- Patients with probable ARVD and negative electrophysiology study could be considered as low risk group.
- ICD therapy plays an important role in primary prevention of sudden cardiac death in patients with ARVD/C.
- ARVC linked to 3p25 is a malignant disease, particularly in males, who frequently die suddenly in early adulthood.
- SCD may be the first symptom in those at high risk.
- ICD should be considered as a primary prevention therapy in familial ARVC linked to 3p25.

Clinical presentation[41]

- Patients with ARVD/C typically present between the second and fifth decades of life with symptoms of palpitation, syncope or SCD associated with ventricular tachycardia.
- These patients may also present with nonspecific chest pain.
- In a concealed form of ARVD/C sudden death, usually during exercise, could be the first clinical presentation.
- Symptomatic ventricular arrhythmias may occur during exercise; 50–60% of patients present with monomorphic ventricular tachycardia with LBBB morphology.
- VT with multiple morphologies may occur.
- An inferior QRS axis during ventricular tachycardia reflects the right ventricular outflow tract as site of origin, while a superior axis reflects the right ventricular inferior wall as site of origin.
- The occurrence of arrhythmic cardiac arrest due to ARVD/C is significantly increased in athletes. Patients with established diagnosis of ARVD/C should not be allowed to participate in competitive sports and/or moderate-to-high intensity level recreational activities
- In certain parts of Italy, ARVD/C has been shown to be the most frequent cause of exercise-induced cardiac death in athletes.
- Patients with advanced disease may present with right ventricular failure with or without arrhythmias. These patients may be eligible for cardiac transplant.

Prognosis

- Both sexes have similar mortality risk with peak occurring in fourth decade.
- ARVD/C may account for up to 5% of sudden deaths in young adults in the United States and 25% of exercise-related deaths in the Veneto region of Italy.
- In the absence of SCD progressive impairment of cardiac function may result in right or biventricular heart failure, usually in 4–8 years.

Treatment[55,56]

- In asymptomatic children identified with ARVC based on clinical or genetic testing, restriction from competitive sports, modification of recreational sports, and yearly evaluation, including echocardiography, SAEKG, and ambulatory monitoring should be recommended.

- Ten percent of ARVC deaths occur during adolescence or earlier, that extremes of exercise are a recognized trigger for arrhythmic events, and that endurance exercise appears to accelerate disease progression.

Antiarrhythmic agents
- There is no data to support the use of antiarrhythmic agents for prevention of SCD.
- Sotalol amiodarone and beta-blockers could be used to reduce the arrhythmia burden and recurrent shocks from the defibrillator.

Radiofrequency Ablation
- Radiofrequency ablation can be considered if antiarrhythmic agents are ineffective or produce side-effects.
- There is no data to suggest that the ablation alone will be effective in preventing SCD.
- Three dimensional mapping system and endocardial electrograms demonstrating low amplitude fractionated and earliest electrogram are effective in targeting the site of origin of VT.
- Long-term success of the ablation is low because of the progressive and diffuse nature of the disease, resulting in multiple arrhythmogenic foci and multiple morphologies of the VT, which may be difficult to abolish.
- Initial success of ablation is 60 to 80%, recurrence rate of approximately 30-80%.
- Commonest complication during ablation is cardiac perforation (10%) probably due to thinning of the RV walls.
- The cumulative VT recurrence-free survival does not differ by procedural success, mapping technique, or repetition of procedures.
- A PVC burden of >20% may result in left ventricular dysfunction.

ICD implant[56]
- It is the treatment of choice for patients who had syncope, sustained VT or aborted cardiac arrest.
- Patients who receive ICD for secondary prevention have higher rate of appropriate ICD therapies[5].
- Electrophysiologic study may not be able to predict, in primary prevention group as to who will receive appropriate shock.
- ICD therapy plays an important role in primary prevention of sudden cardiac death in patients with ARVD/C.
- Possible problems with the use of ICD in patients with ARVD/C include right ventricular perforation during lead implant or during fallow up and increase in pacing threshold due to fibrosis at the tip of the pace sense electrode. This may also result in decrease in R wave amplitude and poor detection of the arrhythmia.
- There may be increase in defibrillation energy requirements.
- As the disease progresses and involves left ventricle, CHF may occur. Its treatment with diuretics, ace inhibitors and β blockers should be considered.

- Intractable heart failure may require cardiac transplant.
- Asymptomatic ARVC patients with malignant family history may be candidate for ICD.
- Patients who receive ICD for syncope or sustained ventricular tachycardia may receive appropriate ICD shock during follow-up.
- Syncope is an important predictor of life-saving ICD intervention.

Brugada syndrome[57-59]

- Its mode of transmission is autosomal dominant.
- Brugada syndrome is due to mutation of the sodium ion channel SCN5A alpha subunit located on chromosome 3. This mutation results in loss of function[3].
- Single amino acid substitution of SCN5A at residue 1623 causes LQT3, however similar mutation at position 1620 causes Brugada syndrome.
- SCN5A mutations account for only 18–30% of clinically diagnosed Brugada patients.
- The syndrome is estimated to be responsible for 4% of all sudden deaths and at least 20% of sudden deaths in patients with structurally normal hearts.
- Loss of AP dome (Plateau) in epicardium but not in endocardium causes ST elevation or early repolarization pattern seen in Brugada syndrome.
- Loss of the dome results in contractile dysfunction because the entry of calcium into the cells is greatly diminished and sarcoplasmic reticulum calcium stores are depleted.
- Delayed activation may be responsible for recording of late potentials.
- Abbreviation of APD occurs due to strong outward currents during plateau phase due to decrease in I_{Na}, inhibition of the I_{Ca} or activation of I_{to} at the end of phase 1.
- Acetylcholine facilitates shortening of plateau by suppressing I_{Ca} or augmenting I_{to}. β-adrenergic agonists restore these changes by increasing I_{Ca}.
- Sodium channel blockers facilitate shortening of plateau by shifting the voltage at which phase 1 begins.
- Loss of Na channel function by mutation or by blockade using drugs may reduce inward currents and leave outward currents unopposed resulting in shortening of APD.
- Increase ST elevation in Brugada syndrome by vagal maneuvers or class I agents and reduction in ST elevation with β adrenergic agonist is consistent with above observations.
- Occurrence of ST elevation in right precordial leads is due to shortening of plateau phase over the right ventricular epicardium where I_{to} is most prominent. These changes are also responsible for ST elevation, phase 2 reentry and episodes of VF in Brugada syndrome.
- Agents that inhibit I_{to} such as 4 amiopyridine (4 AP), quinidine, disopyramide, restore AP plateau phase and electrical homogeneity and abolish arrhythmias.
- Class IA agents such as procainamide and ajmaline that block I_{Na} but not I_{to} exacerbate the electrophysiologic abnormalities of Brugada syndrome.
- Lithium has been shown to be potent Na channel blocker and may unmask Brugada ECG changes.

- Gene mutations that increase the intensity and kinetic of I_{to}, $I_{K,ATP}$ or decrease the intensity and kinetic of I_{Ca} during early phase of AP will result in electrocardiographic changes suggestive of Brugada syndrome.
- Abnormal expression of the genes that modulate autonomic receptor and $I_{K,ATP}$ may also produce Brugada like changes.
- ST-segment elevation in the right precordial ECG leads, a shorter-than-normal QT interval≤360 ms, and a history of sudden cardiac death have been attributed to loss-of-function missense mutation in genes encoding the cardiac L-type calcium channel. Brugada syndrome phenotype is combined with shorter-than-normal QT intervals.
- Quinidine may normalize the QT interval and prevent stimulation-induced ventricular tachycardia.
- Low serum potassium level is a predisposing factor for VF in Brugada syndrome.
- Mutations in SCN5A result in loss of function due to
  1 Failure of the sodium channel to express.
  2 A shift in the voltage and time dependence of sodium channel current (I_{Na}) activation, inactivation, or reactivation.
  3 Entry of the sodium channel into an intermediate state of inactivation from which it recovers more slowly.
  4 Accelerated inactivation of the sodium channel.
  5 Alter functional properties (gating) of the sodium channel protein.
  6 Failure to express in the sarcolemma (trafficking).
- Missense (M) mutations, in which a single amino acid is replaced by an aberrant amino acid, most often disrupt gating of the channel.
- In contrast, truncation (T) mutations, in which the sodium channel protein is truncated because of the presence of a premature stop codon, are usually not inserted into the sarcolemma, and cause haploinsufficiency.
- Mutant sodium channels with gating abnormalities confer no dominant-negative effects on normal sodium channels, T mutations potentially reduce I_{Na} more than M mutations and cause the most severe phenotype.
- Thirty percent of BrS patients have a *SCN5A* mutation (Table 7.11)
- A second locus on chromosome 3, close to but distinct from *SCN5A*, has been linked to the syndrome associated with progressive conduction disease, a low sensitivity to procainamide, and a relatively good prognosis.
- Mutation in the gene *GPD1L* encoding the enzyme glycerol-3-phosphate dehydrogenase-1-like results in BrS.
- A mutation in GPD1L has been shown to result in a reduction of I_{Na}.
- The third and fourth genes associated with the BrS encode the α1- (CACNA1C) and β- (CACNB2b) subunits of the L-type cardiac calcium channel.
- Mutations in the α- and β-subunits of the calcium channel can also lead to a shorter than normal QT interval, creating a new clinical entity consisting of a combined Brugada/SQTS.
- Loss-of-function sodium channelopathies are autosomal-dominant and cause Brugada syndrome and progressive cardiac conduction disease (PCCD).
- PCCD and Brugada syndrome present significant overlap and can coexist in the same family and even in the same individual

Table 7.11 Gene mutations and Brugada syndrome.

Type	Locus on chromosome	Gene	Protein	Affected current	Effect on channel function	Incidence, %
BS1	3p21	SCN5A	Nav1.5	I_{Na}	Loss of function	20
BS2	3p24	GPD1-L	GPD1-L protein	I_{Na}	Loss of function	1
BS3	12p13.3	CACNA1C	Cav1.2	I_{CaL}	Loss of function	7
BS4	10p12.33	CACNB2b	Cavβ2b	I_{CaL}	Loss of function	5
BS5	19q13.1	SCN1B	Navβ1	I_{Na}	Loss of function	1
BS6	11q13–q14	KCNE3	MiRP2	I_{to}	Gain of function	1

- Brugada syndrome is characterized by coved ST elevation and negative T waves in the right precordial leads of the electrocardiogram
- ECG abnormalities are provoked and/or exacerbated by sodium channel blockers.
- Reversal of the transmural gradient of repolarization results in ECG characteristics and transmural dispersion of APs initiates phase 2 reentry, premature ventricular activations, and tachyarrhythmias.
- It is the most common cause of natural death in young Asians. Involving young male adults, with arrhythmogenic manifestation first occurring at an average age of 40 years, with sudden death typically occurring during sleep.
- Account for up to 4% of all SCDs and 20% of unexplained sudden death in the setting of a structurally normal heart
- Brugada syndrome can manifest in early childhood and has been diagnosed in infants as young as 2 days. May be basis for some cases of sudden infant death syndrome.
- BrS is sensitive to body temperature and can lead to T-wave alternans (TWA), VT, and sudden death. Hyperthermia abbreviates AP and facilitates reentry and tachyarrhythmias.
- Blockade of the transient outward current, I_{to}, reduces AP heterogeneity and prevents arrhythmias in the Brugada syndrome model.
- Epicardial activation delay leads to fragmented QRS, a risk marker of prognosis in BrS.
- Brugada syndrome occurs predominantly in male adults and can be affected by heart rate, autonomic nervous activity, fever, and drugs.
- PVT and VF occur spontaneously at night.

- These arrythmis can be triggered by programmed electrical stimulation, pharmacological blockade of the sodium channel or by administration of acetylcholine;
- The membrane density of I_{to}, which is the major contributor of the phase 1 notch, is higher in the right than in the left ventricles, in the epicardium than in the endocardium, and near the base than near the apex of the ventricles.
- Several gene mutations that affect Na^+, L-type Ca^{2+}, or transient outward K^+ channels are identified in patients with Brugada syndrome
- Relationships between genotype and phenotype are not always predictive. Mutations in different genes can express similar Brugada syndrome phenotypes. Conversely, mutations in the same gene can also lead to different syndromes.
- Mutations in the gene encoding the α-subunit of the Na^+ channel (*SCN5A*) that hamper its opening (loss of function) have been identified in 18%–30% of the patients with Brugada syndrome (BS1), and also in patients with progressive cardiac conduction system disease.
- Mutated *SCN5A* can also impede the closure (gain of function) of the Na^+ channel, leading to type 3 LQTS.
- Mutations in the glycerol-3-phosphate dehydrogenase 1-like gene on chromosome 3p22–25 (BS2) and in *SCN1B* on chromosome 19q13.1, which encodes the β-subunit of Na^+ channel (BS5), can also cause Na^+ channel dysfunction, reducing the I_{Na} and resulting in Brugada syndrome.
- These proteins are components of the macromolecular complex of the Na^+ channel and thus modulate Na^+ channel function. The haplotype of the promoter region of SCN5A also prolongs the PR and QRS durations in the ECG of patients with BrS.
- Loss of function mutations in α- and β-subunits of the Ca^{2+} channel gene produces in BS3 and BS4, respectively, resulting in phenotypical expression of Brugada syndrome in combination with short QT intervals and familial sudden cardiac death.
- A mutation of ankyrin-B, which modulates Ca^{2+} and Na^+ currents, and mutations of the delayed rectifier K channel genes (*KCNH2* and *KCNQ1*) have been reported in patients with Brugada syndrome.
- Mutation of *KCNE3*, which encodes the β-subunit of the Kv4.3 channel, enhances the I_{to} and can also lead to BS6.
- While gene mutations provide a proarrhythmic substrate, the adult male dominance of clinical manifestation suggests that gender- and age-related factors (e.g., sex hormones) are triggers for arrhythmia in Brugada syndrome.
- Genotype–phenotype correlations revealed that compared with patients without an *SCN5A* mutation, patients with an *SCN5A* mutation had longer and progressive conduction delays (PQ, QRS, and HV intervals), frequent occurrences of fragmented QRS complex (f-QRS) and ventricular arrhythmias of extra RVOT origin.
- In contrast, most (about 80%) of the patients with Brugada syndrome without an *SCN5A* mutation had ventricular arrhythmias of RVOT origin.

- Patients with a Ca^{2+} channel gene mutation had a short QT interval.
- f-QRS (Fractionated QRS)occurred frequently in patients with Brugada syndrome having episodes of VF and/or *SCN5A* mutations.

Clinical and electrocardiographic features[60-62]

- Brugada syndrome is a heritable arrhythmia syndrome manifesting as syncope or sudden cardiac death due to polymorphic ventricular tachycardia in the absence of ischemia, structural heart disease, or QT prolongation
- Brugada syndrome is diagnosed when an ECG pattern characterized by J-point and ST-segment elevation with negative T wave ("coved" or type 1 Brugada ECG pattern) is observed spontaneously in right precordial leads V1 to V3 or following administration of a sodium channel blocker (ajmaline, flecainide, procainamide), in conjunction with a personal or family history of major ventricular arrhythmic events and/or blood relatives displaying the type 1 ECG pattern.
- High V1 to V3 leads (from the third or second intercostal space), which overlie the right ventricular outflow tract (RVOT), are more sensitive than the conventional V1 to V3 leads for detection of the type 1 Brugada pattern.
- Bipolar precordial lead with a positive electrode overlying approximately the base of the ventricles (e.g., at V2) and a negative electrode in the area of the apex (e.g., at V4 or V5) could detect the diagnostic type 1 Brugada ECG pattern.
- The presence of RBBB is not required for the diagnosis of Brugada syndrome, although mild-to-moderate widening of QRS duration often is observed.
- Two specific types of ST-segment elevation (coved-type and saddleback) are observed in this syndrome, and the pattern and amplitude of ST-segment elevation can be dynamic. Coved-type ST-segment elevation may occur just before and after episodes of VF and is associated with higher incidence of VF and sudden cardiac death.
- Type 1 ST-segment elevation, which is defined as a coved ST-segment elevation $\geq 0.2\,mV$ at the J point with or without a terminal negative T wave, is required to diagnose Brugada syndrome (Figure 7.15).
- Type 2 and type 3 ST-segment elevation, which have a saddleback configuration, are not diagnostic for Brugada syndrome.
- A transient outward potassium current (I_{to})–mediated phase 1 notch of the AP is greater in the epicardium than in the endocardium in many species, including humans.
- A net outward shift in current active at the end of phase 1 AP (principally I_{to} and L-type calcium current [I_{Ca-L}]) can increase the magnitude of the AP notch, leading to loss of the AP dome (all-or-none repolarization) in the epicardium but not in the endocardium, contributing to a significant voltage gradient across the ventricular wall and producing ST-segment elevation in the ECG.
- In the setting of coved-type ST-segment elevation, heterogeneous loss of the AP dome (coexistence of loss of dome regions and restored dome regions) in the epicardium creates marked epicardial dispersion of repolarization, giving rise to premature beats due to phase 2 re-entry, which precipitate VF.

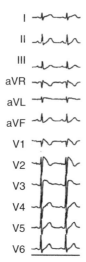

Figure 7.15 Typical ST coving suggestive of Brugada syndrome.

- The Brugada syndrome seems to be a clinical counterpart of the mechanism of all-or-none repolarization in the epicardial cells and phase 2 reentry-induced premature beats between adjacent epicardial cells.
- Higher sensitivity for ECG diagnosis of Brugada syndrome by recordings of higher V1–V2 leads is expected to be due to a higher or wider distribution of abnormal epicardial cells in the right ventricular outflow tract area in some patients with Brugada syndrome.
- There is high incidence of sudden death usually at a mean age of 40 years. These patients have structurally normal hearts. Twenty percent of SCD in patients with structurally normal hearts are due to Brugada syndrome.
- Prevalence is estimated to be 5/10 000.
- Sudden death usually occurs at rest and at night.
- Hypokalemia may contribute to SCD. In certain oriental countries large carbohydrate meal may contribute to hypokalemia. Glucose insulin infusion may unmask Brugada type ECG pattern.
- Elevated temperature is known to prematurely inactivate SCN5A. Febrile illness, use of hot tubs may precipitate VF.
- Fever might impair trafficking of the channel, which is known to be temperature dependent
- Temperature is known to modulate I_{to} by increasing current density and accelerating activation and inactivation, which is expected to increase Brugada pattern.
- Increased vagal tone may unmask the Brugada pattern.
- Approximately 20% of patients with Brugada syndrome may develop supraventricular arrhythmias, including AF. These arrhythmias may result in inappropriate ICD shocks.
- ECG characteristics of Brugada syndrome are dynamic and often concealed, but can be unmasked by potent sodium channel blockers such as ajmaline, flecainide, procainamide, disopyramide, propafenone, and pilsicainide.

- If the epicardial action potential continues to repolarize before that of endo-cardium, the T wave remains positive, giving rise to a saddleback configuration of the ST-segment elevation. Further accentuation of the notch is accompanied by prolongation of the epicardial action potential causing it to repolarize after endocardium, thus leading to inversion of the T wave.
- In Brugada syndrome, there is seasonal peak from spring to early summer and a significant circadian peak from midnight to early morning in terms of the occurrences of VF.
- Other ECG abnormalities include prolongation of PR, QRS, and P duration, and presence of S waves in leads I, II, and III.
- There may be prolongation of the QT interval more in the right precordial leads. This may be due to selective prolongation of action potential duration in right ventricular epicardium.
- Concealed ECG manifestations can be unmasked by sodium channel blockers, during a febrile illness or with vagotonic agents.
- Asymptomatic patients with type I ECG changes do not require drug challenge.
- Diagnosis of Brugada syndrome should be considered if Type 1 ST-segment elevation with or without sodium channel blocking agent and one of the following are present:
  1 Documented ventricular fibrillation and/or polymorphic ventricular tachycardia.
  2 Inducible VT with programmed electrical stimulation.
  3 Syncope.
  4 Nocturnal agonal respiration.
  5 Family history of sudden cardiac death at young age (<45 years).
  6 ST elevation T inversion in precordial leads of family members.
- Type 2 ECG changes are characterized by saddleback type ST-segment elevation of more than 2 mm, a trough and a positive or biphasic T wave.
- Type 3 ECG pattern is considered when saddleback or coved type of ST-segment elevation of <1 mm is present.
- Type 2 and type 3 ECG patterns are not diagnostic of Brugada syndrome.
- Serial ECGs from the same patient may show all three patterns, at different times, spontaneously or after the administration of specific drugs.
- Diagnosis of Brugada syndrome should be considered when a type 2 or type 3 ECG pattern changes to type I pattern after administration of sodium channel blocker.
- One or more of the clinical criteria described above should be present.
- Change from type 3 to type 2 pattern, after administration of Na channel blockers, is considered inconclusive for a diagnosis of Brugada syndrome.
- Rounded or upsloping ST elevation or early repolarization pattern are not suggestive of Brugada syndrome.
- Sixty to 70% of patients with Brugada syndrome show late potentials detected by signal-averaged ECG.
- In the presence of a BS-type ECG pattern, aVR sign (R wave ≥3 mm or R/Q ratio ≥ 0.75 in lead aVR) may reflect more right ventricle conduction delay and

subsequently more electrical heterogeneity, which in turn is responsible for a higher risk of arrhythmia. The aVR sign was defined as R wave ≥0.3 mV or R/Q ≥0.75 in lead aVR.

- Asymptomatic patients whose type 1 ECG only appears after a sodium channel blocker test have a lower arrhythmic risk.
- f-QRS is more frequent in patients with SCN5A mutations and syncope due to VF.
- The presence of J waves in leads V1–V3 (Brugada pattern) and in leads I, aVL, II, III, aVF, and V4–V6 (Aizawa pattern and variant Brugada pattern) is a well-established ECG marker associated with the occurrence of fast polymorphic ventricular tachycardia, ventricular fibrillation (VF), and sudden death in patients without structural heart disease.

Provocative test to unmask Brugada ECG pattern[63,64]

- The test is performed by giving one of the Na channel blockers, Procainamide 10 mg/kg IV over 10 min, or Flecainide 2 mg/kg IV over 10 min, or 400 mg, PO, or ajmaline 1 mg/kg IV over 5 min, or pilsicainide 1 mg/kg IV over 10 min.
- The test should be monitored with a continuous ECG recording and should be terminated when the diagnostic type 1 Brugada ECG changes become evident, premature ventricular beats or other arrhythmias develop, or QRS widens to >130% of baseline.
- Patients with underlying conduction defect may develop AV block.
- Elderly patients or those with preexisting conduction defects (prolong P, PR, QRS) may benefit by temporary pacemaker prior to initiating the test.
- Isoproterenol and sodium lactate may be used to neutralize the effects of Na channel blockers.
- Patients with type 2 or type 3 electrocardiographic changes, who do not convert to type 1 after a provocative test and are not inducible doing electrophysiologic study have a good prognosis.
- Patients with a spontaneously diagnostic pattern have a twofold greater risk of developing a cardiac event than patients with a pattern induced only by a provocative test.
- Patients with no conversion from type 2 or 3 ECG patterns into a type 1 ECG pattern may have good prognosis.
- There is no evidence that EPS would be of value in the stratification of asymptomatic patients with a spontaneously diagnostic pattern.
- In patients with a type 2 or 3 ECG pattern with a negative provocative test result and without a family history of Brugada syndrome, EPS should not be considered for risk stratification.
- EPS has high negative predictive value (almost 100%), whereas its role in positive patients is debatable.
- There is a wide variation in clinical presentation, which ranges from asymptomatic patients to patients resuscitated after sudden cardiac death and variation in ECG pattern, which can range from normal to typical type 1 in the same patient, sometimes over the course of a few hours.

- Circumstances leading to the performance of the test are variable; include asymptomatic patients with a suspicious ECG or a family history of Brugada syndrome or sudden cardiac death to patients with a normal or suspicious ECG who experienced sudden cardiac death or unexplained syncope.
- In patients with an unexplained syncopal episode, identification of Brugada syndrome by provocative test will lead to placement of an ICD.
- In asymptomatic patients, diagnosis of Brugada syndrome will have no effect on patient management, even if electrophysiologic study is considered.
- In asymptomatic patients, the purpose of the test is to confirm the diagnosis and allow subsequent familial screening. This point must be clearly explained to the patient before the test is performed because identification of a disease that is potentially responsible for sudden cardiac death, not only in the patient but also in his/her family members, can lead to psychological distress.
- There are arrhythmic risks from the test.
- Test should be stopped if type 1 Brugada ECG is displayed, if arrhythmias develop, or if QRS widens to greater than 130% of baseline.

Differential diagnosis[65]
- The majority of patients with Brugada syndrome have structurally normal hearts.
- Some patients with arrhythmogenic right ventricle dysplasia may demonstrate ST changes suggestive of Brugada syndrome (Table 7.12).

The following conditions may mimic ECG pattern of Brugada syndrome[31,32] (Box 7.6):

Table 7.12 Differentiating features between ARVD/C and Brugada syndrome.

	Brugada syndrome	ARVD/C
Genetic characteristics	Defect in *SCN5A*	Three genes on 10 locations
ECG changes	1 Dynamic 2 Induced by Na channel blockers.	Persistent & progressive 1 T wave inversion 2 Epsilon waves 3 ↓ R amplitude 4 Unaffected by Na channel blockers.
Right ventricle imaging	No structural abnormality. Wall motion abnormality due to conduction defect may be present.	Structural and wall motion abnormalities are present.
Ventricular arrhythmias	1 Polymorphic VT. 2 Facilitated by vagotonic agents, beta-blockers. 3 Occur during sleep	1 Monomorphic VT with LBB morphology. 2 Facilitated by catecholamines. 3 Occur during exercise.

Drugs responsible for Brugada like ECG pattern (Box 7.7)

Risk stratification[66]
- Currently, risk stratification in Brugada syndrome patients is based on
  1 Spontaneous coved-type ST-segment elevation
  2 Male gender
  3 History of syncope or aborted sudden death
  4 Inducibility of ventricular tachyarrhythmia during programmed ventricular stimulation
  4 Late potentials were found to be the most important noninvasive marker for risk stratification, recurrences, and inducibility of malignant arrhythmias during electrophysiological testing.

Treatment[67,68]
- ICD is the only proven and effective therapy for Brugada syndrome.
- Recommendations for ICD implant in symptomatic patients are outlined in Figure 7.16.
- Recommendations for ICD implant in patients with Na channel block induced Type 1 pattern are outlined in Figure 7.17.
- Although the arrhythmias and sudden cardiac death are associated with bradycardia, the role of chronotropic agents and pacemakers remains undefined.
- Ablation of the ventricular premature beats that trigger VT/VF in Brugada syndrome may decrease the frequency of the arrhythmias and ICD shocks.

Box 7.6

Acute myocardial ischemia or infarction
Acute pericarditis
Arrhythmogenic right ventricular dysplasia
Atypical right bundle-branch block
Central and autonomic nervous system abnormalities
Dissecting aortic aneurysm
Duchenne muscular dystrophy
Early repolarization
Hypercalcemia
Hyperkalemia
Hypothermia
Large pericardial effusions
Left ventricular hypertrophy
Mediastinal tumor compressing on RVOT
Pectus excavatum
Prinzmetal angina
Pulmonary embolism
Thiamin deficiency

Box 7.7 Drugs responsible for Brugada syndrome

1 Antiarrhythmic drugs:
   Flecainide, propafenone, ajmaline, procainamide, disopyramide
2 Calcium channel blockers:
   Verapamil nifedipine, diltiazem
3 Blockers:
   Propranolol, Nadolol.
4 Nitrates:
   Isosorbide dinitrate, nitroglycerine
5 Potassium channel openers:
   Nicorandil
6 Tricyclic antidepressants:
   Amitriptyline, nortriptyline, desipramine, clomipramine
7 Tetracyclic antidepressants:
   Maprotiline
8 Phenothiazines:
   Perphenazine, cyamemazine
9 Selective serotonin reuptake inhibitors:
   Fluoxetine
10 Anaesthetics
   Bupivacaine
11 Miscellaneous:
   Cocaine, alcohol abuse

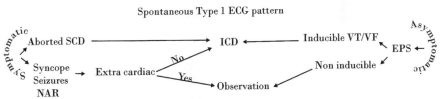

Figure 7.16 Approach to spontaneous type 1 ECG pattern. NAR = nocturnal agonal respiration.

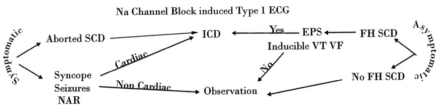

Figure 7.17 Approach to Na channel block induced type 1 ECG pattern (FH = family history).

- Occurrence of spontaneous VF among patients undergoing prophylactic ICD implantation for "asymptomatic Brugada syndrome with inducible VF" seems to be only 1% per year.

Acute and chronic management of electrical storm of VF in Brugada syndrome

- Continuous infusion of isoproterenol (0.002 μg/kg/min) may decrease the J-point amplitude and change coved-type to saddleback-type ST-segment elevation in lead V2. Increasing dose of isoproterenol (0.004 μg/kg/min) may normalize ST-segment elevation in lead V2 and completely suppresses repetitive episodes of VF.
- Isoproterenol infusion may have to be continued for 10 to 20 days.
- Subsequently, the IV infusion can be replaced by the following oral medications.
  - Denopamine (30 mg/day)
  - Quinidine (400 mg/day)
  - Isoproterenol (45 mg/day)
  - Cilostazol (200 mg/day)
  - Bepridil (200 mg/day)
- Isoproterenol, a β-adrenergic agonist, decreases ST-segment elevation and suppresses VF by strongly augmenting I_{Ca-L}.
- Denopamine a α+β-adrenergic stimulant, is effective as a chronic treatment, probably by increasing I_{Ca-L}.
- Quinidine, a class IA sodium channel blocker, has a relatively strong effect in blocking I_{to} and has been proved effective in suppressing a spontaneous episode of VF in patients with Brugada syndrome
- Cilostazol, a phosphodiesterase III inhibitor that increases I_{Ca-L}.
- Quinidine and tedisamil (Class1 antiarrhythmic drugs) block I_{to}, thus restoring APD and provide therapeutic effect.
- Quinidine has been shown to restore epicardial action potential dome, thus normalizing ST segment and preventing phase-2 reentry and polymorphic VT. Large doses of 1200 to 1500 mg are recommended[13].
- Catecholamines by enhancing L type I_{Ca} may also restore action potential dome.
- I_{to} blockers and I_{Ca} enhancers have been shown to normalize ST-segment elevation and control recurrent ventricular arrhythmias (electrical storms) in patients with Brugada syndrome.
- Phosphodiesterase III inhibitor, Cilostazol may normalizes the ST segment by enhancing calcium current (I_{Ca}) and by reducing I_{to} due to its chronotropic effect.
- Tedisamil is a potent I_{to} blocker. Unlike quinidine it does not block inward currents.
- The risk for cardiac arrest for patients with negative EPS is only 1 to 2%.
- Brugada syndrome has been associated with mutations affecting sodium, calcium, and potassium channels subunits.
- Irrespective of the ion channel involved, a prominent I_{to} seems to play a predominant role in arrhythmogenesis.

- Consequently, blocking the I_{to} channel is a logical approach and this can be done with quinidine.
- Use of quinidine for the primary prevention of arrhythmic death in Brugada syndrome is supported by following evidence:
- Quinidine prevents phase II re-entry and VF in the wedge preparation that mimics Brugada syndrome in vitro.
- It may normalize the electrocardiogram in some patients.
- It is extremely effective in preventing the induction of VF in humans during EPS.
- It is very effective for terminating VF storms when other drugs fail.
- Quinidine may prevent spontaneous arrhythmias in high-risk patients with Brugada syndrome during long-term follow-up.
- There is 2 to 8% risk of Torsades de Pointes from quinidine. It reflects the risk for patients with organic heart disease.
- Risk of drug-induced Torsades de Pointes is less in males, and the majority of patients with Brugada syndrome are males.
- Quinidine-induced Torsades de Pointes occur soon after the onset of therapy, and close monitoring during the first 3 days of therapy should prevent proarrhythmic complications.
- Torsades de Pointes occurring long after the onset of therapy is often caused by drug interactions or hypokalemia and meticulous avoidance of such risk factors should reduce the risk of Torsades de Pointes from quinidine in patients with Brugada syndrome to a minimum.

Early repolarization and idiopathic VF[69–72]

- Idiopathic VF occurs in patients without obvious structural heart disease and in the absence of Brugada syndrome, LQTS or other recognized channelopathies.
- Terminal QRS notching, also known as the J wave, may be associated with the development of idiopathic VF (Figure 7.18).

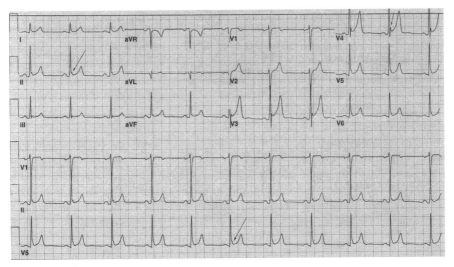

Figure 7.18 J waves.

- J waves are commonly noted in leads V1 through V3 and may appear in inferior leads.
- Transient outward current (I_{to})-mediated prominent action potential notch in epicardium, but not endocardium, provides a voltage gradient, which manifests as J waves.
- J point or ST elevation is not induced in leads V1 through V3 by infusion of sodium channel blockers such as procainamide and disopyramide.
- Prominence of the J wave and resultant VF are bradycardia dependent. The J wave and VF are eliminated by cilostazol.
- Decrease in heart rate spontaneous or drug induced may augment I_{to}.
- Verapamil-induced accentuation of J waves may be due to the decrease in I_{Ca} or bradycardia.
- Elimination of J waves by isoproterenol may be due to the increase in I_{Ca} and the decrease in I_{to} secondary to the increase in heart rate.
- Atrial pacing may suppress J wave due to inhibition of I_{to} related to increase heart rate.
- Procainamide may not have any effect, indicating that sodium channel blockade is not associated with the appearance and/or accentuation of J waves.
- Abolition of J waves by disopyramide may be due to its anticholinergic effects or suppressive effects on I_{to}.
- Cilostazol in a dose of 300 mg/day may suppress the J waves and VF. This effect may be due to suppression of I_{to} secondary to the increase in heart rate and/or increase in I_{Ca}. Elevated intracellular cyclic AMP concentration secondary to inhibition of phosphodiesterase activity by Cilostazol may accentuate I_{Ca}.

Catecholaminergic polymorphic ventricular tachycardia[73,74]

- Catecholaminergic polymorphic ventricular tachycardia (CPVT) is a genetic disease characterized by adrenergically mediated ventricular arrhythmias causing syncope, cardiac arrest, and SCD in young individuals with structurally normal heart and normal QT interval.
- The mean age of onset of symptoms is 8 years, but the first syncope may occur during adulthood.
- Approximately 30% of affected individuals have symptoms before age 10, and close to 60% of patients have at least 1 syncopal episode before age 40.

Genetic abnormalities[75–78]

- The causative genes are located on chromosome 1. Mutations of the cardiac ryanodine receptor gene (*RyR2*) have been implicated in autosomal dominant type, while calsequestrin gene (*CASQ2*) mutations are seen in recessive form.
- Ankyrin-B mutations have been identified in some cases of catecholaminergic polymorphic VT.
- Mutations in Ankyrin-B gene have been linked to the long-QT 4.
- Cardiac RyR2 is located on the sarcoplasmic reticulum (SR) and controls intracellular Ca release and cardiac muscle contraction.
- RyR2 is responsible for calcium-induced calcium release from the SR.

Table 7.13 Genetic mutations in catecholaminergic polymorphic ventricular tachycardia.

Type	Arrhythmia	Inheritance	Location	Gene
CPVT1	Bi DVT	AD	1q42–43	RyR2
CPVT2	BiDVT	AR	1p13–21	CASQ2

AD = autosomal dominant; AR = autosomal recessive.

- Skeletal muscle ryanodine receptor RyR1 mutation is responsible for malignant hyperthermia.
- Cardiac RyR2 receptors are also implicated in the cardiac arrhythmias associated with heart failure, as these are mediated by sympathetic over activity and catecholamine excess.
- Calstabin 2 is a stabilizing subunit of the RyR2 complex. Mutation may result in reduced calstabin 2 binding to RyR2 resulting in abnormal calcium release during exercise, which may trigger ventricular arrhythmias and SCD.
- RyR2 mutations have also been identified in patients with a variant form of arrhythmogenic right ventricular dysplasia (ARVD2).
- Mutations in human cardiac CASQ2, a calcium-binding protein located in the SR, have been linked with recessive form of catecholaminergic polymorphic VT.
- *CASQ2* mutations impair sarcoplasmic calcium storing and calcium-induced calcium release. This may lead to DAD.
- Ankyrin B is required for the assembly of the Na/Ca exchanger, Na/K ATPase, and inositol triphosphate (IP3) receptor in SR of cardiomyocytes.
- Mutations of ankyrin B may result in abnormal Ca dynamics, and catecholaminergic polymorphic VT.
- There are four different genetic mutations that could express as catecholaminergic polymorphic VT (Table 7.13).
  1 RyR2 mutation
  2 Calstabin 2 mutation
  3 CASQ2 mutation
  4 Ankyrin B mutation

Mechanism of arrhythmias in CPVT
- Ventricular arrhythmias occur during exercise or stress testing and fade during the rest. As the work load and the heart rate increase, arrhythmias become more frequent and more complex until polymorphic or bidirectional ventricular tachycardia may occur.
- DAD-induced triggered activity is the initiating mechanism of the typical polymorphic ventricular tachycardia in CPVT.
- In resting ECG, there is no known ECG marker of the syndrome.
- EKG of the patients with *RyR2* mutations may show late-appearing U-waves coinciding with DADs suggesting U-waves as potential ECG markers of

arrhythmia vulnerability. Late-appearing U-waves were distinct from simultaneous double T-waves in the same patients.

- Similar double T-waves or T-wave humps are seen in the long QT syndrome, and the terms T1 and T2 (instead of T and U) are recommended
- T2-waves may be ECG counterparts for early afterdepolarizations (EADs) which mediate triggered activity as the initiating arrhythmia mechanism in the long QT syndrome. Although double T-waves were observed in RyR2 mutation patients, increase in transmural dispersion of repolarization (TDR) may be responsible for ventricular arrhythmias in CPVT.
- T-wave peak to T-wave end (TPE) interval serves as an ECG estimate of TDR.

Ca kinetics[79]

- Normal operation of the heart relies on ordered cycling of intracellular Ca^{2+}.
- On a beat-to-beast basis, Ca^{2+} that enters the cell via voltage-dependent L-type Ca2 channels (left coronary cusp, LCC) during the plateau phase of the action potential triggers the release of Ca^{2+} from the sarcoplasmic reticulum (SR) via Ca2-sensitive Ca^{2+} release channels (also known as cardiac ryanodine receptors, RyR2s).
- This process, known as Ca^{2+}-induced Ca^{2+} release (CICR), amplifies the initial Ca^{2+} entry signal to produce an elevation of cytosolic $[Ca^{2+}]$ ($[Ca^{2+}]c$) which then causes activation of actin-myosin filaments and myocyte shortening, leading to systole
- During relaxation (i.e., diastole), surplus Ca^{2+} in the cytosol is re-sequestered into the SR by the SR calcium adenosine triphosphatase (SERCA), the activity of which is controlled by the phosphoprotein phospholamban (PLB).
- Some of the Ca^{2+} is extruded from the cell by the Na^+/Ca^{2+} exchange (NCX) to balance the Ca^{2+} that enters with ICa.
- Under pathological conditions associated with increased accumulation of Ca2 in the SR (i.e., Ca^{2+} overload), SR Ca^{2+} releases occur spontaneously, rather than as a part of excitation–contraction coupling, causing inappropriately timed Ca^{2+} transients and contractions.
- The propensity of the SR Ca2 stores to discharge spontaneously is a result of self-perpetuating nature of CICR and the tendency of even a small Ca^{2+} release to elicit more release.
- Spontaneous Ca^{2+} releases occur in the form of self-propagating waves of CICR that originate locally (Ca^{2+} sparks), and then spread through the cell via diffusion-coupled CICR.
- Spontaneous Ca^{2+} waves are arrhythmogenic. They induce Ca^{2+}-dependent depolarizing membrane currents by activation of NCX and DAD. Large, DAD evoke extrasystolic action potentials, thereby causing triggered arrhythmia.
- RyR2 modulation by luminal Ca^{2+} involves a group of auxiliary proteins including CASQ2, triadin (TRD), and junctin (JN) complexed with the RyR2 at the luminal side
- Cardiac RyR2, by far the largest protein of the complex, operates as a Ca^{2+} conducting channel.
- CASQ2 is a low-affinity, high-capacity Ca^{2+} binding protein.

- Dominant form is linked to mutations in *RyR2* and the recessive form is linked to mutations in *CASQ*
- *RyR2* mutations may account for majority of the cases of CPVT, *CASQ2* mutations are less common.
- Abnormal SR Ca^{2+} release occurs in digitalis poisoning, metabolic inhibition, ischemia–reperfusion, and chronic heart failure.
- In presence of Ca^{2+} overload, abnormal RyR2 behavior is secondary to the elevation of the SR Ca^{2+} content.
- On exposure to Na^+,K^+–adenosine triphosphatase-inhibiting glycosides, increased accumulation of intracellular $[Na^+]$ results in reduced NCX-mediated Ca^{2+} extrusion and hence increased accumulation of Ca^{2+} in the SR. Elevated intra-SR $[Ca^{2+}]$ then stimulates RyR2 activity, leading to spontaneous Ca^{2+} release and DAD.
- In CPVT, spontaneous Ca^{2+} release and DAD can occur without Ca^{2+} overload and sometimes when SR Ca^{2+} is reduced.
- This arrhythmogenic Ca^{2+} release at reduced SR Ca^{2+} loads is attributable to enhanced responsiveness of RyR2s to luminal Ca^{2+}.
- Sensitization to luminal Ca^{2+} produces a Ca^{2+} overload-like condition that promotes spontaneous Ca^{2+} release not as a result of $[Ca^{2+}]SR$ becoming abnormally high, but rather because of lowering the $[Ca^{2+}]SR$ threshold for spontaneous Ca^{2+} release below the normal baseline level ("perceived" Ca^{2+} overload).
- A similar mechanism may underlie triggered arrhythmia in heart failure and ischemic heart disease, in which SR Ca^{2+} release regulation is compromised because of acquired defects in components of the RyR2 channel complex.
- Mutations in RyR2 and CASQ2 account only for half of the CPVT cases, genetic defects in other Ca^{2+} regulatory proteins may be involved.
- Spontaneous Ca^{2+} release occurs when $[Ca^{2+}]$ SR reaches a certain threshold level it enhances RyR2 and relieves inhibition by CASQ2.
- SR Ca^{2+} content is reduced rather than increased in CPVT.
- Reduced SR Ca^{2+} is expected to inhibit rather than stimulate spontaneous Ca^{2+} release (known as the "Ca^{2+} overload" paradox).
- CASQ2 mutations alter the way the RyR2 channels sense or respond to $[Ca^{2+}]$ SR.
- Arrhythmogenic potential of the RyR2(R4496C) mutation is attributable to the increased $Ca(^{2+})$ sensitivity of RyR2(R4496C), which induces diastolic $Ca(^{2+})$ release and lowers the threshold for triggered activity.
- More than 70 different RyR2 mutations have been reported
- Calsequestrin is a Ca^{2+} buffering protein in the SR and it participates, together with junctin and triadin, in modulating the responsiveness of the RyR2 to luminal Ca^{2+}. Calsequestrin mutations are found in 1 to 2% of CPVT patients.
- Because the parents of homozygous *CASQ2* mutation carriers (who harbor a heterozygous mutation) are usually not clinically affected,
- *CASQ2* mutations may be accountable for cases of adrenergically triggered idiopathic VF in the absence of detectable family history or clinical signs of CPVT.

- BVT may occure with digitalis intoxication. Due to Ca^{2+} overload causing DAD-induced triggered activity.
- CPVT arrhythmias may originate from the specialized conduction system.
- DAD as the origin of CPVT arrhythmias is supported by the clinical evidence of correlation between the coupling interval of ventricular beats and the preceding RR interva (a typical feature of triggered arrhythmias).
- At low luminal $[Ca^{2+}]$ CASQ2 inhibits RyR2 activity, but when $[Ca^{2+}]$ increases the inhibition is relieved with t increased RyR2 activity.
- Autosomal dominant form is linked to RyR2, an intracellular Ca^{2+} release channel found in the sarcoplasmic reticulum, and an autosomal recessive form is caused by a mutation in the CASQ2 calcium storage protein in the SR.
- In the case of the former, a "gain-of-function" mutation causes leakage of Ca^{2+} into the cell. In the latter case, a "loss-of-function" mutation results in more available free Ca^{2+} in the sarcoplasmic reticulum.
- U waves are not often seen in leads I, aVR, and aVL.
- Ca^{2+}/calmodulin-dependent protein kinase II (CaMKII) is a regulator of excitation–contraction coupling,
- CaMKII-mediated phosphorylation of Ca^{2+} cycling
- Chronic activation of CaMKII in diseased hearts leads to abnormal intracellular Ca^{2+} handling, which could promote cardiac arrhythmias.
- The ensuing Ca^{2+} transient leads to myocyte contraction, which quickly ends when Ca^{2+} is removed from the cytoplasm due to SR Ca^{2+} reuptake through the SR Ca^{2+}-ATPase (SERCA2a) and is extruded via the Na^+/Ca^{2+}-exchanger (NCX).
- In healthy hearts, RyR2 remain closed during diastole to facilitate SR refilling before the subsequent systolic Ca^{2+} release. In contrast, heart failure is associated with spontaneous openings of RyR2 during diastole, which can interfere with SR Ca^{2+} loading, decreased systolic Ca^{2+} release and cardiac contractility.
- Clinical observations suggest that CaMKII activation might increase the risk of arrhythmias in patients with CPVT, as arrhythmias typically occur only above specific threshold heart rates (and CaMKII activity is rate dependent).
- Defects in RyR2 regulation may also contribute to triggered activity and arrhythmogenesis in patients with atrial arrhythmias.
- Defects in SR Ca^{2+} release may occur in chronic atrial fibrillation (AF).

Natural history
- The majority of arrhythmic events occur during childhood.
- More than 60% of affected individuals experience a first episode of syncope or cardiac arrest by age 20 years.
- In 13% of patients cardiac arrest is the first manifestation of the disease.
- Approximately 30% of patients have a family history of juvenile SCD and/or stress-related syncope (07/06)[3].

Clinical presentation[73]
- Patients present with exercise or emotional stress induced syncope in the first or second decade. Earlier or later occurrences have also been documented.
- It may be mistaken for epilepsy.

- Catecholaminergic polymorphic VT should be considered as one of the causes of swimming-triggered cardiac events.
- RyR2 mutation is more common in males.
- It is characterized by bidirectional VT, monomorphic and polymorphic VT, and a high risk for sudden cardiac death (30–50% by age 20–30 years).
- DAD-induced triggered activity appears to be the mechanism underlying monomorphic or bidirectional VT.
- Caffeine mimics the defective calcium homeostasis encountered in catecholaminergic polymorphic VT.
- The combination of isoproterenol and caffeine leads to the development of DAD-induced triggered activity arising from the epicardium, endocardium, or M region.
- Alternation of epicardial and endocardial sources of ectopic activity results in bidirectional VT.
- Ectopic activity or VT that arises from the epicardium is associated with an increased T_{peak}–T_{end} interval and TDR due to reversal of the normal transmural activation sequence. It create the substrate for reentry, and programmed electrical stimulation may induce polymorphic VT
- Ventricular arrhyhtmias may occur during sleep.

Differential diagnosis
- Exercise- or emotional stress-induced syncope with polymorphic VT should suggest the diagnosis of catecholaminergic polymorphic VT. Similar presentation may occur in some of the long-QT syndromes.
- Bidirectional VT, one of the hallmarks of catecholaminergic polymorphic VT, has also been described in ATS (LQT7).
- In catecholaminergic polymorphic VT, the ECG is normal and the QT interval is either normal or borderline.
- The heart is structurally normal.
- The arrhythmia can be induced by exercise or by isoproterenol infusion.
- Ambulatory monitoring may reveal exercise induced arrhythmias.
- Electrophysiological studies are of limited value. Arrhythmias are not inducible during programmed electrical stimulation.
- Catecholaminergic polymorphic VT must be differentiated from diseases that can trigger polymorphic VT due to exercise, emotions, or stress, such as LQT1, ATS, arrhythmogenic right ventricular dysplasia, acute and chronic heart failure, and ischemic heart disease (HRJ07/06)[3].
- Gender is an important factor in the etiology, pathogenesis, and cardiac risk stratification of patients with catecholaminergic polymorphic VT and their relatives.
- Most RyR2-positive patients are male.
- Males with RyR2 mutations have earlier onset of clinical symptoms.
- The risk of cardiac events at a young age is significantly higher in males with RyR2 mutations than in females (relative risk = 4.2).
- Most RyR2-negative patients are female.
- Exercise-induced polymorphic VT, even bidirectional VT, may be due to disorders other than catecholaminergic polymorphic VT.

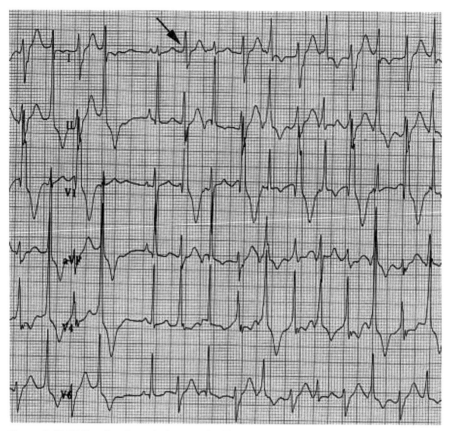

Figure 7.19 Bidirectional VT during treadmill exercise test. Onset at the arrow.

Electrocardiographic features

- The ECG during catecholaminergic polymorphic VT may demonstrate bidirectional VT.
- The resting ECG is usually normal. Frequency of ventricular premature beats increases with exercise, usually when heart rate exceeds 120 bmp.
- The frequency and complexity of the PVCs increases as the heart rate increases and may result in bidirectional VT or polymorphic VT. Syncope may occur. Arrhythmias resolve on discontinuation of exercise or on stopping of isoproterenol infusion (Figure 7.19).
- Supraventricular arrhythmia in the form of isolated atrial ectopic beats, nonsustained supraventricular tachycardia, and short runs of atrial fibrillation may occur during exercise. Atrial fibrillation may precede ventricular arrhythmias.
- The premature beats originate from left ventricle and demonstrate RBBB pattern with alternating right and left axis deviation.
- In ARVD2 premature beats arise from right ventricle and have LB morphology.
- Catecholaminergic polymorphic VT arrhythmias may originate from both the right and the left ventricular outflow tract (more frequently from the left) as

well as the right ventricular apex. No single ECG lead is ideal for making the diagnosis.

- Exercise-induced bigeminy is strongly associated with the presence of significant cardiovascular disease but is far more likely to indicate CPVT than LQTS.
- Induction of BVT or PVT is usually reproducible during graded exercise, which therefore represents the single most important test for diagnosis.
- In some instances, arrhythmias are induced by epinephrine infusion (0.1 to 0.3 µg/kg/min). This test can be used in patients with a negative exercise test in whom syncope/cardiac arrest occurred during exercise or emotion and who present with a normal resting ECG.

Treatment[80,81]

- Beta-blockers are the treatment of choice. Nadolol (1 to 2 mg/kg/day) and propranolol (2.5 to 3.5 mg/kg/day) are commonly used.
- IV propranolol can be used for terminating the tachycardia. Nadolol is effective prophylactically. Asymptomatic PVCs may persist inspite of beta-blockers. Complete suppression of asymptomatic PVCs is not necessary.
- Exercise stress test and Holter monitoring guided titration of the initial beta-blocker dosage (nadolol is started at 1.5–2 mg/kg/day) should be done.
- Beta-blockers also are indicated for all silent carriers of RyR2 mutation.
- Amiodarone is not as effective.
- Calcium channel blocker verapamil is partially successful in suppressing arrhythmias.
- Catheter ablation was reported as unsuccessful.
- If beta-blocker dose is insufficient or missed it may lead to sudden death.
- An ICD implant provides protection against SCD.
- Potential problems of implanting ICD in young patients include inappropriate shocks, regular ICD fallow up and replacement when battery reaches depletion.
- A combination of beta-blockers with an ICD appears to be the ideal therapy.
- The detection interval of the ICD should be extended to avoid shocks for non-sustained VTs. Maximally tolerated dosages of beta-blockers should be continued to minimize the number of ICD shocks.
- The use of volatile anesthetics or succinylcholine may result in malignant hyperthermia in carriers of RyR1 mutations in skeletal muscle. Such complications have not been reported in carriers of cardiac RyR2 mutations or in patients with catecholaminergic polymorphic VT.
- Beta-blockers and calcium blockers could be better than β-blockers alone for preventing exercise-induced arrhythmias in CPVT.
- An ICD is indicated for patients who have failed on beta-blocker therapy or present with syncope.
- Verapamil, not as an alternative but as an addition to beta-blockers, can be used.
- LCSD is known to raise the threshold for ventricular fibrillation LCSD has been used as an effective treatment option for patients with CPVT.

Prognosis

• Mortality in untreated patients is estimated to be 30–50% by the age of 20–30 years.
• Mortality may be reduced to 5–7% per year with the use of beta-blockers, however it is considered unacceptably high.
• Fifty percent of the patients may receive appropriate ICD shocks over 2 year.
• Early diagnosis of CPVT is essential. Undetected it may lead to sudden death early in life. Family screening by genetic studies is useful to identify asymptomatic carriers who may develop symptoms during stress.

Ventricular tachycardia in left ventricular noncompaction[82–87]

• Isolated ventricular noncompaction is a cardiomyopathy caused by intrauterine arrest of compaction of the myocardial fibers and meshwork, leading to multiple prominent trabeculation and intratrabecular recesses in continuity within the ventricular cavity and the characteristically spongy appearance of the myocardium.
• Noncompacted myocardium has been categorized as an unclassified cardiomyopathy by the World Health Organization.
• It may present with triad of heart failure symptoms, arrhythmia, and embolic events.
• Natural history and prognosis of patients with isolated ventricular noncompaction may be better than initially reported.
• The trabecular layer of the developing ventricular walls is known to compact during its development from base to apex, from epicardium to endocardium, and from the septal to the lateral wall.
• Seventy percent of autopsied healthy hearts may show some degree of noncompaction.
• Incidental finding off left ventricular noncompaction in asymptomatic patients may have no clinical significance.
• Diagnosis of isolated ventricular noncompaction is made by echocardiography or cardiac MRI.
• Cardiac MRI is a sensitive tool for identifying LCNC. It raises the question of the prognostic significance of noncompacted myocardium in patients with normal LV function and an apparently normal echocardiogram.
• Areas of noncompaction in the left ventricle are common, especially in the lateral and apical regions.
• Petersen's criteria for pathologic noncompaction Cutoff value of noncompacted to compacted ratio greater than 2.3 to distinguish pathologic isolated ventricular noncompaction, with sensitivity, specificity, positive predictive value, and negative prediction value of 86%, 99%, 75%, and 99%, respectively.
• On the basis of echocardiographic studies, its prevalence has been estimated at 0.05% in the general population, and the finding of a ratio of >2.0 between the thickness of the non-compacted and compacted myocardial layers in systole is considered diagnostic. Echocardiography poses problems in assessing the LV apex, known to be the most commonly non-compacted area.

- It can be associated with neuromuscular disorders and can co-exist with other cardiac malformations.
- Left ventricular noncompaction may demonstrate autosomal dominant pattern.

7.6 Ventricular tachycardias in structurally normal heart

Idiopathic VTs[88]
- These VTs occur in the absence of structural heart disease.
- Idiopathic VT can be classified on the following basis:
  1 Anatomic origin: RVOT or LVOT VT, left ventricular VT, fascicular VT.
  2 Response to pharmacologic agents: adenosine or verapamil sensitive.
  3 Morphologic features: Bundle branch pattern, QRS morphology.
  4 Mechanistic features: Triggered activity, re-entry, automaticity.
  5 Response to exercise: RVOT VT, LVOT VT, left ventricular VT.
- Multiple characteristics may be present in a given VT. Description on the basis of anatomic location best describes the clinical features and therapeutic options for a given VT.

RVOT VT
- The majority of the VTs in the absence of structural heart disease arise from RVOT.
- It arises from RVOT. It is adenosine sensitive, exercise induced LBB morphology and inferior axis VT.
- It could present as nonsustain repetitive monomorphic VT (Gallavardin VT).
- It is caused by cAMP mediated triggered activity (DAD). It is sensitive to (inhibited by) adenosine. Response to adenosine is specific for catecholamine-mediated DAD.
- Verapamil is also effective in terminating triggered activity induced VT.
- Nicorandil, ATP sensitive potassium channel opener may also suppress or terminate adenosine sensitive VT.
- Without preceding catecholamines stimulation adenosine has no effect on ion channels in ventricular myocardium.

Mechanism[89]
- Mechanism appears to be calcium-dependent triggered activity, and no discrete anatomic abnormalities have been identified.
- The area from which these arrhythmias could originate spans from the RV inflow region to the anteroseptal aspect of the RVOT under the pulmonic valve.
- It may extends leftward to include the cusp region of the aortic valve and the anterior left ventricle (LV) in front of the aortic valve, both endocardially and epicardially, and aortomitral continuity and superior mitral annulus.
- Proximity of the outflow tract to the epicardial fat pads containing the ganglionated plexuses may explain the response to exercise, autonomic and hormonal changes.

- A consistent characteristic of outflow tract tachycardia is that acceleration of heart rate facilitates its initiation. This can be achieved by:
  1 Incremental pacing from either the ventricle or atrium (provided that conduction to the ventricles is not limited by AV nodal Wenckebach in the case of the latter)
  2 Iinfusion of a catecholamine alone or during concurrent rapid pacing.
- Termination of the arrhythmia is dependent on either direct blockade of the dihydropyridine receptor by calcium channel blockers or agents or maneuvers that lower cyclic adenosine monophosphate (cAMP) levels.
- Examples of the latter include activation of the M2-muscarinic receptor (with edrophonium or vagal maneuvers), competitively inhibiting the β-adrenergic receptor (beta-blocker), or activation of the A1-adenosine receptor (adenosine).
- Adenosine's antiarrhythmic properties on ventricular myocardium are due to its antagonism of the stimulatory effects of β-adrenergic activation on intracellular calcium.
- Adenosine's cellular effects in the ventricle are mediated by and initiated upon its binding to a G-protein-coupled receptor (A1-adenosine receptor). The GTP–α complex decreases cAMP levels through its inhibition of adenylyl cyclase This blunts arrhythmogenic effects of cAMP-dependent, protein kinase A (PKA)-mediated phosphorylation of specific ion channels and regulatory proteins.
- As a result, adenosine reverses the stimulatory effects of PKA phosphorylation on the L-type Ca^{2+} current (I_{CaL}), reducing the transient inward current (Iti).
- Adenosine may inhibit cAMP-dependent phosphorylation of the ryanodine receptor (RyR) and phospholamban.
- Adenosine has no effect on unstimulated ventricular currents during basal conditions,
- Potassium current I_{KAdo}, the predominant current that mediates adenosine's antiarrhythmic activity in supraventricular tissue, is not expressed in ventricular myocardium.
- In outflow tract VT, catecholamine stimulations increases intracellular Ca^{2+} and potentiates development of DAD. This process is mediated through activation of the β-adrenergic receptor and stimulatory G protein Gs, triggering sequential activation of adenylyl cyclase, cAMP, and cAMP-dependent PKA.
- PKA phosphorylates the L-type Ca^{2+} channel, RyR, and phospholamban, among other proteins. Each of these events can contribute to the generation of DADs.
- Normal activation of RyR is dependent on the influx of ICaL.
- Adenosine has no effect on EADs
- DAD elicited by a cAMP-independent pathway are also adenosine insensitive, an example of which is triggered activity initiated by ouabain-induced inhibition of Na^+/K^+-ATPase.
- DAD and Iti, which are dependent on catecholamine-activated currents, are abolished by adenosine.
- Automatic VT initiation is facilitated by catecholamines, and the arrhythmia shows sensitivity to beta-blockade.

- The arrhythmia is unresponsive to calcium channel blockers and does not initiate or terminate in response to programmed stimulation.
- Adenosine may suppress but not terminate the arrhythmia.
- Suppression represents a transient effect (between 5 and 20 seconds), with spontaneous reemergence of VT immediately following washout of adenosine. Termination is a longer-lasting effect; reinitiation of the arrhythmia is not spontaneous but frequently requires an intervention, such as programmed stimulation.
- Triggered activity or automaticity are likely causes of VT with focal origin.
- Idiopathic outflow tract (OT)-VTs have a focal origin.
- Termination of idiopathic RVOT tachycardias by an intravenous bolus of adenosine or infusion of calcium channel blockers, or by vagotonic manoeuvres is consistent with triggered activity as the likely mechanism for some of these tachycardias.
- These tachycardias can be difficult to induce at electrophysiology testing; rapid burst pacing and/or isoproterenol infusion is often required. Aminophylline, calcium infusion, and atropine may also be useful.

Anatomy of RVOT
- The boundaries of RVOT region are defined superiorly by the pulmonic valve and inferiorly by the RV inflow tract and the top of the tricuspid valve, laterally by RV free wall, and medialy by the interventricular septum
- The RVOT region wraps around the root of the aorta and extends leftward. The top of the RVOT may be convex or crescent shaped, with the posteroseptal region directed rightward and the anteroseptal region directed leftward.
- The anteroseptal aspect of the RVOT is located in close proximity to the left ventricular epicardium, adjacent to the anterior interventricular vein and in proximity to the left anterior descending coronary artery.
- The aortic valve cusps are within the crescent-shaped septal region of the RVOT and are inferior to the pulmonic valve.
- The posteroseptal aspect of the RVOT is adjacent to the region of the right coronary cusp, and the anterior septal surface is adjacent to the anterior margin of the right coronary cusp or the medial aspect of the left coronary cusp.
- The aortic valve is parallel to the pulmonic valve and perpendicular to the mitral valve. In some patients, the aortic valve may have a more vertical tilt and parallel the mitral valve. The location, rotation, and horizontal position of the heart in the chest cavity influence surface ECG characteristics.
- The outflow tract is the tube-like portion of the right ventricular cavity, above the supraventricular crest.
- Its thickness is variable, ranging from approximately 3 to 6 mm,
- Thinnest part (1 mm or less) is at the level of muscular infundibulum near the wall of the pulmonary trunk.
- Septal component of right ventricular outflow tract is in proximal part, at the branch point of the septomarginal trabeculation. Above this area, the right ventricular outlet curves to pass anterior and cephalad to the left ventricular outlet,

- Perforation in the septal part is more likely to go outside the heart than into the left ventricle
- Coarse muscular trabeculations are characteristic of the right ventricular apex, other trabeculations are present in the RVOT.
- Region immediately beneath the pulmonary valve tends to be smooth.
- In normal hearts, the right ventricle is composed of two layers of myocardial fibers, superficial and subendocardial, with different fiber orientations and not separated by fibrous sheaths.
- A thick middle layer is found only in the left ventricle.
- Subepicardial layer of the right ventricular outflow tract constitutes two-thirds of the wall thickness and is comprised of fibers that run horizontally to encircle the infundibulum.
- Subendocardial layer consists mainly of longitudinal fibers.

Clinical features
- It is common in women.
- Age at onset varies from 10 to 70 years.
- The commonest symptom is palpitation, however 10% of patients may present with syncope.
- Prognosis is good and spontaneous resolution may occur in 20% of patients.
- Outflow tract tachycardia is a stable, organized arrhythmia that is associated with a uniform ECG morphology and manifests with a left bundle branch block, inferior-axis configuration.
- Aarrhythmia may occur during exercise or it may occur at rest.
- Episodes tend to increase in frequency and duration during exercise and emotional stress. Thus, an exercise test may provoke focal OT-VT either during exercise or in the recovery phase.
- In a significant number of patients, exercise suppresses the arrhythmia.

Electrocardiographic features[90–92]
- Electrocardiogram during sinus rhythm is normal, however, during tachycardia it shows LBBB and inferior axis (Figure 7.20, Table 7.11).
- Precordial QRS transition begins in lead V3 and more typically occurs in lead V4.
- Tachycardias originating from the top of the tricuspid valve in the inflow area of the RVOT, which is lower and to the right in the outflow tract, will have a positive QRS deflection in lead aVL, QRS amplitude in lead II > lead III, and typically a very positive QRS complex in lead I.
- On the septal side the QRS complex is negative in lead I at site anterior and leftward and positive at site posterior and rightward. On the free-wall side QRS transition is later, QRS duration is wider with notching, and decreased amplitude in the inferior leads and lateral precordial leads.
- The most common site of origin for RVOT tachycardias is the left septal side of the outflow tract just underneath the pulmonic valve. These tachycardias produce large positive QRS complexes in leads II, III, and aVF and large negative complexes in leads aVR and aVL.

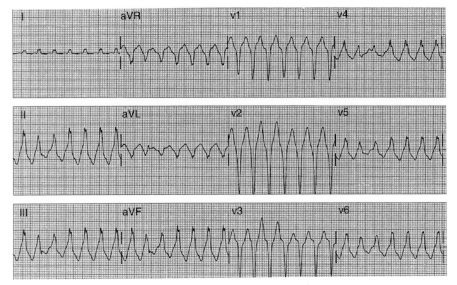

Figure 7.20 RVOT VT demonstrating LB morphology and inferior axis.

- The QRS morphology in lead I is multiphasic and has a net QRS vector of zero or only modestly positive.
- The frontal plane axis, precordial QRS transition, QRS width, and complexity of the QRS in the inferior leads can pinpoint the origin of VT in RVOT.
- The VT may originate at the leftward edge of the septal aspect of the outflow tract just under the pulmonic valve. This extreme "leftward" aspect of the RVOT produces a negative QRS complex in lead I, consistent with how far this aspect of the RVOT wraps around the aortic root and is located to the left of the apical septum.
- Ventricular tachycardia arising from RVOT typically shows an R/S transition zone in the precordial leads at V4, whereas an R/S transition at V1 or V2 indicates an LV origin.
- Runs of nonsustained monomorphic VT may occur during increase sympathetic tone.
- On the basis of the QRS morphology in standard leads and precordial transition, the site of the origin of the RVOT VT can be speculated (Table 7.14)
- Premature beats or the first beat of VT usually has a relatively long coupling interval to the preceding QRS-complex.
- Echocardiogram is usually normal. Rarely, it may show RV enlargement or PMV
- Exercise may reproduce VT in 25 to 50% of the patients. Its induction is dependent on critical heart rate.
- SAEGK, cardiac MRI and RV biopsy are normal.
- Multiple distinct VT morphologies are very rare and should raise the suspicion that a scar-related VT.

Table 7.14 Localization of the origin of RVOT VT from QRS morphology during VT or pace map.

QRS morphology	Anterior septal	Posterior septal	Anterior free wall	Posterior free wall[4]
Lead I	Negative QRS	Positive QRS	Negative QRS	Positive QRS
R wave Lead II,III & aVF	Tall and Narrow	Tall and narrow	Broader shorter & notched.	Broader shorter & notched.
Precordial transition	Early	Early	Late. R/S >1 by V4	Late. R/S >1 by V4
QRS duration (ms)	<140	<140	>140	>140

- Although idiopathic focal OT-VT has a benign course, potentially malignant forms of VT that resemble idiopathic focal OT-VT may also arise from the OT region, including VT in ARVC.
- All patients presenting with OT-VT require an evaluation for organic heart diseases or genetic syndromes associated with sudden death.
- The ECG during sinus rhythm is usually normal, but ~10% of patients with OT-VT show complete or incomplete RBBB.
- T-wave inversion in the anterior precordial leads suggests ARVD.
- A Brugada type ECG, findings of reduced LV or RV function, PMVT or multiple VT morphologies, a history of recurrent syncope, or a family history of SCD mandate further detailed evaluation.
- An exercise test and cardiac imaging (usually at least echocardiography) should be done in all patients.

Electrophysiologic features
- Tachycardia can be initiated and terminated by programmed stimulation. It cannot be entrained. It can be induced by atrial pacing. Burst pacing is also effective in inducing the VT.
- Tachycardia is terminated with adenosine, valsalva maneuvers, carotid sinus pressure, edrophonium, Verapamil and beta-blockers.
- Effects of vagal stimulation and acetylcholine are mediated by M2 muscarinic cholinergic receptors which produces same cascade as adenosine.
- Isoproterenol by increasing cAMP, atropine by inhibiting the effects of acetylcholine and aminophylline by antagonizing the effects of adenosine facilitate induction of the arrhythmias.
- Arrhythmias in the presence of arrhythmogenic right dysplasia (ARVD) morphologically may resemble RVOT VT. In patients with ARVD electrocardiogram may show conduction delay and ST-T wave changes in anterior

precordial leads. MRI shows fatty infiltration in right ventricle wall and wall motion abnormalities[6].

- Septal origin in the RVOT is suggested by QRS duration <140 ms, whereas free-wall origin is suggested by QRS duration ≥140 ms associated with notches in the downslope of QRS in inferior leads (II, III, aVF).
- Deeper S waves in aVR than in aVL indicate rightward inferior origin, while deeper S waves in aVL than in aVR indicate leftward superior origin.
- Idiopathic VT originating from the RVOT shows a monomorphic pattern with nonsustained VT separated by several sinus beats and frequent VPCs.
- Idiopathic VT is generally catecholamine sensitive and is often induced with exercise or infusion of catecholamine, such as isoproterenol and epinephrine.
- Given the proximity of the RVOT and the right aortic cusp, slight anatomical deviations of these 2 structures may cause ambiguous ECG findings.

Treatment
- No treatment is required for asymptomatic patients.
- Beta-blockers, Ca channel blockers, class I and class III antiarrhythmic drugs are found to be effective in half of the patients.
- Acute termination of the tachycardia can be achieved by vagal maneuvers, IV adenosine and IV verapamil.
- For symptomatic patients treatment of choice remains radiofrequency ablation.
- Ablation focus is discrete. Commonest site of the origin for VT is septal wall.
- Earliest activation during tachycardia at ablation site may precede by 20 to 40 ms before the onset of the surface QRS.
- Identical match during pace map in 11 of the 12 leads is also helpful in identifying the suitable ablation site.
- Pace mapping is performed in sinus rhythm at VT cycle length.
- Unipolar electrograms demonstrate QS pattern at the site of earliest activation.
- Intracardiac echocardiogram may help delineate RVOT boundaries.
- Three dimensional mapping has increased the success rate of the ablation.
- During ablation there may be acceleration of the tachycardia before termination.
- Successful ablation can be achieved in 90% of the patients. Recurrence rate is 10%.
- Catheter ablation is effective in this setting. However, late recurrences with similar or different morphology may arise in half of patients after initially successful treatment. Antiarrhythmic drug therapy is a valid initial therapeutic option as it is effective in about half of patients.
- Premature ventricular complexes with the same morphology as VT are an acceptable target if VT is not inducible. In the absence of spontaneous or inducible clinical arrhythmia, catheter ablation should be avoided.
- Precise localization for ablation is guided by activation mapping, pace mapping, or a combination of both methods.
- Mapping of the great cardiac vein is recommended before epicardial mapping by pericardial puncture.

- In reported case series, acute success rate of RF catheter ablation of RVOT VT is 65–97% and typically exceeds 80%; recurrence of arrhythmia has been reported in up to 5% after acutely successful ablation.
- Failure is usually due to inability to induce the arrhythmia for mapping. Complications are rare, but perforation and tamponade are reported and ablation of foci near the His bundle region can result in heart block.
- Complications include RBBB (2%), cardiac perforation and tamponade.
- The leftward posterior aspect of the RVOT is only 4 mm from the left main coronary artery, such that there is a theoretical risk of coronary artery injury with ablation in that aspect of the RVOT and pulmonary artery, that would likely be increased with the use of high-power, irrigated ablation.
- PA-VT/PVCs should always be considered when the ECG suggests RVOT-VT/PVCs and RF catheter ablation in the RVOT results in both a failed ablation and a change in QRS morphology. PA-VT/PVCs often originate from the septal side of the PA.

LVOT VT

- Its presence is suggested by RBBB morphology in V1 or LBBB morphology with early transition in V2.
- LVOT VT originates from superior basal segment of the septum inferior to AO valve. It may also originate from aorto-mitral continuity, medial aspect of mitral annulus, aortic coronary cusp (commonly from left coronary cusp) and epicardium along the anterior cardiac veins.
- The majority of septal outflow tract tachycardias arise from right side 10% may arise from LV side of the septum.
- This tachycardia is sensitive to adenosine.

Electrocardiographic features
- Electrocardiogram shows dominate R in V1 V2, early R-wave progression and transition by lead V3.
- Axis is inferiorly directed.
- Left bundle morphology VT from the aortic cusp region and top of the LV septum has a precordial transition that is earlier than from the RVOT region. The R wave is positive by lead V2 or V3 with VT from the right coronary cusp and by lead V1 or V2 from the left coronary cusp.
- Left coronary cusp VT and VT originating from the endocardium or epicardium just in front of the left coronary cusp is often associated with a W- or M-shaped pattern in lead V1 and thus is difficult to classify as a true left or right bundle branch block pattern.
- Similar to RVOT tachycardias, VT from the left coronary cusp and usually the right coronary cusp has a tall QRS in the inferior leads if the valve remains parallel to the pulmonic valve.
- The tall QRS morphology in the inferior leads is because the muscular septum is activated in a similar fashion from both the right and left septal perivalvular structures.

- The left coronary cusp tends to have a QS or rS complex in lead I, whereas the right coronary cusp has greater R-wave amplitude in lead I based on how posterior and rightward the right coronary cusp is positioned.
- VT originating from the aortomitral continuity on the endocardium, produce a qR complex in lead V1 and an Rs/rs complex in lead I. With VT originating from the anterior mitral annulus, the R wave in lead I diminishes and a broad, positive R wave is seen in lead V1.
- VT from left ventricular epicardial sites, anterior to the aortic valve, is frequently similar to patterns from the left coronary cusp. These tachycardias appear to cluster at perivascular sites of the left ventricular epicardium, with the majority at the junction of the great cardiac vein/anterior interventricular vein and proximal anterior interventricular vein.
- QRS tend to have LB morphology in lead V1, and slurring in the initial portion of the QRS,
- Left ventricular epicardial VT in this region commonly have a QS morphology in lead I and may show a characteristic QRS transition pattern break, with the QRS in lead V2 being less positive or having a smaller R wave than in both lead V1 and V3. This pattern break is noted for VT with a LBBB or slightly more leftward positioned VT with a RBBB QRS morphology
- Later transitions at V3 and V4 are suggestive of VTs arising from the right ventricular outflow.
- LVOT VT arising from the epicardium demonstrates positive concordance in precordial leads and negative QRS complex in LI and aVL. Pace map tends to be suboptimal.

Electrophysiologic characteristics (Table 7.15)
- Earliest electrogram potentials tend to be low amplitude and far field.
- Epicardial mapping from coronary venous system or pericardium may be required.
- The pace mapping from the aortic cusp region can be difficult because of the paucity of muscle fibers and often requires good contact, stability, high current strength, and placement into the base of the sinus.
- The noncoronary cusp is notable for atrial capture during pace mapping as it abuts the interatrial septum and may be the source of atrial arrhythmias.
- Coronary artery angiograms must be performed to delineate the proximity of the ablation catheter to artery. Left coronary angiograms should be repeated after the ablation.
- Left main coronary artery trauma may occur during ablation of LVOT VT originating from left coronary sinus of Valsalva.
- Location of the ostium of the left main coronary artery should be identified by placing a catheter or guide wire during ablation.
- Pace mapping is performed in regions of interest based on analysis of the 12-lead ECG during VT, with attention to an exact match for all 12 ECG leads. Activation mapping with unipolar and bipolar recordings is used to corroborate the pace map finding when recurrent ventricular premature depolarizations (VPDs) or VT is observed.

Table 7.15 Causes and differentiating features of the tachycardia with LBBB morphology.

	ECG	EP features	Entrainment	Adenosine sensitivity	Structural heart disease
RVOT VT	LB Inf.axis	AVD. No His	No	Yes	No
ARVD	LB Inf/sup axis	AVD No His	Yes	No	Yes
Atriofascicular	LB Sup. axis	His after V	Yes	Yes	No
BB reentry	LB Sup. axis	Long HV	Yes	No	Yes
Septal VT in CAD	LB Inf./Sup. axis	AVD No His	Yes	No	Yes
VT post repair of Fallot.	LB Inf. axis	AVD No His	Yes	No	Yes
SVT LBBB	LB Inf. axis	Normal AH and HV	From atrium	Yes	No

AVD = AV dissociation; Inf. = inferior; Sup. = superior.

- Intracardiac echocardiography can be used to assess catheter tip position in the aortic cusp region and to confirm anatomic location and proximity to coronary anatomy.
- Prior to ablation in the aortic cusp region and in the left ventricular endocardium/epicardium in front of the aortic valve, angiography usually is performed to assess proximity to the coronary circulation. The area anterior to the aortic valve and next to the proximal anterior interventricular vein is adjacent to the left main/left anterior descending coronary artery bifurcation, and caution must be exercised when ablating in this area.
- Standard 4-mm-tip radiofrequency ablation is effective.

Supravalvular atrial and ventricular arrhythmias (Table 7.16)
- Ventricular myocardial sleeves may extend into the great arteries.
- NCC is closely and almost entirely related to atrial tissue, particularly the interatrial septum.
- The junction of the NCC and RCC is directly opposite the commissure between the septal and anterior tricuspid valve leaflets. This is the location of the penetrating bundle of His.
- The RCC, particularly anteriorly, directly underlies the RVOT (posterior infundibulum). A large portion of the LCC and the NCC is directly continuous with the anterior leaflet of the mitral valve (the aortic mitral continuity) but may occasionally have ventricular myocardial extensions in this location.
- Posterior RVOT is in close proximity to to the origin and course of the left main coronary artery.
- LVOT myocardium routinely extends as a crescent above the line of attachment of the RCC.

Table 7.16 Supravalvar arrhythmias – anatomic correlates.

Valve/cusp	Atrial relation	Ventricular relation	Electrograms recorded	Relevant arrhythmia
NCC of aortic valve	Immediate anterior neighbor of the interatrial septum)	None directly	Large atrial electrograms with fragmented near-field electrograms during tachycardia	Atrial tachycardia; accessory pathways traversing the NCC
RCC	Overlying right atrial appendage and SVC RA junction	Posterior infundibular portion of RVOT	Large ventricular electrogram more posteriorly atrial electrograms from overlying appendage; His bundle electrograms at RCC/NCC commissure	Ventricular tachycardia; vantage point for posterior RVOT; supravalvar myocardium; atrial tachycardia posteriorly; accessory pathway traversing the cusp
LCC	Typically none unless aortic mitral continuity has myocardial fibers	Typically none unless fibers in aortic mitral continuity and extending above the LCC	Far-field ventricular electrogram with atrial electrograms posteriorly	Ventricular tachycardia
Pulmonary valve anteriorly	Overlying left atrial appendage	Left ventricular myocardium inferiorly and continuity with RVOT	Large ventricular electrogram, possibly small far-field atrial electrogram from appendage proximity	Ventricular tachycardia; accessory pathway connecting to the infundibulum
Pulmonary valve posteriorly	Portion of anterior left atrium and possibly a second posterior lobe of left atrial appendage	RCC lies posteriorly and on the right with the LCC and left main coronary artery immediately posterior to the posterior supravalvar pulmonary artery	Large ventricular electrogram, spikes or near-field signals distinct from nearby ventricular activation	Ventricular tachycardia

- Most of the NCC and parts of the LCC lack ventricular myocardium, as in this region fibrous continuity with the anterior leaflet of the mitral valve exists.
- The RVOT passes anterior and then to the left of the RCC of the aortic valve.
- The NCC is immediately anterior to the interatrial septum.
- Both left and right atrial myocardium is adjacent to this cusp as the interatrial septum forms.
- In some patients, the posterior portion of the RCC can be related to the interatrial septum or to the anteroseptal portion of the annular, anteroseptal portion of the right atrium.
- The right atrial appendage overlies the lateral ascending aorta just above the RCC.
- The LCC is typically not anatomically related to either the right or left atria.
- The left atrial appendage overlies the anterior and leftward portions of the RVOT and pulmonary annulus.

Relation to the annuli and conduction system
- Commissure between the NCC and LCC is positioned along the area of the aortic mitral continuity. Here the immediate relationship is with the anterior mitral valve leaflet with typically no myocardium intervening.
- The commissure between the NCC and RCC is located immediately adjacent to the commissure of the anterior and septal leaflets of the tricuspid valve. The joining of these commissures forms the membranous portion of the interventricular septum and is the location of the penetrating bundle of His and, more distally, the origin of the left bundle branch.
- The compact AVN node is located more posteriorly and inferiorly to this commissure. The fast pathway input to the AVN, is located directly posterior to this commissure and is thus related to the anterior portions of the NCC.
- Ablation of the interatrial septum from the NCC of the aortic valve and the deep midmyocardial portion of the posterior RVOT from the RCC of the aortic valve can be attempted.
- Frequent symptomatic PVCs and sustained ventricular tachycardia either RVOT or LVOT in origin have been ablated above the pulmonic valve or in the RCC or LCC
- RVOT is anterior to the LVOT, and as the conus tapers to the level of the pulmonary valves, the RVOT is to the left of the LVOT and aortic valve. This anatomic fact has to be appreciated during mapping procedures.
- During mapping of PVCs the site of earliest activation is noted anteriorly and as leftward as the operator can reach with the catheter when mapping on the right side, it may be incorrectly perceived that the true site of origin is in the LVOT. If far-field and relatively early signals are seen rightward and posterior in the RVOT, a possible origin above the aortic valve should be considered.
- Because of the leftward and cephalad orientation of the pulmonary annulus relative to the aortic annulus, injury to the left main coronary artery may occur when ablating posteriorly in a supra pulmonary valve location
- Ventricular myocardium is not seen above the NCC and LCC, and, in fact, myocardium is absent typically 1–2 cm below the line of attachment of these cusps.

- There is fibrous continuity among the aortic valve, the anterior leaflet of the mitral valve, and the central fibrous body of the heart in this location.
- The classic QRS vector in RVOT tachycardia shows a left bundle branch block pattern, inferior axis, and QS complexes in both leads aVR and aVL. There is an entirely negative QS complex in lead V1 and usually no discernible R wave.
- In the presence of incomplete RBBB pattern may signify left ventricular origin, however two other situations need to be considered
  1 Tachycardia origin above the pulmonary valve.
  2 Focus being located on the posterior RVOT.
- Because the pulmonic valve is the leftmost part of the RVOT, the vector from early activation above the pulmonary valve is initially toward lead V1, a right and anterior chest lead.
- Epicardial mapping is rarely needed for ablating aortic root tachycardia.
- In posterior RVOT tachycardia, initial vector causes the small R wave toward lead V1, an anteriorly placed lead.
- Mapping the posterior wall of the RVOT can be difficult.
- From the femoral approach clockwise rotation is required to get the catheter into the RVOT. This may allow the anterior portion of the RVOT to be mapped. Counterclockwise rotation may be required to reach the posterior wall however that results in a poor contact and or catheter displacement.
- Earliest recorded near-field signal for a focus originating in the posterior RVOT may be from a catheter placed in the supravalvar RCC of the aortic valve (located just behind the posterior RVOT). Further, not only mapping but ablating posterior RVOT tachycardia can be accomplished both from the RVOT and from a catheter in the anterior supra-aortic valve region.
- When the R wave is all positive, with a typical RBBB pattern in V1, the origin of arrhythmia is invariably in the left ventricle.
- Any site in the left ventricle (mitral annulus, apex, free wall, epicardial) will be associated with a right bundle branch block pattern.
- Considering outflow tract arrhythmia with a right bundle branch block pattern inferior axis, some specific anatomic correlations should be made
- Damage to the coronary artery during outflow tract ablation may occur. This may occur when ablating in the aortic cusps, anatomically the coronary arteries are closer to the posterior RVOT.
- In the proximal part of the RVOT near the free wall, the right coronary artery is 4–5 mm away and separated by a variable amount of fat. The left main coronary artery is immediatly posterior to the RVOT and pulmonary valve.
- Because of the cephalocaudal separation of the pulmonic and aortic valve, the pulmonic valve is very close to the origin of this coronary artery.
- Anterior interventricular coronary veins are located on the interventricular septum and near the base are close to the epicardial surface of the leftward portion of the RVOT. Occasionally, smaller tributaries may drain the tissue between the RVOT and LVOT, and these veins can be used to map or ablate foci in this region.

- The anterior and lateral portions of the RVOT are fairly thin. Although foci may occur on the epicardial surface of the RVOT in these locations, ablation from the endocardium is usually effective.
- The posterior RVOT (infundibulum) is much thicker, but the epicardial surface of the posterior infundibulum is the LVOT, and thus ablation may be effective from either the left or the right side for arrhythmias arising deep in the myocardium of the posterior RVOT.
- There is no true epicardial location for the supravalvular aortic region because central anatomic location of the aortic valve and because the "epicardial" anterior structure to the RCC or anterior LCC is the posterior RVOT. There is no role for epicardial mapping to try and ablate epicardial supravalvular aortic foci.
- The NCC is the most posterior of the three aortic cusps. The most anterior portion of this cusp is the commissure with the RCC. As noted, this is the location of the membranous septum at which the His bundle is located. Thus, mapping or ablation in the NCC is unlikely to record a His bundle electrogram or ablate this structure. However, as the fast pathway and anteroseptal atrial myocardium are posterior to the His bundle, a catheter placed in the rightward portion of the NCC will map and potentially ablate these structures.
- Find a large atrial electrogram when the catheter is located in the NCC and little or no atrial electrograms with large ventricular electrograms when mapping the RCC.

Clues for atrial tachycardia origin above the valve
- The electrocardiogram shows narrow P waves that tend to be positive in V1 (whereas anterior tricuspid valve and right atrial appendage tachycardias are typically all negative in V1).
- Short P-R interval is sometimes noted with atrial tachycardia arising in supra-valvar locations.
- Relatively simultaneous activation of the His bundle, fast pathway, septal mitral annulus, and superior ostial coronary sinus regions is seen. The possibility of deep myocardial focus in the anterior portion of the interatrial septum and ablation in the NCC should be considered.
- Ablation near the commissure with the RCC may injure the fast pathway, and thus cryoablation should be considered. Another important clue is the finding of far-field electrograms on the right interatrial septum just behind the superior portion of the tendon of Todaro that precede local activation (the near-field electrogram) by 20–40 ms. This should also alert the operator to the presence of either an NCC atrial tachycardia or a septal mitral annular tachycardia.

Left ventricular VT (intrafascicular tachycardia): fascicular VT
- It originates near left posterior fascicle in the region of inferoposterior left ventricle septum.
- It is common in men. There is no structural heart disease and baseline electrocardiogram tends to be normal.

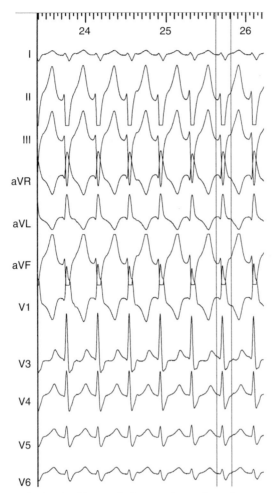

Figure 7.21 Left ventricular VT RB morphology and superior axis.

- During tachycardia ECG shows RBBB morphology and left superior axis (Figure 7.21).
- Presents as exercise-related VT between the ages of 15 and 40 years.
- These arrhythmias do not involve the His bundle, are verapamil sensitive, and occur in patients without structural cardiac disease.
- Most appear to have a mechanism of reentry involving either false tendons or long loops of fascicular tissue.
- The mechanism is reentry in or near portions of Purkinje fascicles of the left bundle. More than 80% of these VTs have exits near the posterior fascicles of the left bundle, causing a superior frontal plane axis.
- Sites of ablation are guided by inscription of fascicular potentials from the left anterior lateral region of the left ventricle.
- The rarest form of fascicular tachycardia (upper septal VT) presents as a narrow complex rhythm that involves simultaneous anterograde activation of the

left anterior and posterior fascicles with retrograde conduction over a separate fascicle inserting into the LBB.

- Purkinje fibers may survive acute ischemia and be involved in both triggered and reentrant arrhythmias.
- Occasionally, VT has an inferior axis, suggesting an exit in the vicinity of the anterior fascicle. potentials in diastole during VT and sinus rhythm are present in the inferoseptal region that appears to indicate a slow conduction region that is sensitive to verapamil.
- Ablation targets sharp potentials near the circuit exit or the diastolic potentials.
- Mechanical trauma from catheter manipulation often terminates VT and prevents reinitiation. Ablation then targets the site of mechanical termination, low amplitude, or diastolic sinus rhythm potentials, or creates a line of lesions through this region.
- Overall success rate of ablation was >95%.
- Although complications related to left heart catheterization and are expected, no serious complications were reported. Left posterior hemiblock has been observed when a line of RF lesions was placed through the posterior septal region.
- It can be induced by atrial pacing. Tachycardia is verapamil sensitive.
- Symptoms during tachycardia include palpitations, dizziness and syncope.
- Tachycardia can be induced by exercise and emotional distress.
- It may originate from superior fascicle in 5 to 10% of patients. In these cases ECG shows RBBB morphology and right inferior axis.
- The RS interval during VT is 60–80 ms.
- QRS is relatively short and the morphology is sharp when compared with muscle or scar related VT.
- SAECG tends to be normal.
- It is verapamil sensitive.
- Tachycardia may originate from the false tendon.
- It does not result in SCD.
- Reentrant monomorphic VT originating from the left posterior Purkinje fibers, which is analogous to idiopathic left VT, can develop in the acute or chronic phase of MI. Catheter ablation is highly effective in eliminating this VT without affecting left ventricular conduction.

Electrophysiologic characteristics of left ventricular VT
- A short VH interval is recorded during the tachycardia. Sharp high frequency fascicular potential precedes earliest ventricular activation by 30 to 40 msec during VT. These may represent Purkinje potentials.
- HPS potential can be recorded during sinus rhythm (Figure 7.22).
- The mechanism of the tachycardia is reentry. Antegrade limb appears to be slowly conducting verapamil sensitive Purkinje tissue and retrograde limb is Purkinje tissue from posterior fascicle.
- Antegrade His capture may occur during atrial pacing without affecting VT cycle length. Sinus beats and PVCs can capture ventricle without resetting the tachycardia. These findings suggest small reentrant circuit.

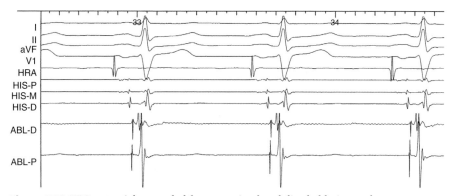

Figure 7.22 HPS potentials recorded from proximal and distal ablation catheter electrodes.

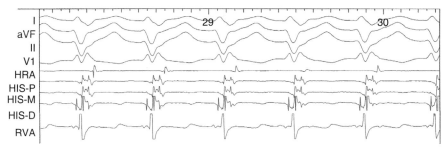

Figure 7 .23 Retrograde activation of His during VT.

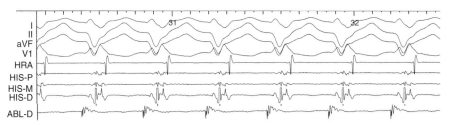

Figure 7.24 Fractionated electrograms recorded at the site of earliest activation from the distal electrodes of the ablation catheter.

- His bundle is not a required component of VT circuit, because the retrograde H is recorded 20 to 40 msec after the earliest activation (Figure 7.23).
- Tachycardia can be induced by pacing or programmed stimulation from atrium or ventricle with or without isoproterenol infusion. Inverse relation between initiating PVC and first beat of the VT has been described.
- Continuous or mid diastolic activity may be recorded from ablation site.
- Fractionated electrograms may be recorded at the site of earliest activation (Figure 7.24).

- The area of slow conduction in VT zone depends on inward calcium current. This may explain sensitivity of the tachycardia to verapamil but not to adenosine or Valsalva maneuvers.
- It may respond to adenosine if catecholamine stimulation is required to induce the tachycardia.
- Tachycardia can be entrained by pacing from RVOT. The tachycardia can be entrained by atrial pacing,

Treatment
- IV verapamil can be used for acute termination and oral verapamil for chronic therapy of left ventricular VT.
- Ablation should be considered when antiarrhythmic therapy fails. Pace map may not be helpful in identifying the ablation site. Presence of earliest Purkinje potential is crucial for the success of the ablation even more important than the earliest QRS activation site.
- Identification and ablation of purkinje potentials during sinus rhythm, in patients in whom tachycardia can not be induced, may provide satisfactory outcome.
- Ablation may be successful either over the exit site in the posteroinferior left ventricle septum or at a site of inscription of a discrete presystolic potential, which may be recorded at a distance of 2 to 3 cm from the exit site and is defined by a mid-diastolic potential.
- Complications may include mitral and/or aortic regurgitation.

Interfascicular VT
- Re-entrant circuit involves superior and inferior division of LB.
- RBBB with a variable frontal plane QRS axis depending on the tachycardia circuit. Tachycardia could present as RBBB and left posterior fascicular block if the antegrade conduction occurred over left anterior fascicle and retrograde conduction over left posterior fascicle. Presence of RBBB and left anterior fascicular block will occur if the circuit was reversed.
- RBBB morphology is similar during sinus rhythm and during tachycardia.
- During tachycardia there is reversal in the activation sequence of His and LB and HV interval is shorter during VT than in sinus rhythm because the upper turnaround point is at the LBB.
- Block in either fascicle results in termination of the tachycardia.
- Demonstrating that the fascicular potentials drive the ventricular response and that the His bundle is passive and can be dissociated from the tachycardia is diagnostic.
- Cure of interfascicular reentry involves ablation of the fascicle involved in the tachycardia circuit.

Papillary muscle VT (Table 7.17)
- VT could arise from anterolateral or posteromedial left ventricular papillary muscle.
- During electrophysiologic study and radiofrequency ablation papillary muscle involvement is established by intracardiac echocardiography.

Table 7.17 Differentiating features between fascicular VT and te papillary muscle VT.

Electrocardiographic features	Papillary muscle VT	FascicularVT
EKG	Absent	rsR' pattern in V1
	Absent	Q in leads I and aVL with superior axis Q waves in leads II, III and aVF with inferior axis
	Relatively wider QRS width during arrhythmia 150 msec	Relatively narrower QRS width during arrhythmia 127 msec
Electrophysiologic features		
	Purkinje potential to QRS interval shorter	Purkinje potential to QRS intervals longer
	Less likely	Purkinje potential at effective site
	Matching pace map at effective site	Unlikely
	Low Voltage ventricular EGM	High-voltage ventricular EGM

Cellular electrophysiology of Purkinje cells
- The transient outward current I_{to} is more prominent in Purkinje cells than in myocytes, Inward rectification current IK1 and the L-type Ca^{2+} current are more prominent in myocytes.
- Normal Purkinje cells do not show automaticity and are overdrive suppressed by sinus node activity.
- Purkinje fiber automaticity is enhanced by digitalis. It inhibits Na^+/K^+ ATPase activity resulting in cytosolic Ca^{2+} overload.
- Ca^{2+} waves have been shown to occur in normal Purkinje cells even without electrical stimulation.
- Purkinje cells are capable of generating both automatic and triggered rhythms
- His bundle and Purkinje fibers express both Cx40 and Cx43, as opposed to ventricular myocardium, which predominantly expresses Cx43.
- The cellular architecture of Purkinje fibers explains the rapid conduction in the HPS (2–3 m/s) compared with cardiac muscle (0.2–0.4 m/s).
- Trifascicular system Thin left anterior fascicle, which connects the left bundle branch to region of the anterolateral papillary muscle, a broader left posterior fascicle, which inserts midway between the base and apex near the base of the posterior papillary muscle, and a separate septal fascicle.

- ECG criteria of left anterior fascicular block seldom shows isolated focal block in the anterior fascicle. It acted as a surrogate for diffuse endocardial fibroses involving the left-sided specialized conduction system.
- The diffuse nature of fascicular involvement may play a role in fascicle-to-fascicle re-entry.

Short coupled torsades

- Syndrome of polymorphic VT associated with a short-coupling interval (245 ± 28 ms) between PVCs and conducted complexes in patients without ischemic, structural cardiac disease or ion channel abnormalities.
- The arrhythmia may not be provoked by isoproterenol, but the coupling interval may increase and long-term arrhythmia control may be achieved with verapamil therapy. Torsades de points due to congenital or acquired long QT syndrome is associated with much longer coupling interval and an abnormal QT interval.
- Catheter ablation of PVCs responsible for initiating polymorphic ventricular tachycardia may abolish the arrhythmia.

Mechanism of short-coupled torsades

- Initiating PVCs have very short coupling intervals.
- The trigger complex frequently gives rise to bursts of polymorphic VT
- It appears to be focal because ablation of the trigger (and possibly associated diseased Purkinje tissue) results in tachycardia cure.
- Catecholamines are not an arrhythmia provocateur, and verapamil may have a beneficial effect.
- Possible mechanisms for the short-coupled trigger include:
  - Spontaneous Ca^{2+} waves emanating from the Purkinje tissue or contiguous muscle
  - Phase 2 reentry in tightly coupled muscle–Purkinje junctions
  - Marked conduction slowing and reentry in diseased Purkinje fibers
  - The effects of verapamil tend to favor involvement of Ca^{2+} in initiation of the trigger.
  - Short-coupled PVCs, may be a reflection of delayed afterdepolarizations, which lead to arrhythmias.

Aortic cusp ventricular tachycardias

- VT originating from extension of ventricular myocardium above the aortic annulus that required ablation from within the sinuses of Valsalva accounted for 15 and 20% of idiopathic OT-VTs
- Electrocardiographic characteristics of aortic cusp ventricular tachycardia or PVCs include: (Figure 7.25)
- For right coronary cusp VT
  1 Left bundle morphology. Small broad R-wave in V1 V2
  2 Early transition.
  3 S wave in lead I
  4 R wave in lead II, III and AVF
  5 No S wave in V6

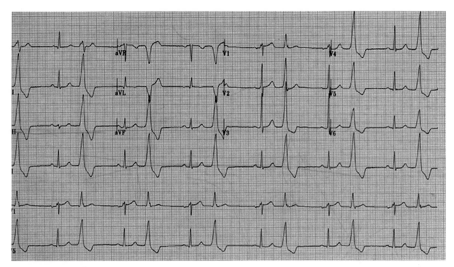

Figure 7.25 Left coronary cusp PVCs.

- For left coronary cusp VT
  1 M or W pattern in V1.
  2 rS in LI.
- For noncoronary cusp
  1 Presents as supraventricular tachycardia. Atrial capture when paced from here.
- The majority are ablated from the left coronary cusp, followed in frequency by the right coronary cusp, the junction between the right and left coronary cusp, and rarely the non-coronary cusp.
- The majority are ablated from the LCC, followed in frequency by the RCC, the junction between the RCC and LCC, and rarely the NCC.
- Activation mapping typically shows a two-component electrogram with the earliest deflection preceding the QRS complex by an average of 39 ms, but sometimes >50 ms. Pace mapping in the aortic sinus may require high output and is less likely to reproduce the VT QRS compared with pace mapping for endocardial VTs.
- Acute occlusion of the left main or right coronary arteries is a major concern.
- The proximity of the coronary ostia to the ablation site must be defined by coronary angiography or ICE.
- Sites of successful ablation are typically >8 mm below the coronary artery ostia.
- Injury to the aorticvalve is theoretically possible.
- Titration of energy beginning at low power is reasonable.
- Epicardial ablation may increase the risk of Phrenic nerve injury given that the PN is in direct contact with the epicardial surface. The anatomic location of the PN is frequently determined by eliciting diaphragmatic stimulation with bipolar pacing at high-voltage output.
- Methods for separating the PN from the epicardial surface include introduction of a balloon catheter or air in the pericardial space

7.7 Miscellaneous forms of ventricular arrhythmias

Bidirectional VT

- It is a fascicular tachycardia. QRS complex is narrow with RBBB pattern and alternating left and right axis deviation in frontal plane giving rise to bidirectional appearance in limb leads.
- Twelve lead electrocardiogram is required to make the diagnosis.
- It is descriptive term where the causes and mechanism of the tachycardia may be different.
- It is often associated with digitalis toxicity in the presence of structural heart disease. It has also been observed in the presence of herbal aconite poisoning and familial hypokalemic periodic paralysis (Table 7.18).
- Aconitine results in persistent activation of the Na channel and may mimic LQT3.
- Mechanism of the digitalis induced bidirectional VT appears to be triggered activity due to delayed after depolarization.
- It carries poor prognosis.
- Digoxin specific Fab fragment administration is the treatment of choice for digitalis induced tachycardia.

Accelerated idioventricular rhythm (AIVR)[51]

- AIVR is characterized by more than three consecutive ventricular beats at less than 100 bpm but faster than the intrinsic ventricular escape rhythm.
- It may be associated with isorhythmic AV dissociation and fusion beats at onset and termination.
- Gradual onset and termination may occur depending on the intrinsic sinus rate.
- AIVR may occur in a normal heart or in the presence of structural heart disease such as myocardial ischemia and infarction, Myocarditis, cardiomyopathy, digitalis and cocaine toxicity.
- AIVR commonly occurs following myocardial reperfusion. QRS may be multiform.
- The mechanism of the AIVR appears to be abnormal automaticity.
- AIVR is generally benign. It does not require treatment.

Table 7.18 Causes of bidirectional VT.

Causes of bidirectional VT	Therapeutic options
Catecholaminergic polymorphic ventricular tachycardia	Beta-blockers, ICD
Digoxin toxicity	Digoxin antibodies
Familial hypokalemic periodic paralysis.	Potassium replacement
Herbal aconite poisoning	IV lidocaine
Andersen–Tawil Syndrome	ICD

- In patients with diminished cardiac function loss of atrial contribution may cause symptoms. Increasing sinus rate by atropine may resolve AIVR.
- Occurrence of AIVR in the presence of acute MI does not increase the incidence of VF or mortality.

Parasystole[52]

- Parasystole results from automatic and protected focus.
- Normal or abnormal automaticity, triggered activity due to EAD or DAD can cause parasystole.
- Parasystole is characterized by
  ○ Varying coupled interval.
  ○ Fusion beats.
  ○ Mathematically related interectopic intervals which may vary due to autonomic influences.
- Parasystole is classified as:
  ○ Continuous without exit block.
  ○ Continuous with exit block.
  ○ Intermittent.

Propofol-related infusion syndrome (PRIS)

- Constellation of otherwise unexplained cardiac failure, metabolic acidosis, rhabdomyolysis, and renal failure in the setting of prolonged high-dose propofol therapy.
- Patients with PRIS often develop malignant arrhythmias leading to sudden cardiac death. High-dose propofol, especially in the presence of concomitant therapy with catecholamines or corticosteroids, is suspected of acting as a trigger for PRIS.
- Propofol impairs mitochondrial function by uncoupling oxidative phosphorylation, energy production, and oxygen utilization. It antagonizes beta-adrenoceptor binding, inhibits the cardiac L-type calcium current, and potentiates its myocardial depressive effects by superimposing the cardiomyocytolytic effects of catecholamines.
- Although propofol can contribute to proarrhythmic properties by blocking mitochondrial fatty acid utilization with accumulation of un-utilized free fatty acids, the mechanisms leading to malignant arrhythmias and sudden cardiac death in patients with PRIS remain unclear.
- ECG abnormalities in precordial leads V1 to V3 in the setting of high-dose propofol infusion similar to that described in Brugada syndrome have been observed.
- Genetic analysis of these patients did not reveal mutations in the *SCN5A* gene, and the result of a flecainide challenge test was negative. Neither significant change in repolarization nor propofol-induced ST segment elevation was observed even in the PRIS-like conditions of hyperkalemia and acidosis.
- Patients with PRIS are at risk for lethal ventricular arrhythmias with development of ECG abnormalities and that propofol anesthetic should be promptly withdrawn.

- Propofol infusion at high doses (>5 mg/kg/hr) should be discouraged for long-term sedation (>48 hours) in the intensive care setting.

Mechanically induced ventricular fibrillation (commotio cordis)[93,94]

- Sudden cardiac death secondary to relatively innocent chest wall impact is known as commotio cordis.
- Sudden death occurs when VF is initiated by relatively innocent chest wall impact.
- These recreational players are often young (mean age 14 years) and male (>95%).
- Impact objects are solid implements. Striking directly over the cardiac silhouette.
- Baseball, lacrosse, softball, and hockey account for the majority of the sports. Chest wall protection does not prevent sudden death.
- Resuscitation is possible with early cardiopulmonary resuscitation and defibrillation.
- Impacts occurring 0–40 ms before the peak of the T wave cause VF, and the impacts are most lethal during the 10- to 30-ms window.
- Impacts at other times in the cardiac cycle may cause transient heart block, left bundle branch block, or ST elevations, but these abnormalities are self-limited.
- Of these three abnormalities, ST elevations appear independent of the timing of the strike, but transient heart block and bundle branch block are more common with QRS strikes.
- Stiffness of the impact object directly correlated with the probability of VF occurring with chest wall impact, the impact energy increases to 40 mph,
- The initial 3–5 s is an undulating polymorphic ventricular tachycardia with a cycle length of 200–250 ms.
- Chest wall thumping produces ventricular depolarization and effective myocardial contraction in asystole.
- Chest wall blows produce a ventricular depolarization
- Shocks with energies that lie between the lower and upper limits of vulnerability will cause VF.
- In electrically induced VF, this critical energy window of vulnerability to VF is thought to be based on whether complete or incomplete depolarization of the ventricle occurs.

Cardiac sarcoidosis[95,96]

- In cardiac sarcoidosis patients, CAVB develops mainly during the active phase of the disease.
- Early treatment with corticosteroids might improve AV conduction disturbance. However, sustained VT is not closely linked with disease activity and frequently develops in the advanced stage of disease.
- The disease process in cardiac sarcoidosis often involves a specific area in the basal right ventricle predisposing to peritricuspid reentry.

- Sarcoidosis is a systemic inflammatory disease of unknown etiology that is characterized by the formation of noncaseating granulomas and subsequent tissue scarring.
- It primarily affects the lungs, reticuloendothelial system, and skin.
- Clinical evidence of myocardial involvement is present in approximately 5% of patients with systemic sarcoidosis, but myocardial involvement has been reported in 20 to 27% at autopsy.
- Clinical manifestations of cardiac sarcoidosis include CHF, ventricular tachyarrhythmia, supraventricular arrhythmia, AV conduction block, and sudden death. Cardiac involvement of sarcoidosis is associated with a mortality rate greater than 40% at 5 years, and many of the deaths are caused by ventricular tachyarrhythmias.
- The results of antiarrhythmic therapy for life-threatening ventricular tachyarrhythmias in patients with cardiac sarcoidosis often are disappointing
- Steroids have been used in patients with cardiac sarcoidosis and have been reported to improve prognosis, but their effect on VT is unclear.
- Placement of an ICD is recommended for all patients with cardiac sarcoidosis who present with VT refractory to medication.
- Catheter ablation has been attempted in cardiac sarcoidosis patients with frequent VT episodes, but the results have been disappointing.
- The success rate of VT ablation in patients with cardiac sarcoidosis was much lower than that in patients with ischemic heart disease
- Patients have less severe left ventricular dysfunction;
- Induced VT smay have LBBB morphology, which usually indicates origination from the right ventricle. Because the right ventricular wall is thinner than that of the left ventricle, the effect of ablation is more likely to extend to the epicardium.
- Success rate was higher for VTs with LBBB morphology than for those with RBBB morphology.
- Cardiac involvement by sarcoid may manifest as impaired AV conduction, ventricular arrhythmias, and sudden death.
- Twenty-five percent of patients with systemic sarcoidosis may have myocardial involvement.
- It involves a small area of the heart and may remain clinically silent.
- Eight percent of the scar-related VTs in nonischemic heart disease may be due to cardiac sarcoidosis.
- Although most patients with systemic sarcoid have preserved ejection fraction, advanced cardiac involvement can lead to reduced systolic function.
- VT may be the initial manifestation of cardiac involvement of sarcoid disease.
- Cardiac biopsy initially may be negative in 50% of the patients.
- It may be mistaken for arrhythmogenic right ventricular dysplasia.
- Electrophysiologic study may reveal evidence of scar-related reentry resulting in monomorphic VTs with multiple morphologies with both right bundle branch block and left bundle branch block QRS configuration.

- The majority (>90%) of the patients demonstrate areas of low-voltage scar in the right ventricle, 50% may have left ventricular and 25% may have epicardial involvement.
- In patients with cardiac sarcoid, ventricular tachycardia (VT) is associated with significant morbidity and is an independent predictor of mortality.
- Current management for VT includes immunosuppressive therapy, defibrillator implantation, antiarrhythmic therapy, radiofrequency ablation and transplantation.

References

1 Ideker RE, Walcott GP, Epstein AE, Plumb VJ, Kay N. Ventricular fibrillation and defibrillation – what are the major unresolved issues? *Heart Rhythm.* 2005;2(5): 555–558.

2 Josephson ME, Callans DJ. Using the twelve-lead electrocardiogram to localize the site of origin of ventricular tachycardia. *Heart Rhythm.* 2005;2(4):443–446.

3 Stevenson WG, Khan H, Sager P, et al. Identification of reentry circuit sites during catheter mapping and radiofrequency ablation of ventricular tachycardia late after myocardial infarction. *Circulation.* 1993;88(4 Pt 1):1647–1670.

4 Bogun F, Kim HM, Han J, et al. Comparison of mapping criteria for hemodynamically tolerated, postinfarction ventricular tachycardia. *Heart Rhythm.* 2006;3(1):20–26.

5 Anon. A comparison of antiarrhythmic-drug therapy with implantable defibrillators in patients resuscitated from near-fatal ventricular arrhythmias. The Antiarrhythmics versus Implantable Defibrillators (AVID) Investigators. *N. Engl. J. Med.* 1997;337(22): 1576–1583.

6 Wood MA. Percutaneous pericardial instrumentation in the electrophysiology laboratory: a case of need. *Heart Rhythm.* 2006;3(1):11–12.

7 Gersh BJ, Maron BJ, Bonow RO, et al. 2011 ACCF/AHA guideline for the diagnosis and treatment of hypertrophic cardiomyopathy: a report of the American College of Cardiology Foundation/American Heart Association Task Force on Practice Guidelines. *J. Thorac. Cardiovasc. Surg.* 2011;142(6):e153–203.

8 Selvi Rani D, Nallari P, Dhandapany PS, et al. Cardiac troponin T (TNNT2) mutations are less prevalent in indian hypertrophic cardiomyopathy patients. *DNA Cell Biol.* 2011. Available at: http://www.ncbi.nlm.nih.gov/pubmed/22017532. Accessed January 18, 2012.

9 Watkins H, McKenna WJ, Thierfelder L, et al. Mutations in the genes for cardiac troponin T and alpha-tropomyosin in hypertrophic cardiomyopathy. *N. Engl. J. Med.* 1995;332(16):1058–1064.

10 Hedley PL, Haundrup O, Andersen PS, et al. The KCNE genes in hypertrophic cardiomyopathy: a candidate gene study. *J Negat Results Biomed.* 2011;10:12.

11 Maron BJ, Shen WK, Link MS, et al. Efficacy of implantable cardioverter-defibrillators for the prevention of sudden death in patients with hypertrophic cardiomyopathy. *N. Engl. J. Med.* 2000;342(6):365–373.

12 Nishimura RA, Ommen SR. Hypertrophic cardiomyopathy, sudden death, and implantable cardiac defibrillators: how low the bar? *JAMA.* 2007;298(4):452–454.

13 Nannenberg EA, Michels M, Christiaans I, et al. Mortality risk of untreated myosin-binding protein C-related hypertrophic cardiomyopathy: insight into the natural history. *J. Am. Coll. Cardiol.* 2011;58(23):2406–2414.

14 Streitner F, Kuschyk J, Dietrich C, et al. Comparison of ventricular tachyarrhythmia characteristics in patients with idiopathic dilated or ischemic cardiomyopathy and defibrillators implanted for primary prevention. *Clin Cardiol.* 2011;34(10):604–609.

15 Sliwa K, Forster O, Zhanje F, et al. Outcome of subsequent pregnancy in patients with documented peripartum cardiomyopathy. *Am. J. Cardiol.* 2004;93(11):1441–1443, A10.

16 Caceres J, Jazayeri M, McKinnie J, et al. Sustained bundle branch reentry as a mechanism of clinical tachycardia. *Circulation.* 1989;79(2):256–270.

17 Tester DJ, Will ML, Haglund CM, Ackerman MJ. Compendium of cardiac channel mutations in 541 consecutive unrelated patients referred for long QT syndrome genetic testing. *Heart Rhythm.* 2005;2(5):507–517.

18 Priori SG. From genes to cell therapy: molecular medicine meets clinical EP. *J. Cardiovasc. Electrophysiol.* 2005;16(5):552.

19 Priori SG. Inherited arrhythmogenic diseases: the complexity beyond monogenic disorders. *Circ. Res.* 2004;94(2):140–145.

20 Shimizu W, Noda T, Takaki H, et al. Diagnostic value of epinephrine test for genotyping LQT1, LQT2, and LQT3 forms of congenital long QT syndrome. *Heart Rhythm.* 2004; 1(3):276–283.

21 Vyas H, Hejlik J, Ackerman MJ. Epinephrine QT stress testing in the evaluation of congenital long-QT syndrome: diagnostic accuracy of the paradoxical QT response. *Circulation.* 2006;113(11):1385–1392.

22 Keating MT. The long QT syndrome. A review of recent molecular genetic and physiologic discoveries. *Medicine (Baltimore).* 1996;75(1):1–5.

23 Aiba T, Shimizu W. Molecular screening of long-QT syndrome: risk is there, or rare? *Heart Rhythm.* 2011;8(3):420–421.

24 Krishnan Y, Zheng R, Walsh C, Tang Y, McDonald TV. Partially dominant mutant channel defect corresponding with intermediate LQT2 phenotype. *Pacing Clin Electrophysiol.* 2012;35(1):3–16.

25 Koopmann TT, Alders M, Jongbloed RJ, et al. Long QT syndrome caused by a large duplication in the KCNH2 (HERG) gene undetectable by current polymerase chain reaction-based exon-scanning methodologies. *Heart Rhythm.* 2006;3(1):52–55.

26 Tester DJ, Medeiros-Domingo A, Will ML, Ackerman MJ. Unexplained drownings and the cardiac channelopathies: a molecular autopsy series. *Mayo Clin. Proc.* 2011;86(10): 941–947.

27 Mohler PJ, Schott J-J, Gramolini AO, et al. Ankyrin-B mutation causes type 4 long-QT cardiac arrhythmia and sudden cardiac death. *Nature.* 2003;421(6923):634–639.

28 Tsuboi M, Antzelevitch C. Cellular basis for electrocardiographic and arrhythmic manifestations of Andersen-Tawil syndrome (LQT7). *Heart Rhythm.* 2006;3(3): 328–335.

29 Plaster NM, Tawil R, Tristani-Firouzi M, et al. Mutations in Kir2.1 cause the developmental and episodic electrical phenotypes of Andersen's syndrome. *Cell.* 2001; 105(4):511–519.

30 Splawski I, Timothy KW, Sharpe LM, et al. Ca(V)1.2 calcium channel dysfunction causes a multisystem disorder including arrhythmia and autism. *Cell.* 2004;119(1):19–31.

31 Giustetto C, Schimpf R, Mazzanti A, et al. Long-term follow-up of patients with short QT syndrome. *J. Am. Coll. Cardiol.* 2011;58(6):587–595.

32 Topilski I, Rogowski O, Rosso R, et al. The morphology of the QT interval predicts torsade de pointes during acquired bradyarrhythmias. *J. Am. Coll. Cardiol.* 2007;49(3):320–328.

33 Sy RW, van der Werf C, Chattha IS, et al. Derivation and validation of a simple exercise-based algorithm for prediction of genetic testing in relatives of LQTS probands. *Circulation.* 2011;124(20):2187–2194.

34 Vincent GM. Risk assessment in long QT syndrome: the Achilles heel of appropriate treatment. *Heart Rhythm.* 2005;2(5):505–506.

35 Priori SG, Napolitano C, Schwartz PJ, et al. Association of long QT syndrome loci and cardiac events among patients treated with beta-blockers. *JAMA.* 2004;292(11): 1341–1344.

36 Mönnig G, Köbe J, Löher A, et al. Implantable cardioverter-defibrillator therapy in patients with congenital long-QT syndrome: a long-term follow-up. *Heart Rhythm.* 2005;2(5):497–504.

37 Vincent GM. Role of DNA testing for diagnosis, management, and genetic screening in long QT syndrome, hypertrophic cardiomyopathy, and Marfan syndrome. *Heart.* 2001;86(1):12–14.

38 Fenichel RR, Malik M, Antzelevitch C, et al. Drug-induced torsades de pointes and implications for drug development. *J. Cardiovasc. Electrophysiol.* 2004;15(4): 475–495.

39 Gross GJ. IK1: the long and the short QT of it. *Heart Rhythm.* 2006;3(3):336–338.

40 Anttonen O, Junttila MJ, Maury P, et al. Differences in twelve-lead electrocardiogram between symptomatic and asymptomatic subjects with short QT interval. *Heart Rhythm.* 2009;6(2):267–271.

41 Marcus FI, Zareba W, Calkins H, et al. Arrhythmogenic right ventricular cardiomyopathy/dysplasia clinical presentation and diagnostic evaluation: results from the North American Multidisciplinary Study. *Heart Rhythm.* 2009;6(7):984–992.

42 Calkins H. Arrhythmogenic right ventricular dysplasia. *Trans. Am. Clin. Climatol. Assoc.* 2008;119:273–286; discussion 287–288.

43 Kiès P, Bootsma M, Bax J, Schalij MJ, van der Wall EE. Arrhythmogenic right ventricular dysplasia/cardiomyopathy: screening, diagnosis, and treatment. *Heart Rhythm.* 2006;3(2):225–234.

44 Palmisano BT, Rottman JN, Wells QS, DiSalvo TG, Hong CC. Familial evaluation for diagnosis of arrhythmogenic right ventricular dysplasia. *Cardiology.* 2011;119(1): 47–53.

45 Basso C, Bauce B, Corrado D, Thiene G. Pathophysiology of arrhythmogenic cardiomyopathy. *Nature Reviews. Cardiology.* 2011. Available at: http://www.ncbi.nlm.nih.gov/pubmed/22124316. Accessed January 12, 2012.

46 Kaplan SR, Gard JJ, Protonotarios N, et al. Remodeling of myocyte gap junctions in arrhythmogenic right ventricular cardiomyopathy due to a deletion in plakoglobin (Naxos disease). *Heart Rhythm.* 2004;1(1):3–11.

47 Marcus FI, McKenna WJ, Sherrill D, et al. Diagnosis of arrhythmogenic right ventricular cardiomyopathy/dysplasia: proposed modification of the task force criteria. *Circulation.* 2010;121(13):1533–1541.

48 Wu S, Wang P, Hou Y, et al. Epsilon wave in arrhythmogenic right ventricular dysplasia/cardiomyopathy. *Pacing Clin Electrophysiol.* 2009;32(1):59–63.

49 Peters S, Trümmel M, Koehler B, Westermann KU. The value of different electrocardiographic depolarization criteria in the diagnosis of arrhythmogenic right ventricular dysplasia/cardiomyopathy. *J Electrocardiol.* 2007;40(1):34–37.

50 Pfluger HB, Phrommintikul A, Mariani JA, Cherayath JG, Taylor AJ. Utility of myocardial fibrosis and fatty infiltration detected by cardiac magnetic resonance imaging in the diagnosis of arrhythmogenic right ventricular dysplasia – a single centre experience. *Heart Lung Circ.* 2008;17(6):478–483.

51 Abbara S, Migrino RQ, Sosnovik DE, et al. Value of fat suppression in the MRI evaluation of suspected arrhythmogenic right ventricular dysplasia. *AJR Am J Roentgenol.* 2004;182(3):587–591.

52 Marcus FI, Zareba W, Sherrill D. Evaluation of the normal values for signal-averaged electrocardiogram. *J. Cardiovasc. Electrophysiol.* 2007;18(2):231–233.

53 Kapplinger JD, Landstrom AP, Salisbury BA, et al. Distinguishing arrhythmogenic right ventricular cardiomyopathy/dysplasia-associated mutations from background genetic noise. *J. Am. Coll. Cardiol.* 2011;57(23):2317–2327.

54 Hulot J-S, Jouven X, Empana J-P, Frank R, Fontaine G. Natural history and risk stratification of arrhythmogenic right ventricular dysplasia/cardiomyopathy. *Circulation.* 2004;110(14):1879–1884.

55 Woźniak O, Włodarska EK. Prevention of sudden cardiac deaths in arrhythmogenic right ventricular cardiomyopathy: how to evaluate risk and when to implant a cardioverter-defibrillator? *Cardiol J.* 2009;16(6):588–591.

56 Hodgkinson KA, Parfrey PS, Bassett AS, et al. The impact of implantable cardioverter-defibrillator therapy on survival in autosomal-dominant arrhythmogenic right ventricular cardiomyopathy (ARVD5). *J. Am. Coll. Cardiol.* 2005;45(3):400–408.

57 Schimpf R, Veltmann C, Wolpert C, Borggrefe M. Arrhythmogenic hereditary syndromes: Brugada Syndrome, long QT syndrome, short QT syndrome and CPVT. *Minerva Cardioangiol.* 2010;58(6):623–636.

58 Carey SM, Hocking G. Brugada syndrome – a review of the implications for the anaesthetist. *Anaesth Intensive Care.* 2011;39(4):571–577.

59 Antzelevitch C, Pollevick GD, Cordeiro JM, et al. Loss-of-function mutations in the cardiac calcium channel underlie a new clinical entity characterized by ST-segment elevation, short QT intervals, and sudden cardiac death. *Circulation.* 2007;115(4):442–449.

60 Wilde AAM, Antzelevitch C, Borggrefe M, et al. Proposed diagnostic criteria for the Brugada syndrome. *Eur. Heart J.* 2002;23(21):1648–1654.

61 Brugada P, Brugada J. Right bundle branch block, persistent ST segment elevation and sudden cardiac death: a distinct clinical and electrocardiographic syndrome. A multicenter report. *J. Am. Coll. Cardiol.* 1992;20(6):1391–1396.

62 Antzelevitch C, Brugada R. Fever and Brugada syndrome. *Pacing Clin Electrophysiol.* 2002;25(11):1537–1539.

63 Nogami A, Nakao M, Kubota S, et al. Enhancement of J-ST-segment elevation by the glucose and insulin test in Brugada syndrome. *Pacing Clin Electrophysiol.* 2003;26(1 Pt 2):332–337.

64 Fish JM, Antzelevitch C. Role of sodium and calcium channel block in unmasking the Brugada syndrome. *Heart Rhythm.* 2004;1(2):210–217.

65 Wang K, Asinger RW, Marriott HJL. ST-segment elevation in conditions other than acute myocardial infarction. *N. Engl. J. Med.* 2003;349(22):2128–2135.

66 Morita H, Takenaka-Morita S, Fukushima-Kusano K, et al. Risk stratification for asymptomatic patients with Brugada syndrome. *Circ. J.* 2003;67(4):312–316.

67 Hermida J-S, Denjoy I, Clerc J, et al. Hydroquinidine therapy in Brugada syndrome. *J. Am. Coll. Cardiol.* 2004;43(10):1853–1860.

68 Viskin S. Inducible ventricular fibrillation in the Brugada syndrome: diagnostic and prognostic implications. *J. Cardiovasc. Electrophysiol.* 2003;14(5):458–460.

69 Noda T, Shimizu W, Tanaka K, Chayama K. Prominent J wave and ST segment elevation: serial electrocardiographic changes in accidental hypothermia. *J. Cardiovasc. Electrophysiol.* 2003;14(2):223.

70 Tikkanen JT, Anttonen O, Junttila MJ, et al. Long-term outcome associated with early repolarization on electrocardiography. *N. Engl. J. Med.* 2009;361(26):2529–2537.

71 Wang K, Asinger RW, Marriott HJL. ST-segment elevation in conditions other than acute myocardial infarction. *N. Engl. J. Med.* 2003;349(22):2128–2135.

72 Haïssaguerre M, Derval N, Sacher F, et al. Sudden cardiac arrest associated with early repolarization. *N. Engl. J. Med.* 2008;358(19):2016–2023.

73 Sy RW, Gollob MH, Klein GJ, et al. Arrhythmia characterization and long-term outcomes in catecholaminergic polymorphic ventricular tachycardia. *Heart Rhythm.* 2011;8(6):864–871.

74 Ylänen K, Poutanen T, Hiippala A, Swan H, Korppi M. Catecholaminergic polymorphic ventricular tachycardia. *Eur. J. Pediatr.* 2010;169(5):535–542.

75 Medeiros-Domingo A. [Genetic of catecholaminergic polymorphic ventricular tachycardia: basic concepts]. *Arch Cardiol Mex.* 2009;79 Suppl 2:13–17.

76 Priori SG, Chen SRW. Inherited dysfunction of sarcoplasmic reticulum Ca^{2+} handling and arrhythmogenesis. *Circ. Res.* 2011;108(7):871–883.

77 Priori SG, Napolitano C, Tiso N, et al. Mutations in the cardiac ryanodine receptor gene (hRyR2) underlie catecholaminergic polymorphic ventricular tachycardia. *Circulation.* 2001;103(2):196–200.

78 Tester DJ, Kopplin LJ, Will ML, Ackerman MJ. Spectrum and prevalence of cardiac ryanodine receptor (RyR2) mutations in a cohort of unrelated patients referred explicitly for long QT syndrome genetic testing. *Heart Rhythm.* 2005;2(10):1099–1105.

79 Maier LS. CaMKII regulation of voltage-gated sodium channels and cell excitability. *Heart Rhythm.* 2011;8(3):474–477.

80 van der Werf C, Zwinderman AH, Wilde AAM. Therapeutic approach for patients with catecholaminergic polymorphic ventricular tachycardia: state of the art and future developments. *Europace.* 2011. Available at: http://www.ncbi.nlm.nih.gov/pubmed/21893508. Accessed January 18, 2012.

81 van der Werf C, Kannankeril PJ, Sacher F, et al. Flecainide therapy reduces exercise-induced ventricular arrhythmias in patients with catecholaminergic polymorphic ventricular tachycardia. *J. Am. Coll. Cardiol.* 2011;57(22):2244–2254.

82 Fazio G, Corrado G, Zachara E, et al. Anticoagulant drugs in noncompaction: a mandatory therapy? *J Cardiovasc Med (Hagerstown).* 2008;9(11):1095–1097.

83 Takano H, Komuro I. Beta-blockers have beneficial effects even on unclassified cardiomyopathy such as isolated ventricular noncompaction. *Intern. Med.* 2002;41(8):601–602.

84 Bozić I, Fabijanić D, Carević V, Polić S. Echocardiography in the diagnosis and management of isolated left ventricular noncompaction: case reports and review of the literature. *J Clin Ultrasound.* 2006;34(8):416–421.

85 Stöllberger C, Blazek G, Dobias C, et al. Frequency of stroke and embolism in left ventricular hypertrabeculation/noncompaction. *Am. J. Cardiol.* 2011;108(7):1021–1023.

86 Bhatia NL, Tajik AJ, Wilansky S, Steidley DE, Mookadam F. Isolated noncompaction of the left ventricular myocardium in adults: a systematic overview. *J. Card. Fail.* 2011;17(9):771–778.

87 Salemi VMC, Rochitte CE, Lemos P, et al. Long-term survival of a patient with isolated noncompaction of the ventricular myocardium. *J Am Soc Echocardiogr.* 2006;19(3):354. e1–354.e3.

88 Dixit S, Gerstenfeld EP, Callans DJ, Marchlinski FE. Electrocardiographic patterns of superior right ventricular outflow tract tachycardias: distinguishing septal and free-wall sites of origin. *J. Cardiovasc. Electrophysiol.* 2003;14(1):1–7.

89 Tandri H, Bluemke DA, Ferrari VA, et al. Findings on magnetic resonance imaging of idiopathic right ventricular outflow tachycardia. *Am. J. Cardiol.* 2004;94(11):1441–1445.

90 Tanner H, Wolber T, Schwick N, Fuhrer J, Delacretaz E. Electrocardiographic pattern as a guide for management and radiofrequency ablation of idiopathic ventricular tachycardia. *Cardiology*. 2005;103(1):30–36.

91 Tada H, Ito S, Naito S, et al. Prevalence and electrocardiographic characteristics of idiopathic ventricular arrhythmia originating in the free wall of the right ventricular outflow tract. *Circ. J*. 2004;68(10):909–914.

92 Morin DP, Mauer AC, Gear K, et al. Usefulness of precordial T-wave inversion to distinguish arrhythmogenic right ventricular cardiomyopathy from idiopathic ventricular tachycardia arising from the right ventricular outflow tract. *Am. J. Cardiol*. 2010;105(12):1821–1824.

93 Maron BJ, Estes NAM 3rd. Commotio cordis. *N. Engl. J. Med*. 2010;362(10):917–927.

94 Maron BJ, Doerer JJ, Haas TS, Estes NAM 3rd, Link MS. Historical observation on commotio cordis. *Heart Rhythm*. 2006;3(5):605–606.

95 Yeboah J, Lee C, Sharma OP. Cardiac sarcoidosis: a review 2011. *Curr Opin Pulm Med*. 2011;17(5):308–315.

96 Youssef G, Beanlands RSB, Birnie DH, Nery PB. Cardiac sarcoidosis: applications of imaging in diagnosis and directing treatment. *Heart*. 2011;97(24):2078–2087.

Answers to self-assessment questions

7.0 Ventricular Arrhythmias

1 A

7.1 VT in the presence of CAD

1 B
2 C
3 C

7.3 Hypertrophic and dilated cardiomyopathy

1 D
2 A
3 D
4 C
5 D
6 C

7.4 BBRVT

1 C
2 D
3 A

7.5 Channelopathies

LQTS

1 D
2 C

3 A
4 B
5 B
6 A
7 D

ARVD/C

1 D
2 C
3 C

Brugada syndrome

1 B
2 B
3 B

CPVT

1 C
2 A

7.6 VT Normal heart

1 C
2 D
3 A
4 B

7.7 Miscellaneous VT

1 D
2 C

CHAPTER 8

Sudden cardiac death and risk stratification

Self-assessment question

1 A 57-year-old man developed chest pain while playing tennis. Five minutes later he collapsed, Cardiopulmonary resuscitation was provided by his tennis partners until an ambulance crew arrived six minutes later. Electrocardiogram showed ventricular fibrillation, and external defibrillation restored sinus rhythm. He was admitted to the hospital.

The next day coronary angiogram revealed significant (>75%) stenosis of major epicardial coronary arteries. Left ventriculogram showed ejection fraction of 55% and no regional wall motion abnormalities. Serial electrocardiograms showed transient T wave inversion. Serum troponin I level peaked at 2. Which of the following is most appropriate at this time?

A Electrophysiologic study

B Implantation of a cardioverter-defibrillator

C Coronary artery bypass grafting and implantation of a cardioverter-defibrillator

D Coronary artery bypass grafting without implantation of a cardioverter-defibrillator

---

Essential Cardiac Electrophysiology: The Self-Assessment Approach, Second Edition. Zainul Abedin.
© 2013 Blackwell Publishing Ltd. Published 2013 by Blackwell Publishing Ltd.

8.1 Sudden cardiac death[1]

- Sudden cardia death (SCD) is defined as death, due to cardiac arrhythmias, that occurs within one hour of symptoms.
- In patients presenting with out of hospital cardiac arrest the initial rhythm could be ventricular tachycardia (VT), ventricular fibrillation (VF), pulseless activity, or asystole, depending on the duration from arrest.
- If the time elapsed is less than 4 minutes, 90% of the patients will show VF and 5% will have asystole. As the time interval increases, the proportion of asystole as the detected rhythm increases.
- Post cardiac arrest survival depends on the time elapsed since arrest. Presence of asystole or pulseless cardiac contractions indicates long duration since cardiac arrest and survival of less than 5%.
- In the presence of acute ischemia or myocardial infarction (MI) the cause of SCD is VF. Less than 30% of these patients with SCD have inducible monomorphic VT in EP lab.
- Patients with previous MI, abnormal signal-averaged electrocardiogram (SAECG) and low ejection fraction (EF) tend to present with monomorphic VT (Table 8.1).
- Ten percent of SCD patients may be discharged alive from the hospital.
- Early resuscitation and return of spontaneous circulation (RSC) is predictive of better survival.
- In patients with severe congestive heart failure (CHF) SCD may be due to bradyarrhythmias.
- approximately 10% to 15% of autopsy negative sudden infant death syndrome (SIDS) cases stem from cardiac channelopathies,
- Clinical risk factors identified thus far are prior sudden cardiac arrest (SCA), the presence of coronary artery disease (CAD)/ MI, and left ventricular dysfunction (EF ≤35%).

Table 8.1 Causes of sudden cardiac death.

CAD	Cardiomyopathies	Repolarization abnormalities	Infiltrative disorders	Arrhythmia induced
Ischemia	Idiopathic	LQTS	Sarcoidosis	WPW
MI	Hypertrophic	Proarrhythmia	Amyloidosis	Idiopathic VF
	RV dysplasia	Electrolyte	Tumors	Torsades
	Myocarditis	Brugada		Bradycardia asystole
	Valvular heart disease	CPVT1		
	Congenital heart disease			

CPVT1 = Catecholaminergic polymorphic VT. LQTS = long QT syndrome.

- Low EF has poor sensitivity in identifying patients at risk of sudden cardiac death. Small numbers of SCD victims have undergone previous cardiac evaluation.
- The commonest cause of SCD is CAD accounting for 65% of all SCD.
- Primary electrical diseases (e.g., congenital long QT syndrome, Brugada) and structural cardiomyopathies (e.g., hypertrophic cardiomyopathy, arrhythmogenic right ventricular dysplasia), contribute a small fraction of overall numbers of SCDs.
- Familial history of SCD is a risk factor for SCD, independent of risk for CAD or MI.
- The commonest cause of the autopsy negative sudden unexpected death in young may be due to channelopathies induced arrhythmias[1].
- SCD claims an estimated 300 000 to 350 000 lives each year in the United States.
- VF is the most common mechanism of cardiac arrest, occurring in up to two-thirds of patients in this setting off myocardial ischemia.
- Noninvasive markers of autonomic dysfunction, such as heart rate variability, baroreflex sensitivity, and (more recently) heart rate turbulence may identify patients at increased risk for death.
- Interventions that favorably impact autonomic function, such as beta-blockers, angiotensin-converting enzyme inhibitors, aldosterone antagonists, statins, omega-3 fatty acids, and cardiac resynchronization therapy, are associated with improved survival.
- Beta-blockers are most crucial in patients with structural heart disease.

SCD in young athletes
- Current pre-participation cardiovascular screening has not been effective in detecting potentially lethal cardiac abnormalities that place young athletes at risk for SCD.
- In approximately 80% of SCD, the athlete is asymptomatic until the SCA, with death being the initial event.
- The underlying cardiac pathology in young athletes with SCD is hypertrophic cardiomyopathy in 25% coronary artery anomalies in 14% of cases.
- Commotio cordis, involving a blunt, nonpenetrating blow to the chest leading to a ventricular arrhythmia in a structurally normal heart, accounts for approximately 20% of SCD in young athletes.
- In the setting of out-of-hospital cardiac arrest, the time from arrest to defibrillation is the major factor affecting survival, with survival rates declining 7% to 10% for every minute defibrillation is delayed.
- Despite witnessed collapse, immediate CPR, and prompt AED use, the survival rate after SCA in young athletes is lower than expected given the young age, physical conditioning, and overall good health of the athletes (HRJ07/06).[1]

Epidemiology and pathogenesis of SCD during sports
- There is male predominance (male-to-female ratio 10:1) and significant upward trend with increasing age.
- Females more likely to survive sudden cardiac arrest than males.

- Sports-related fatalities ranges from 1:15 000 to 1:50 000.
- Prevalence of fatal events in high school and college athletes (age range 13–24 years) in the United States is estimated at <1:100 000 participants per year.
- The majority of athletes who die suddenly have previously unsuspected structural heart diseases.
- Atherosclerotic CAD accounts for the majority of fatalities in older athletes (adults >35 years).
- In young athletes, substrates include congenital and inherited heart disorders, cardiomyopathies, including hypertrophic cardiomyopathy, arrhythmogenic right ventricular cardiomyopathy/dysplasia, myocarditis, long QT syndrome, Brugada syndrome, Lenègre disease, short QT syndrome, pre-excitation syndrome (Wolff–Parkinson–White syndrome), CAD.
- There is no evidence of deleterious cardiac effects of previous top-level endurance athletic activity.

Circadian rhythms

- Output of the afferent limbs of the autonomic nervous system varies during the day. During the night, the parasympathetic limb prevails, whereas early morning hours are associated with increased sympathetic activity resulting in higher levels of circulating catecholamine, cortisol, and serotonin.
- Seasonal variation in QTc interval exists; the QTc interval being longest in October. No significant variation was seen for women.
- The QT interval in normal subjects exhibits diurnal variation.
- Sudden cardiac death rates exhibit diurnal variation, with peak incidence between 6 a.m. and noon in both men and women.
- Sudden cardiac death incidence peaks in humans within the first 3 hours after awakening
- Autonomic tone has been shown to influence ventricular refractoriness and QT interval, with both sympathetic and parasympathetic effects.
- Transplanted hearts do not exhibit diurnal variation in QT interval, which suggests autonomic influence on ventricular repolarization.
- SCD incidence also exhibits seasonal (circannual) variation, with peak rates in winter months, (December through February), and a nadir in summer months (June through August). Similar winter peak in SCD has been observed in women and men.
- Implantable cardioverter-defibrillators eliminate this winter peak, suggesting that ventricular tachyarrhythmias account for the SCD.
- The winter peak in of the incidence of SCD is seen equally in the northern and southern hemispheres.
- The sympathetic nervous system acts as a trigger of ventricular tachyarrhythmias and SCD in patients.
- Beta-adrenergic blockade decreases sudden cardiac death mortality in patients following myocardial infarction.
- Left cardiac sympathetic denervation, involving ablation of the left stellate ganglion, decreases the incidence of ventricular tachyarrhythmias in patients with MI.

- REM sleep is associated with enhanced sympathetic neural activity and surges in heart rate. 20% of sudden cardiac deaths occur at night as patients sleep, raising the possibility that diurnal increases in neural activity may play a role.

Clinical presentation of SCD
- In 25% of patients with CAD, SCD may be the first manifestation.
- Causes of SCD are listed in Table 8.1.
- Left ventricular function is the most important predictor of SCD. EF of less than 30% is associated with three- to fivefold increase in SCD.
- Premature ventricular contractions (PVC) and nonsustained VT (NSVT) are predictors of SCD but suppression of these arrhythmias may not improve survival.
- Abnormal results of the SAECG, heart rate variability, baroreceptor sensitivity and electrophysiologic study have a low positive predictive value and therefore are not useful in making treatment decisions.

Mechanisms
- Lethal ventricular arrhythmias occur in the presence of substrate such as scar or hypertrophy and initiating factors such as ischemia, autonomic dysfunction, hypoxia, acidosis, electrolyte, gene expression and ion channel abnormalities.
- Increase in sympathetic activity, in patients with ischemic heart disease and CHF, is associated with increased risk of SCD.
- Denervation of the sympathetic nerve may occur due to MI, which may result in super-sensitivity to circulating catecholamines distal to MI. This may shorten refractory period and cause arrhythmias.
- A decrease in parasympathetic activity may also lower threshold for occurrence of ventricular arrhythmias.
- The onset of acute ischemia in the setting of prior MI results in VF.
- Thromboxane A2 and serotonin may cause coronary artery spasm and ischemia.
- In normal ventricle, sympathetic stimulation shortens action potential duration and the QT interval as seen in ECG and can reduce the dispersion of repolarization.
- In pathologic states associated with reduced repolarization reserve such as heart failure and long QT syndrome, sympathetic stimulation induces arrhythmias, by enhancing the dispersion of repolarization or by generating after-depolarizations.
- Parasympathetic stimulation modestly prolongs ventricular refractoriness and the QT interval in the normal heart, reflected by a longer QT interval during vagal stimulation in animal studies and during sleep in humans.
- Angiotensin II promotes the elaboration of cytokines, growth factors, and fibrosis by myofibroblasts.
- Aldosterone and endothelin peptides are profibrotic.
- Myocardial norepinephrine release is promoted by angiotensin II, and norepinephrine further activates the renin–angiotensin system (RAS).

- Angiotensin II enhances release of aldosterone from the adrenal cortex.
- Aldosterone has potent sodium-retaining properties and can induce myocardial hypertrophy and fibrosis. Like angiotensin II, aldosterone regulates cardiac ion channels.
- Chronic exposure of ventricular myocytes to aldosterone reduces I_{to} and increases I_{CaL}.
- Aldosterone antagonism inhibits fibrosis, reduces myocardial norepinephrine content, and increases VF threshold.
- Treatment with the aldosterone receptor antagonists spironolactone or eplerenone has been demonstrated to reduce SCD in heart failure patients.
- Majority have coronary atherosclerosis with a recent plaque rupture or erosion resulting in acute coronary thrombosis or evidence of prior MI but no acute coronary thrombosis.
- Healed infarction is found in at least one fourth of cases.
- Cardiac arrest is the initial manifestation of heart disease in approximately 50% of cases. Such patients are likely to have single-vessel coronary disease and normal or mildly abnormal left ventricular systolic function than cardiac arrest victims with prior MI. Although heart failure increases risk for both sudden and nonsudden death, a history of heart failure is present in only approximately 10% of arrest victims.
- Low EF identifies patients at increased risk for cardiac arrest, the majority of sudden deaths occur in patients with EF >30%.
- One of the genetic variants associated with SCD risk in population-based studies is a nonsynonymous single nucleotide polymorphism (SNP) resulting in an amino acid substitution (Gln27Glu, rs1042714) in *ADRB2* gene, which encodes the β2-adrenergic receptors (β2AR), an important mediator of the cardiovascular response to sympathetic activation.

Clinical evaluation and treatment
- Following an episode of SCD, an evaluation should be performed to determine the extent of the underlying heart disease and assessment of reversible factors such as ischemia, sever hypokalemia, use of proarrhythmic drugs.
- The risk of reoccurrence of SCD is 20% in first year.
- If the VF occurs in the setting of acute ischemia or MI and subsequent evaluation shows normal EF, the reoccurrence rate of VF is approximately 2%.
- The treatment of choice is an implantable cardioverter-defibrillator (ICD).
- In the Antiarrhythmic Versus Implantable Defibrillator trial (AVID), 2-year survival in patients treated with amiodarone was 74.7% and it was 81.6% in patients randomized to ICD therapy.
- Ischemia should be identified and treated before ICD implant.
- These patients should be treated with beta-blockers and angiotensin-converting enzyme (ACE) inhibitors.
- Amiodarone and ablation can be considered for recurrent ICD shocks.
- Electrical discharges at a low-energy setting (microjoule in magnitude) can terminate both VT as well as the prefibrillatory arrhythmia characterized by ultrarapid, regular coarse waves – ventricular flutter. However, the moment

the waveform fractionates to small chaotic undulations, the electrical energy for restoring sinus rhythm increases by more than 1000-fold.

- At the onset of VF, there is a grace period of about 1–2 minutes when thumpversion is effective. Coarse and relatively large waves of depolarization define this period electrocardiographically. Once the waves are diminutive, thumpversion is ineffective.

8.2 Risk stratification for sudden cardiac death[2]

- Ten percent of all deaths, in the western population are cardiac and 50% of all cardiac deaths are sudden.
- Seventy-five percent of the arrhythmic deaths are due to VT or VF and 25% are due to bradyarrhythmias or asystole. The commonest terminal arrhythmia is VF and more than 90% of the victims of SCD have CAD, although acute MI at the time of the SCD is uncommon.
- After initial episode of VT or VF the possibility of reoccurrence is approximately 30% in next 24 months. This risk is even higher in the presence of left ventricular dysfunction.
- The following have been identified as risk factors for SCD:
  1 Ejection fraction <35%
  2 QRS duration >0.12 second
  3 History of heart failure (New York Heart Association class III or IV)
  4 Age >70 years.
  5 Atrial fibrillation
  6 Nonsustained VT
  7 Inducible VT.
- Patients with EF <30% but no other risk factor have a low predicted mortality risk (<5% over a 2-year period)
- Risk stratification is an attempt to identify specific and sensitive markers that could assess the probability of occurrence or reoccurrence of morbid ventricular arrhythmias and elimination of those risk factors thus will improve outcome. This goal has not been achieved.
- Frequent PVCs in a post MI patient are a well established independent risk factor of mortality, yet suppression of this arrhythmia does not result in improved survival (CAST and CHF-STAT trials).
- Reduction in arrhythmic death does not imply reduction in total mortality.
- A combination of multiple risk predictors, each with low sensitivity or specificity, may not provide useful predictive information applicable to individual patient.
- Not all post MI patients suffer from ventricular arrhythmias.
- Risk assessment provides probability association of risk factors and events. It does not, in absolute terms, distinguish between patients who will or will not suffer from arrhythmias.
- The RAS, kallikrein–kininogen and ACE2 systems, where ACE plays a central role, influence arrhythmias and SCA risk.
- In population studies, higher renin levels are associated with increased risk of cardiovascular disease mortality.

- Blocking these pathways with ACE inhibitors, angiotensin receptor blockers, or aldosterone inhibitors decreases risk of SCA.

12 Lead ECG

- Left bundle branch block, as well as nonspecific intraventricular conduction delay (IVCD), but not right bundle branch block, are associated with increased total mortality risk.
- No link between bundle branch block and inducible monomorphic VT has been shown.
- QRS duration and bundle branch block are not associated with the occurrence of ventricular tachyarrhythmias.
- Left ventricular hypertrophy (LVH) on the ECG or on echocardiogram is independently associated with sudden death,
- Prolonged QT interval in post MI setting is associated with increased risk of SCD.
- Variation in QT interval over time also has been correlated with occurrence of SCD.
- Elevated resting heart rate is an independent risk factor for cardiac mortality.
- Enhanced adrenergic activity is arrhythmogenic and that efferent vagal tone is cardioprotective by opposing adrenergic influences through presynaptic inhibition of norepinephrine release and an action at the receptor level mediated by second messenger mechanisms.
- Respiratory sinus arrhythmia constitutes an important measure of cardiovascular health. This rhythmic change in heart rate during breathing is mediated through the Hering–Breuer reflex, which acts through the medullary cardiovascular regulatory centers.
- During inspiration, cardiac efferent vagal tone is inhibited and sympathetic efferent tone is enhanced, resulting in heart rate accelerations. During expiration, reciprocal changes in autonomic balance occur that slow heart rate.
- Respiratory sinus arrhythmia appears to provide a "measure of biologic cardiac age" as it is depressed with advancing age, reflecting decreases in cardiac and vascular elasticity and compliance or in the capacity of the pacemaker to be activated.

Heart rate recovery after exercise

- Heart rate recovery after exercise, another marker of vagus nerve responsiveness, has proved to be predictive of cardiovascular mortality and sudden cardiac death in relatively low-risk cohorts including asymptomatic individuals.
- The reduction in heart rate during the first 30–60 seconds after exercise appears to be caused by reactivation of the parasympathetic nervous system but subsequently by withdrawal of sympathetic tone.
- However, because the exponential deceleration in heart rate after exercise persists during blockade of both limbs of the autonomic nervous system with atropine and propranolol, that heart rate recovery may result to a significant degree from autonomically independent alterations in venous return with the attendant changes in stretch of atrial receptors of pacemaker tissue.

- A 2% reduction in death was associated with each 1-bpm reduction in resting heart rate and each 5-bpm increase in heart rate was associated with an 8% increase in cardiovascular death as well as increases in hospital admission for heart failure, myocardial infarction, and coronary revascularization.
- Ivabradine is a current-dependent blocker of the I_f current, the main determinant of the slope of diastolic depolarization in the sinoatrial node. It is a specific, use-dependent agent with substantial heart rate-reducing effects. Ivabradine does not alter myocardial contractility or coronary vasomotor tone.

Family history of SCD
- Family history of SCD is an independent risk factor for sudden death.
- A parental history of early (age <65 years) SCD is associated with an ~2.7-fold greater risk than among similarly aged subjects.
- Family history of SCD is also a significant risk factor among individuals with acute MI.
- Nonsynonymous variant (S1103Y) in the cardiac sodium channel gene *SCN5A* has been associated with increased SCD risk in adults and infants.
- Insertion/deletion polymorphism in the α2B-adrenergic receptor gene (*ADRA2B*) and common variants in the β2-adrenergic receptor gene (*ADRB2*) may predispose to SCD.
- *NOS1AP* is associated with QT interval duration and SCD risk in general populations. *NOS1AP* encodes a nitric oxide synthase (NOS) adaptor protein (designated CAPON) that is expressed widely in human tissues including brain and heart but was not previously known to influence cardiac function generally or myocardial repolarization specifically.
- Overexpression of CAPON in ventricular myocytes caused shortening of action potentials that could be explained largely by a significant reduction in peak L-type calcium current density.
- Myocytes overexpressing CAPON exhibited greater stability in protein levels of NOS1, and inhibition of this enzyme reversed the effects on action potential duration and calcium current density.

PVC as risk factor
- Five to 10% of post-MI patients have NSVT. Twenty percent have greater than 10 PVC/h. Complex and frequent ectopy is an independent predictor of mortality and presence of decreased ejection fraction of <30% is associated with a fourfold increase in mortality within 2 years of MI.
- Suppression of PVC has not improved survival; it may even worsen the outcome.
- Frequent ectopy or NSVT is insensitive, failing to identify 47–94% of SCA victims.
- The single period of highest risk for total and arrhythmic mortality is the first 6 months after acute MI.
- After MI, patients with EF <30–35% account for no more than 50% of SCA.

NSVT

- NSVT may be detected in 5% of the general population with normal hearts and those with CAD with normal left ventricle function.
- It may occur during or after exercise. It does not signify adverse prognosis under these circumstances.
- In early post MI period occurrence of NSVT does not predict inducibility of sustained VT. However, if the EF is less than 40%, the 2 year mortality is 10%.
- In patients with NSVT, EF <40% and inducible VT, the risk of sudden death is 50% in 2 years and 6% in whom VT is noninducible.
- The possibility of inducing VT in patients with CAD, EF <40% and asymptomatic NSVT is 30%.
- The number of episodes and the length of NSVT have no association with mortality.
- NSVT is not an independent predictor of SCD in patients with dilated cardiomyopathy, hypertrophic cardiomyopathy or hypertension.

Signal average ECG (SAECG)[3]

- Late potentials are due to depolarization of the tissue within MI region, that outlast normal QRS due to slow conduction.
- Late potentials are likely to be detected more often in patients with inferior MI than anterior MI due to activation sequence of the ventricles where normally the base of the ventricle is last to be depolarized.
- In the presence of bundle branch block and conduction delays the late potentials may be buried within the prolonged QRS duration.
- There are three parameters that are commonly used to characterize abnormal late potential (Figure 8.1):
  ○ Total QRS duration is greater than 114 ms.
  ○ Root mean square voltage of terminal 40 ms (RMS40) is less than 20 μV. This reflects relative amplitude of late potential.
  ○ Duration of low amplitude signal (signal whose initial value is less then 40 μV) is greater than 38 ms.
- The positive predictive value of SAECG is 20% and negative predictive value is 97%.
- QRS duration is more sensitive then RMS or LAS (low amplitude signal).
- It is a useful tool in the assessment of the patient with syncope, where a negative SAECG will make the diagnosis of ventricular tachycardia as a cause of syncope less likely.
- he negative predictive value has been very good, averaging over 90%.

Heart rate variability[4]

- Excess of sympathetic tone (or deficient parasympathetic tone) has been correlated with increased mortality post-MI as well as increased propensity for VF during acute ischemia.
- Sympathetic–parasympathetic balance has been measured by a number of parameters. The first to be evaluated was heart rate variability (HRV), the amount of beat-to-beat variation in resting sinus rate over time. HRV has been

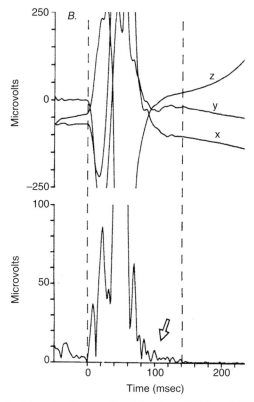

Figure 8.1 Criteria for late potentials are the following: (1) filtered QRS complex duration longer than 114–120 ms; (2) less than 20 microV of root mean square signal amplitude in the last 40 ms of the filtered QRS complex; and (3) terminal filtered QRS complex remains below 40 mV for longer than 39 ms.

expressed in various ways, derived from both short-term (2–8-minute) and long-term (24-hour) ECG recordings. Most data are based on 24-hour recordings. HRV directly measures autonomic effects on sinus node function but is assumed to reflect effects on the ventricles.

- Autonomic nervous system tone has been studied by analyzing HRV.
- Underlying principle is that the pattern of beat-to-beat control of the sinoatrial node reflects autonomic influences on the cardiovascular system.
- Parasympathetic influences exert rapid dynamic control by release of acetylcholine, which affects muscarinic receptors, and are therefore reflected in the high-frequency component of HRV.
- Sympathetic nerve activity, through the influence of norepinephrine on beta-adrenergic receptors, has a slower influence and is manifest in the lower frequency components.
- Thus, HRV is an indirect measure of autonomic function, as it reflects influences on the sinoatrial node but not on the ventricular myocardium.
- Variability of individual cardiac cycle is measured.

- It is measurement of RR interval during normal sinus rhythm (NN interval).
- Premature beats and other rhythms are excluded using QRS morphology criteria. Variance of the NN interval can be presented in time domain as follows:
- SDNN – standard deviation of NN interval.
- SD ANN – standard deviation of average NN interval.
- RMSSD – root mean square of differences between neighboring NN interval.
- pNN50 – percentage of NN intervals differing by more than 50 ms from the immediately proceeding NN interval.
- Length of ECG recording has bearing on HRV measurement. Long-term recordings (Holter) provide more reliable information.
- Varying QRS voltage, tall T waves and recording artifacts may be mistaken for QRS and may affect interpretation.

Frequency domain

- Using frequency domain for HRV analysis requires identification of very low frequency (VLF) of less than 0.04 Hz, low frequency (LF) of 0.04–0.15 Hz, high frequency (HF) of 0.15–0.4 Hz and ultralow frequency (ULF) of <0.0033 Hz.
- These frequency distributions provide information about the degree of autonomic modulation rather then autonomic tone.
- Long term (24-h) recording of ECG for HRV shows responsiveness of autonomic tone to environment.
- Efferent vagal activity is a major contributor to the HF component.
- LF component of the heart rate power spectra reflects baroreflex function rather than cardiac sympathetic innervation.
- High values of LF during day and high values of HF at night have been recorded.
- HF and LF components account for 5% of total power while ULF and VLF account for 95% of the power of spectral analysis.

Use of HRV in risk stratification post-MI

- HRV is depressed following MI due to increased sympathetic activity.
- Depressed HRV predicts increase mortality in post-MI patients.
- In post MI patients, 24 hours SDNN of less than 50–70 ms indicates high risk for arrhythmic death.
- Abnormal HRV has been observed in patients with diabetic neuropathy.
- In patients with CHF reduction of HRV is due to increased sympathetic tone rather than decrease in vagal tone. In these patients SDNN of less than 100 ms and peak O_2 consumption of less than 14 ml/kg/min is predictive of poor prognosis and one year mortality of 37%.
- According to the observations from Defibrillators in Non-Ischemic Cardiomyopathy Treatment Evaluation (DEFINITE) trial, patients with nonischemic dilated cardiomyopathy and preserved HRV SDNN >113 ms have an excellent prognosis (3 year 0% mortality).
- Patients with severely depressed HRV and patients who are excluded from HRV analysis because of atrial fibrillation and frequent ventricular ectopy (an average of 10 PVCs per hour on a 24-h Holter recording) have the highest mortality (17%).

- State of anxiety and anger decreases HRV.
- Sleep related vagal activation is lost in post MI patients.
- Beta-blockers increase HRV.
- The fundamental principle underlying these analyses is that higher-frequency, beat-to-beat variation in heart rate results from respiratory cycles, with increased HRV reflecting greater relative degrees of parasympathetic tone.

Baroreflex sensitivity (BRS)
- Normal reflex is decreased in heart rate in response to an increase in blood pressure.
- Lesser degrees of reduction of heart in response to increase in blood pressure reflect relative excess of sympathetic tone.
- BRS has also been expressed by measure of heart rate turbulence (HRT), the derangement in sinus rate following a ventricular premature depolarization.
- Protective effect of the baroreceptor mechanism has been attributed to the antifibrillatory influence of vagus nerve activity, which presynaptically inhibits norepinephrine release and maintains low heart rate during myocardial ischemia.
- The latter effect improves diastolic coronary perfusion, minimizing the ischemic insult.
- BRS can also be monitored noninvasively from routine ambulatory electrocardiograms using the tool of HRT, which measures heart rate fluctuations after a single ventricular premature beat (VPB), which reflect the fall and recovery of blood pressure.
- These reactions of the cardiovascular system to a VPB are direct functions of baroreceptor responsiveness, as reflex activation of the vagus nerve controls the pattern of sinus rhythm.
- In low-risk patients, sinus rhythm exhibits a characteristic pattern of early acceleration and subsequent deceleration after a VPB. By contrast, patients at high risk exhibit an essentially flat, nonvarying response to the VPB, indicating an inability to activate vagus nerves and to enable their cardioprotective effect.
- Increased carotid pressure prolongs RR interval.
- BRS is decreased in patients following MI.
- Patients with decreased BRS do not tolerate VT and present with syncope and hypotension.
- Pressure sensitivity receptors are located in the carotid sinus and wall of aortic arch.
- Afferent impulses from the carotid sinus through the glossopharyngeal nerve and impulses from aortic arch through the vagus nerve travel to the mid brain.
- Increased systemic arterial pressure activates baroreceptors resulting in decreased sympathetic and increased vagal activity, which decreases heart rate, contractility, and vasoconstriction.
- A fall in blood pressure decreases baroreceptor firing and causes increased sympathetic and decreased vagal activity.
- Baroreceptors interact in concert with multiple inputs from mechanoreceptors, chemoreceptors, and cardiopulmonary receptors. Additional inputs come from posture, exercise, and respiration.

- Under normal circumstances, through baroreceptors, vagal tone in activated and sympathetic tone is inhibited.
- Monitoring of spontaneously occurring blood pressure and heart rate changes is a closed loop where in addition to baroreceptors all other reflexes are active.
- Open loop assessment of the BRS is done by external pharmacological or mechanical stimulus such as an increase in blood pressure.
- When pharmacologic agents are used all baroreceptors are stimulated.
- Phenylephrine, an α-agonist, is injected (as a bolus) at a dose of 1–4 μg/kg to increase blood pressure by 20–40 mmHg. Changes in RR interval (HR) are plotted against the preceding systole blood pressure and expressed as milliseconds of increase in RR with 1 mmHg increase in BP.
- The test is repeated at least three times and average slope of the correlation between HR and BP is obtained.
- In normal subjects average value of BRS is 15 + 9 ms/mmHg.
- Phenylephrine produces direct α-adrenergic stimulation of sinus node; however, this does not interfere with BRS assessment.
- RR interval shortens with lowering of BP with nitroglycerine or nitroprusside.
- BRS slopes tend to be higher with an increase in blood pressure than with a decrease in blood pressure. This indicates that response to rise and fall in blood pressure are asymmetrical.
- BRS decreases when sympathetic tone is dominant and increases when parasympathetic tone is dominant.
- The normal BRS slope suggests effective vagal reflex and normal sympathetic activity.
- A flat BRS response suggests decreased vagal response or increased sympathetic tone.
- BRS is altered in the presence of hypertension and is reduced with increasing age.

Neck chamber technique for assessment of BRS
- Increased neck chamber pressure is sensed as a decrease in arterial pressure by baroreceptors. This initiates vagal withdrawal and increase sympathetic activity.
- BRS slope by neck chamber and phenylephrine may differ because with the neck chamber technique the stimulus is localized to carotid baroreceptors only.
- In a neck suction technique negative pressure is applied for 10 seconds at −7 to −40 mmHg. This simulates an increase in BP and prolongs RR interval.

Spontaneous BRS
- Continuous monitoring of BP and heart rate in time or frequency domain is determined. This provides information about autonomic tone on continuous basis.
- A BRS value of 3 ms/mmHg or less is suggestive of poor prognosis and increased cardiac mortality (ATRAMI trial).
- There is a weak correlation between BRS and HRV suggesting that the two methods express different functions of the autonomic tone.

- Low EF and decreased BRS is associated with increase in cardiac mortality.
- In patients with low EF and normal BRS or decreased BRS and normal EF, the mortality was same but less then when both EF and BRS were decreased.
- Measures to increase vagal tone and restore autonomic balance may decrease mortality in patients with low EF.
- BRS declines more rapidly after age 65 whereas HRV is a more reliable indicator of autonomic tone in patients older than 65 years.

T wave alternans (TWA)[5]

- Elevated heart rate can be an important factor in generating arrhythmogenic T-wave alternans (TWA).
- This phenomenon, defined as a beat-to-beat fluctuation in the amplitude and shape of the T wave, can occur when the capacity of the sarcoplasmic reticulum to reuptake calcium from the cytosol is disrupted.
- This mechanism has been demonstrated with fluorescent dyes, which indicate that calcium transients alternate in synchrony with action potential duration alternans. The elicitation of discordant TWA, wherein neighboring cells alternate out of phase, can establish steep electrical gradients that are highly conducive to life-threatening arrhythmias.
- These arrhythmogenic effects are compounded when heart rates are excessively high, particularly in patients with ischemic heart disease, MI, or heart failure. However, TWA magnitude is also affected by heart rate-independent influences, including enhanced sympathetic nerve activity, exercise, and changes in myocardial substrate associated with ischemic and nonischemic heart disease.
- Electrical alternans observed on a surface ECG, in patients with pericardial effusion, can affect P, QRS and T waves. It appears to be due to a rocking motion of heart inside the pericardium that results in change of electrical axis and QRS morphology in every other beat. This is a mechanical phenomenon without electrophysiologic changes. It does not increase the risk of ventricular arrhythmias.
- TWA is an electrical alternans involving the T waves. It is the result of myocardial repolarization changes.
- TWA visible on surface ECG is seen in the presence of ischemia, long QT syndrome and electrolyte abnormalities. It is associated with increased risk of ventricular arrhythmia and sudden cardiac death.
- Microvolt TWA is detected by computer using a spectral method.
- One hundred and twenty-eight beats are analyzed. Magnitude of alternans in even and odd beats is measured in microvolts compared with mean alternans.
- Average power spectrum of even odd mean beats is computed.
- Alternans ratio (K) is a ratio of alternans amplitude and standard deviation of the background noise.
- $K > 3$ is considered abnormal.
- Abnormal TWA correlates with inducibility of ventricular arrhythmia during electrophysiologic study with sensitive of 80% and specificity of 85%.
- Exercise-induced TWA increases with increasing heart rate.
- Sustained alternans is defined as 1.9 μV alternans with an alternans ratio of greater than 3 that lasts for at least 1 minute during a threshold heart rate.

- Ectopy, noise, pedaling, respiration and heart rate variation may produce artifacts and affect TWA.
- Patients who develop TWA at very high heart rate are at low risk of developing ventricular arrhythmias.
- Occurrence of TWA at a threshold heart rate of less than 110 bpm identifies high risk patients with high degree of predictability.
- The mechanism of TWA appears to be dispersion of refractoriness. In some regions of the myocardium refractoriness may exceed cycle length. Recovery from refractoriness may occur in every other beat resulting in alternans.
- TWA testing did not predict arrhythmic events or mortality in patients with heart failure and left ventricular systolic dysfunction.
- Vagus nerve stimulation, blockade of beta-adrenergic receptors, sympathetic denervation, and spinal cord stimulation, which reduce susceptibility to ventricular tachyarrhythmias, have been shown to decrease TWA magnitude.
- Beta-adrenergic blockade with metoprolol, an agent known to reduce SCD, substantially reduces TWA magnitude without affecting its prognostic utility.
- TWA has a high negative predictive value ≥98%.

Left ventricular ejection fraction (LVEF)
- LVEF is a strong independent predictor of SCD, arrhythmia reoccurrence and total mortality.
- Each 5% decrease in ejection fraction, increases the risk of SCD or arrhythmic death by 15%.

Programmed electrical stimulation (PES)
- In patients with low EF (30%) survival rate in inducible group is similar to those who are not inducible. Positive predictive value of low EF for arrhythmic death is low (11%) but for total cardiac mortality it is superior.
- In patients with previous MI, low EF and nonsustained VT, PES may identify a high risk group.
- Noninducibility in patients with coronary artery disease and EF of >40% identifies low risk group.
- Mechanism of monomorphic VT tends to be scar-related re-entry. It is often inducible and demonstrates late potential.
- Cardiac arrest survivors may have inducible polymorphic VT.
- In the AVID study patients who presented with asymptomatic VT had same prognosis as those with symptomatic or syncopal VT.
- Myocardial ischemia may result in PMVT (polymorphic VT) and VF.
- Revascularization reduces the risk of SCD but does not affect the occurrence or inducibility of monomorphic VT (MVT).
- The negative predictive valve of SAECG is 95% even in patients with low EF and NSVT. This observation makes it an excellent tool for evaluating patients with syncope where arrhythmic cause is low probability. When arrhythmic cause is strongly suspected negative SAECG is not sufficient to exclude VT as cause of syncope.

Table 8.2 Components of arrhythmia mechanism.

Substrate	Triggers	Electrical stimulus
Scar	Autonomic imbalance	PVC
Long QT	Ischemia	
	Electrolyte abnormality	
	Repolarization abnormality	

- In post MI patients with normal ejection fraction the incidence of SCD is 1.5% in one year.
- If ejection fraction is less than 40% and VT/VF is noninducible then the incidence of SCD is 5%. It increases to 40% if arrhythmia is inducible.
- In the MADIT study, 2 year mortality was 14% in spite of defibrillator implant indicating that treatment of arrhythmia alone may not prolong life[6].
- In 5% of SCD victims due to VF, the heart is normal. There is high incidence of reoccurrence.
- In AVID the absolute benefit of risk reduction in the defibrillator group was 7%, resulting in prolongation of life by 3.2 months over a period of 3 years[7].

Syncope as a risk factor for SCD
- In patients with dilated cardiomyopathy (DCM), syncope is a strong predictor of SCD.
- NSVT, SAECG and PES do not reliably predict future arrhythmic events or SCD. Degree of LV dysfunction is a strong predictor of mortality in DCM.
- In patients with DCM, who present with NYHA II, the annual mortality is 10%. Half of those are due to SCD. In patients with functional class IV, the annual mortality is 50% and 15–20% is due to SCD; the rest are due to brady-arrhythmias or pulseless cardiac activity.
- In asymptomatic patients with hypertrophic cardiomyopathy presence of previous cardiac arrest, syncope, presyncope and NSVT indicates increased risk of SCD.
- Fallowing a repair of Fallot tetralogy SCD may occur in 5% of patients. PES does not provide predictive information.
- The presence of LVH increases the incidence of SCD by threefold.
- In patients with ventricular arrhythmia substrate and triggers may change (Table 8.2).
- Risk stratification using currently available methodology should be delayed >1 month after MI.

Primary prevention of SCD
- Ace inhibitor and beta-blockers may reduce the mortality by 30–35% in patients with decreased EF.
- In patients who meet the MADIT I criteria (previous MI, EF less than 35%, nonsustained VT and inducible VT) ICD implant reduced the mortality.
- In MADIT II study (previous MI, EF <30%) ICD implant reduced the mortality from 19% to 14%.

SCD following repair of CHD
- Sudden death could be due to atrioventricular block, atrial flutter with 1:1 conduction or VT.
- Atrial arrhythmias are very common after Mustard, Senning or Fontan procedures.
- In children who have suffered from cardiac arrest, commonest associated condition is surgically repaired Fallot's tetralogy.
- Patients with Fallot's tetralogy have a ventricular septal defect (VSD) and infundibular pulmonary stenosis. Surgical repair requires closure of the VSD by a patch, resection of muscle from right ventricular outflow tract and repair of pulmonary annulus. This procedure is performed through ventriculotomy.
- This approach leaves scar in right ventricle and results in pulmonary insufficiency and right ventricular dysfunction. This may lead to re-entrant ventricular tachycardia arising at the site of ventriculotomy or VSD patch.
- PVCs and complex ventricular arrhythmias are common after surgical repair of Fallot.

Factors influencing occurrence of ventricular arrhythmias
- Age at initial repair. If the initial repair was performed after the age of 10 years the likelihood of ventricular arrhythmia occurrence is very high.
- Time since repair. As more time elapses since repair the incidence of arrhythmia increases.
- The presence of residual RVOT obstruction, pulmonary insufficiency, right ventricular hypertension and dysfunction are associated with increased tendency for arrhythmias.
- Patients with QRS width of more than 180 ms have increased risk of spontaneous and inducible VT or SCD.
- A stress test might identify patients with exercise induced arrhythmias.
- Incidence of mortality is 0.25 to 1.6% after a successful repair.

Treatment
- Radiofrequency ablation can be considered for atrial arrhythmias and well tolerated VT.
- ICD is the treatment of choice for patients with sustained VT or resuscitated cardiac arrest.
- Patients with right to left shunt may have increased tendency for thromboembolic complications. These patients should not undergo transverse lead ICD or pacemaker implant without consideration for anticoagulation.
- Following a repair of the congenital heart defect there is higher incidence of sinus node dysfunction, AV block and atrial flutter.
- Prophylactic ICD could be considered for patients who fallowing a repair of Fallot's tetralogy demonstrates pulmonary insufficiency, abnormal right ventricular hemodynamics, frequent nonsustained ventricular arrhythmias and syncope even if the electrophysiologic study is negative.
- For asymptomatic patient electrophysiologic study, antiarrhythmic drug therapy or insertion of ICD is not recommended.

References

1 Myerburg RJ, Castellanos A. Emerging paradigms of the epidemiology and demographics of sudden cardiac arrest. *Heart Rhythm.* 2006;3(2):235–239.
2 Cutler MJ, Rosenbaum DS. Risk stratification for sudden cardiac death: is there a clinical role for T wave alternans? *Heart Rhythm.* 2009;6(8 Suppl):S56–61.
3 Marcus FI, Zareba W, Sherrill D. Evaluation of the normal values for signal-averaged electrocardiogram. *J. Cardiovasc. Electrophysiol.* 2007;18(2):231–233.
4 Rashba EJ, Estes NAM, Wang P, et al. Preserved heart rate variability identifies low-risk patients with nonischemic dilated cardiomyopathy: results from the DEFINITE trial. *Heart Rhythm.* 2006;3(3):281–286.
5 Bloomfield DM, Hohnloser SH, Cohen RJ. Interpretation and classification of microvolt T wave alternans tests. *J. Cardiovasc. Electrophysiol.* 2002;13(5):502–512.
6 Moss AJ, Hall WJ, Cannom DS, et al. Improved survival with an implanted defibrillator in patients with coronary disease at high risk for ventricular arrhythmia. Multicenter Automatic Defibrillator Implantation Trial Investigators. *N. Engl. J. Med.* 1996;335 (26):1933–1940.
7 Anon. Antiarrhythmics Versus Implantable Defibrillators (AVID)–rationale, design, and methods. *Am. J. Cardiol.* 1995;75(7):470–475.

Answer to self-assessment question

1 D

CHAPTER 9

Cardiac arrhythmias in patients with neuromuscular disorders

Self-assessment questions

1 Which one of the following conditions is least likely to present with prominent R wave in lead V1?
   A Posterior MI
   B RBBB
   C Duchenne muscular dystrophy
   D Friedreich ataxia

2 Which one of the following is likely to present with bidirectional VT?
   A Emery–Dreifuss muscular dystrophy
   B Hypokalemic periodic paralysis
   C Kugelberg–Welander syndrome
   D Friedreich ataxia

3 Which one of the following conditions is unlikely to present with BBR-VT?
   A Myotonic dystrophy
   B Hypertrophic cardiomyopathy
   C Ebstein anomaly
   D Anderson–Tawil syndrome

Essential Cardiac Electrophysiology: The Self-Assessment Approach, Second Edition. Zainul Abedin.
© 2013 Blackwell Publishing Ltd. Published 2013 by Blackwell Publishing Ltd.

9.1 Muscular dystrophies

Duchenne and becker dystrophies[1-3]

- Both are X linked recessive disorders, due to abnormality in dystrophin gene[1].
- In Duchenne dystrophy dystrophin is absent which results in loss of myocytes and fibrosis
- In Becker's dystrophy dystrophin is present in reduced amount leading to a more benign course.
- Heart muscle is involved in both dystrophies.
- Isolated X-linked cardiac muscle dystrophin abnormality may lead to dilated cardiomyopathy without skeletal muscle involvement.
- Duchenne dystrophy becomes symptomatic before the age of 5 years. Cardiac involvement becomes evident by the age of 10.
- It involves posterobasal and posterolateral wall of the left ventricle. This results in prominent R wave in V1 and Q wave in lateral precordial leads. Similar EKG changes may occur in Becker dystrophy.
- The severity of cardiac involvement does not correlate with degree of skeletal muscle involvement.
- Cardiac arrhythmias such as persistent and labile sinus tachycardia, atrial arrhythmia and short PR interval are common.
- Abnormal signal-averaged electrocardiogram (SAECG) is recorded in one-third of the patients.
- Mortality is high; 25% of the deaths are due to arrhythmias (sudden cardiac death, SCD) or congestive heart failure (CHF).

Myotonic dystrophy[4-6]

- It is an autosomal dominant disease. The gene abnormality is found in chromosome 19. Gene abnormality is due to an unstable trinucleotide (CTG) repeat.
- Impaired glucose utilization may be related to abnormal protein kinase function.
- It is characterized by reflex myotonia, weakness, atrophy of distal muscles, early balding, gonadal atrophy, cataract, mental retardation and cardiac involvement
- Cardiac involvement in muscular dystrophy is manifested by degeneration of conduction system including the sinoatrial and atrioventricular (AV) nodes and the His Purkinje system.
- Slowing of conduction results in abnormal SAECG.
- The heart may be involved before skeletal muscle.
- It is common in French Canadians and rare in African blacks.
- Symptoms appear at 20 to 25 years of age and are due to weakness of the muscles of the face, neck and distal extremities. Death occurs at 45 to 50 years of age.
- Myotonia (delayed relaxation of muscle) is the hallmark of the disease. It can be demonstrated in thenar muscles and tongue.
- In an asymptomatic person EMG or genetic testing can make the diagnosis.

- In successive generations the symptoms occur earlier and with increasing severity. This may be related to amplification of CTG repeat.
- Cardiac involvement is manifested by arrhythmias, cardiomyopathy and PMV.
- ECG shows conduction abnormalities and AV blocks.
- Atrial arrhythmias occur in 10% of the patients.
- Sudden death may occur due to asystole (complete AV block) or ventricular arrhythmias such as bundle branch re-entry ventricular tachycardia (VT).
- ECG abnormalities include rhythm other than sinus, PR ≥ 240 ms, QRS duration ≥ 120 ms or 2° or 3° AV block.
- Patients with these ECG abnormalities tend to be older, have more severe skeletal-muscle impairment, heart failure, left ventricular systolic dysfunction, and atrial tachyarrhythmia
- Clinical and genetic characteristics of other dystrophies are described in Table 9.1.

Treatment
- A permanent pacemaker is indicated for patients presenting with syncope.
- PR interval of greater than 240 ms was predictive of future cardiac events such as atrial fibrillation, complete AV block, syncope and SCD. In these high-risk patients prophylactic permanent pacemaker should be considered.
- Ablation should be considered for bundle branch re-entry VT.
- Anesthesia may increase the risk of AV block and other arrhythmias.

9.2 Other neuromuscular disorders

Familial periodic paralysis[7]
- Mutation in alpha 1 unit of dihydropyridine sensitive Ca channel for hypolalemia and in alpha subunit of *SCN4A* for hyperkalemia.
- Clinical presentation with episodic weakness triggered by cold, post exercise or carbohydrate ingestion.
- Bidirectional VT may occur independent of muscle weakness.
- LQTS may be seen.

Treatment
- Normalize K,
- Hyperkalemia.
- Beta-blockers, imipramine for bidirectional VT.

Friedreich ataxia[8,9]
- It is a progressive spinocerebellar degeneration manifested by ataxia, dysarthria, sensory loss and skeletal deformities.
- It is an autosomal recessive disorder. Gene codes for amino acid protein Frataxin and is located on chromosome 9.
- It is associated with concentric left ventricular hypertrophy, rarely asymmetric septal hypertrophy without myocardial fiber disarray. A deposit of calcium salts and iron has been noted.

Table 9.1 Clinical and genetic characteristics of the muscular dystrophies.

Dystrophy	Genetics	Clinical presentation	Arrhythmia manifestation	Treatment
Emery–Dreifuss	X linked abnormality in STA gene codes for protein Emerin	Contractures of elbow, Achilles tendon, posterior cervical muscles	Atrial fibrillation, flutter, Atrial stand still, junctional bradycardia, AV Block	Permanent pacemaker
Limb girdle	Autosomal recessive	Cardiomyopathy Limb girdle weakness	In dominant form atrial and ventricular arrhythmia	
Fascioscapulohumeral	Autosomal dominant. chromosome 4q35	Muscle weakness	Sinus bradycardia, prolonged QRS duration Significant arrhythmia rare	
Periodic paralysis Hypo- or hyperkalemic	Mutation in alpha1 unit of dihydropyridine sensitive Ca channel for hypokalemia and in alpha subunit of SCN4A for hyperkalemia	Episodic weakness, triggered by cold, post exercise or carbohydrate ingestion	Bidirectional VT. VT may occur independent of muscle weakness LQTS may be seen	Normalize KMexiletine for hyperkalemia Beta-blockers Imipramine for bidirectional VT
Mitochondrial encephlomyopathy	Mutation mitochondrial DNA Maternally transmitted	Ophthalmoplegia (Kearns–Sayer KS), myopathy, encephalopathy epilepsy, acidosis	KS AV block, short PR and prolonged HV Leber optic neuropathy short PR and pre-excitation	Pacemaker
Kugelberg–Welander syndrome	Autosomal recessive. chromosome 5q	Atrophy weakness proximal muscles	Atrial fibrillation, atrial standstill, AV block.	Pacemaker symptomatic treatment.

- Degeneration and fibrosis of cardiac nerve, ganglia and conduction system may occur.
- Symptoms appear between the ages of 15 and 25 years
- Electrocardiogram and echocardiogram confirm the presence of LVH.
- Atrial arrhythmias are common. Conduction abnormalities are rare.

Guillain–Barré syndrome
- It is an acute inflammatory demyelinating neuropathy.
- It occurs five to seven days fallowing a viral infection, immunization or surgery
- Arrhythmias are due to autonomic neuropathy and characterized by sinus tachycardia. AV block and ventricular arrhythmias may occur.
- Plasmapheresis, IV immunoglobulin and temporary pacing for AV block should be considered.

Subarachnoid hemorrhage
- Acute cerebrovascular diseases such as subarachnoid hemorrhage are associated with marked ECG repolarization changes. These are characterized by peak inverted T waves and prolong QT interval.
- Ventricular fibrillation may occur.
- Beta-blockers or ganglion blockers can be used for ventricular arrhythmia.

Seizure related arrhythmias
Partial seizures arising from the temporal lobe may cause tachycardia, some patients may exhibit bradycardia or ictal asystole during a seizure.
- This may contribute to seizure-related injury and possibly to sudden unexplained death in epilepsy, found in 7 to 17% of the epileptic population.

Fabry disease[10]
- Fabry disease is a genetic disorder caused by a deficiency of α-galactosidase A.
- Sudden cardiac death due to ventricular arrhythmias may occur.
- Cardiac manifestations in Fabry disease include progressive hypertrophic infiltrative cardiomyopathy, valvular abnormalities, and arrhythmias.
- Monomorphic VT may occur in Fabry cardiomyopathy.

References

1 Wang Q, Yang X, Yan Y, et al. Duchenne or Becker muscular dystrophy: A clinical, genetic and immunohistochemical study in China. *Neurol India.* 2011;59(6):797–802.

2 Pérez Riera AR, Ferreira C, Ferreira Filho C, et al. Electrovectorcardiographic diagnosis of left septal fascicular block: anatomic and clinical considerations. *Ann Noninvasive Electrocardiol.* 2011;16(2):196–207.

3 Kyriakides T, Pegoraro E, Hoffman EP, et al. SPP1 genotype is a determinant of disease severity in Duchenne muscular dystrophy: predicting the severity of Duchenne muscular dystrophy: implications for treatment. *Neurology.* 2011;77(20):1858; author reply 1858–1859.

4 Groh WJ, Lowe MR, Zipes DP. Severity of cardiac conduction involvement and arrhythmias in myotonic dystrophy type 1 correlates with age and CTG repeat length. *J. Cardiovasc. Electrophysiol.* 2002;13(5):444–448.

5 Merino JL, Peinado R, Sobrino JA. Sudden death in myotonic dystrophy: the potential role of bundle-branch reentry. *Circulation.* 2000;101(5):E73.

6 Russo V, Rago A, Politano L, et al. The effect of atrial preference pacing on paroxysmal atrial fibrillation incidence in myotonic dystrophy type 1 patients: a prospective, randomized, single-bind cross-over study. *Europace.* 2011. Available at: http://www.ncbi.nlm.nih.gov/pubmed/22135319. Accessed January 21, 2012.

7 Ai T, Fujiwara Y, Tsuji K, et al. Novel KCNJ2 mutation in familial periodic paralysis with ventricular dysrhythmia. *Circulation.* 2002;105(22):2592–2594.

8 Ribaï P, Pousset F, Tanguy M-L, et al. Neurological, cardiological, and oculomotor progression in 104 patients with Friedreich ataxia during long-term follow-up. *Arch. Neurol.* 2007;64(4):558–564.

9 Rahman F, Pandolfo M. Cardiomyopathy in Friedreich's ataxia. *Acta Neurol Belg.* 2011;111(3):183–187.

10 Higashi H, Yamagata K, Noda T, Satomi K. Endocardial and epicardial substrates of ventricular tachycardia in a patient with Fabry disease. *Heart Rhythm.* 2011; 8(1):133–136.

Answers to self-assessment questions

1 D
2 B
3 D

CHAPTER 10

Syncope

Self-assessment questions

1 A 70-year-old woman is referred to you because of an episode of syncope that occurred last week while sitting at the dining table. She did not have any nausea sweating or other prodromal symptoms. Fallowing the episode she did not have any residual symptoms. Physical examination is unremarkable. ECG shows LBBB. Echocardiogram showed LVH and EF of 45%. Which of the following is the most appropriate recommendation?
   A Head up tilt test.
   B Electrophysiologic study
   C 24 hour Holter monitor
   D EEG and carotid duplex examination

2 Visual prodromal symptom (gray out feeling) prior to syncope is the result of
   A Hypoperfusion of visual cortex
   B Vasoconstriction in brain stem
   C Collapse of retinal blood vessels
   D Lack of perfusion to posture maintaining skeletal muscles.

3 A 37-year-old woman has been aware of fatigue, lightheadedness, precordial pain and aching sensation in "coat hanger "distribution on assuming upright posture. She does not have any nausea or sweating. On physical examination supine blood pressure is 106/60 mmHg. Heart rate is 85 bpm. These symptoms are most likely due to which one of the following?
   A Orthostatic hypotension
   B Prodromal symptoms of vasovagal syncope
   C Prodromal symptoms of cardiac syncope
   D Fainting lark phenomenon

Essential Cardiac Electrophysiology: The Self-Assessment Approach, Second Edition. Zainul Abedin.
© 2013 Blackwell Publishing Ltd. Published 2013 by Blackwell Publishing Ltd.

4 Which of the following factors predict the likelihood of recurrence of syncope during follow up after a positive tilt test?

A Occurrence of syncope within 5 minutes of 80 degree tilt

B History of injury during clinical syncope

C Hypotension and bradycardia during head up tilt test without syncope

D Frequency and the number of syncopal spells preceding positive tilt test.

5 A 19-year-old army recruit fainted while running. Heart rate or blood pressure was not recorded during that episode. During exercise test patient exercised for 11 minutes and achieved heart rate of 180 bpm. Syncope did not occur either during or right after the exercise test. Does this exclude the possibility of exercise induced neurocardiogenic syncope?

A True

B False

6 You are asked to see a 21-year-old male who has had two episodes of rapid palpitations associated with near-syncope in the past 8 weeks. He underwent repair of tetralogy of Fallot at age 3. Which of the following is the most likely mechanism of this patient's near-syncope?

A Ventricular tachycardia from the left ventricular outflow tract

B Ventricular tachycardia from the right ventricular outflow tract

C Ventricular tachycardia from the left ventricular septum

D Ventricular tachycardia from the right ventricular apex

10.1 Syncope

Syncope is a transient, self-limited loss of consciousness (LOC) that usually leads to falling due to loss of postural tone, with a relatively rapid onset and a spontaneous, complete, and relatively rapid recovery.

Pathophysiology[1]

- LOC is due to a global reversible reduction of blood flow to reticular activating area located in brain stem. It results in syncope within 10 seconds.
- It can be provoked by reflex (vasovagal) responses, cardiac arrhythmias, autonomic failure or any condition that reduces cerebral blood flow (CBF) and cerebral oxygenation.
- Many of the premonitory symptoms of a vasovagal syncope are indicative of cerebral hypoperfusion.
- Vagal stimulation during vasovagal syncope may be responsible for the release of pancreatic polypeptide, which could be responsible for gastrointestinal symptoms associated with syncope.
- The visual prodromal symptoms are due to reduction in blood flow to the retina through the ophthalmic arteries.
- The brain and the brain stem are protected by the pressure-equalizing effects provided by the cerebrospinal fluid (CSF). Absence of such pressure equalizing mechanisms and presence of intraocular pressure result in a collapse of retinal blood vessels and perfusion. This occurs before the LOC (gray out feeling).
- Syncope is often associated with the upright position.
- On passive or active assumption of the upright position, a gravitational displacement of blood to the dependent area of the body occurs. This results in a fall of venous return. Orthostatic stress (active standing, or passive standing during tilt test), may result in 0.5 to 1 liter of blood pooling into the abdomen and lower extremities. Orthostatic pooling of venous blood begins immediately and is completed within 3–5 min.
- The Bezold–Jarisch reflex is initiated by excessive venous pooling, resulting in decrease in ventricular volume and an increase in ventricular contractility. This activates receptors located in the inferoposterior portions of the left ventricle, leading to paradoxical withdrawal of sympathetic output to the vasculature and the heart and increase in parasympathetic activity. Marked vasodilatation, hypotension, bradycardia, and the LOC occur.
- Other triggers that may result in hypotension and bradycardia include serotonin and adenosine.
- On standing upright there is 25 to 30 mmHg drop in mean arterial pressure (MAP) within 30 seconds to 1 min.
- This transient fall in MAP explains the feeling of lightheadedness that even healthy humans sometimes experience shortly after standing up. This may result in syncope.
- The rapid short-term adjustments to orthostatic stress are mediated by autonomic nervous system.

- Muscle activity ("the muscle pump") prevents reduction in the central blood volume and prevents hypotension. Lack of "pump" activity, during upright position may result in syncope.
- During vasovagal syncope there is a withdrawal of muscle sympathetic activity resulting in loss of vasomotor tone leading to hypotension and syncope.

The fainting lark
- This is a voluntary self-induced instantaneous syncope. It is a result of gravitational acute arterial hypotension, raised intrathoracic pressure by Valsalva and cerebral vasoconstriction in response to hypocapnia due to hyperventilation.

Cardiac syncope
- This is due to bradycardia or tachyarrhythmias that result in hypotension and cerebral hypoperfusion.
- Onset is often sudden and there are no prodromal symptoms of autonomic activation. The syncopal episode may develop either in erect or supine position. There is no pulse.
- Prolonged asystole may provoke myoclonic movements and urinary and fecal incontinence.
- Recovery is rapid with a return of the pulse, flushing of the face, and usually full orientation.

Syncope due to orthostatic hypotension in patients with autonomic failure[2]
- Orthostatic hypotension is defined as a fall in systolic blood pressure ≥20 mmHg and/or a fall in diastolic blood pressure ≥10 mmHg within 3 minutes of standing.
- The resulting cerebral hypoperfusion can cause lightheadedness, visual blurring, dizziness, generalized weakness, fatigue, cognitive slowing, leg buckling, coat-hanger headache, and gradual or sudden LOC.
- Autonomic failure results in symptomatic orthostatic hypotension.
- Orthostatic hypotension is characterized by 20 mmHg drop in systolic blood pressure within 3 minutes of assuming erect posture.
- Postural orthostatic hypotension is defined as increase in heart rate by 28 bpm and hypotension within 5 minutes of standing.
- Symptoms include lightheadedness and blurring of vision. A neck ache radiating to the occipital region of the skull and to the shoulders ("coat hanger" distribution) often precedes the loss of consciousness. The mechanism of this unique symptom of postural hypotension may be ischemia of postural muscles.
- Impaired muscle perfusion may result in lower back and buttock ache.
- A decrease in myocardial perfusion may result in angina pectoris.
- Symptoms develop within minutes on standing or walking and resolve on lying down. These symptoms are prodromal and may alert the patient to lie down to restore cerebral perfusion. If the erect posture is maintained, consciousness gradually fades and the patient falls slowly. Sudden postural attacks may

occur. Patients with autonomic failure do not exhibit symptoms and signs of autonomic activation like sweating or a vagally induced bradycardia.
- A number of disorders of autonomic failure can result in orthostatic hypotension.
- Autonomic dysfunction can be acute (often in young individuals following a febrile illness),
- Chronic forms of autonomic failure are more common and include:
  1 Pure autonomic failure
  2 Bradbury–Eggleston syndrome, characterized by symptomatic orthostatic hypotension, constipation, urinary retention, inability to sweat, and impotence;
  3 Multiple system atrophy (Shy–Drager syndrome), characterized by symptomatic orthostatic hypotension, urinary and rectal incontinence, external ocular palsy, rigidity, tremor, inability to sweat, and impotence;
  4 Enzyme deficiencies (e.g., dopamine-β-hydroxylase deficiency),
  5 Medications, and
  6 Systemic illnesses (e.g., diabetes mellitus, amyloidosis, renal failure, malignancy)

Treatment
- Lifestyle modifications such as avoidance of excessively hot environments, carbohydrate-rich meals, alcohol, sudden postural changes.
- Nonpharmacologic measures include exercise training, isometric counterma-neuvers, elastic support stockings.
- Water drinking for pressor effect.
  ○ Ingestion of ~500 ml of water can result in an 11 mmHg increase in systolic blood pressure in older individuals and up to a 40 mmHg increase in systolic blood pressure in older individuals with autonomic failure.
  ○ Volume needed is relatively large, and the peak effect on blood pressure is not observed for 30 to 35 minutes.
- Impedance threshold device:
  ○ The device imparts an inspiratory resistance of −7 cmH$_2$O.
  ○ Moderate increase in impedance to inspiration would force intrathoracic pressure to more negative values (resulting in a "vacuum") and enhance venous return from the extrathoracic blood pool, which could ameliorate the orthostatic hypotension.
  ○ It improves symptoms, dramatic blood pressure responses to the inspiratory impedance device were observed in older individuals.
  ○ Device could worsen hemodynamics in some patients.
- Pharmacologic interventions includes, fludrocortisone, midodrine clonidine, desmopressin, ephedrine, erythropoietin, L-dihydroxyphenylserine (DOPS), methylphenidate, octreotide, pyridostigmine, and yohimbine.
  ○ Limited by suboptimal efficacy and a multitude of side effects.
  ○ Supine hypertension is common in patients with orthostatic hypotension and often is a limiting factor to the routine use of these medications.

Table 10.1 Causes of syncope.

Cardiac	Vascular	Neurologic	Metabolic
AV block	Subclavian steal	Seizures	Hyperventilation
Sick sinus syndrome	Autonomic neuropathy	Migraine	Hypoglycemia
Pacemaker failure	Drug-induced hypotension	TIA/CVA	Hypoxia
SVT	Hypovolemia	Hysteria/panic	Alcohol
VT	Carotid sinus sensitivity		
Aortic stenosis	Vasovagal		
Aortic dissection	Situational (cough,		
Cardiac tamponade	micturition, swallow)		
IHSS			
Mitral stenosis			
Pulmonary emboli			

AV = atrioventricular. CVA = cerebrovascular accident. IHSS = idiopathic hypertrophic subaortic stenosis. SVT = supraventricular tachycardia. TIA = transient ischemic attack. VT = ventricular tachycardia.

- Some patients with POTS have inappropriately high plasma angiotensin II levels, with low estimated ACE2 activity.

Prognosis and natural history[3,4]
- Vasovagal syncope often presents in clusters. Multiple events occur in a relatively short period of time and followed by long periods of quiescence.
- The frequency of syncopal events may also decrease after head-up tilt-table testing.
- Syncope due to cardiac causes is associated with high (30%) one year mortality.
- In 35% of patients with syncope, the etiology remains unclear.

Causes of syncope
1 In young people syncope is likely to be due to neurocardiogenic origin and in elderly person, sick sinus, hypersensitive carotid, heart block, medication, and hypotension may be responsible (Table 10.1).
2 History of cardiac disease, family history of sudden death, medication may help identify the cause of syncope.
3 Prodromal symptoms are likely to precede vasovagal syncope.
4 Disorientation, LOC of more than 5 minutes, tongue biting, nystagmus, headache after syncope are likely to be due to seizure.

Diagnostic tests

Electrocardiogram
1 ECG identifies a direct cause of syncope in only 5% of patients.
2 ECG may help identify long QT syndrome (LQTS), Wolff–Parkinson–White syndrome, AV block, myocardial infarction (MI), Brugada syndrome, left

ventricular hypertrophy, T wave inversion in right precordial leads and incomplete right bundle branch block pattern suggestive of right ventricular dysplasia as a cause of syncope.

3 In the presence of normal ECG cardiac cause of syncope is unlikely.

4 Signal average ECG, Holter monitor and event recorders have low yield in determining the cause of the syncope (less than 20%).

Echocardiogram
- It should be obtained in patients with abnormal physical examination and ECG. Echocardiogram may help identify myxoma or aortic stenosis as a cause of syncope.
- In the absence of heart disease by history, physical examination, and electro-cardiogram, the diagnostic yield of echocardiography is low
- The yield from neurologic imaging studies is low.

Exercise stress testing
- It should be considered if ischemic heart disease is suspected or if there is a history of exertional syncope and echocardiography excludes significant obstructive valvular cardiac lesion.
- Clinical variables associated with primary arrhythmia as a cause of syncope include:
  1 Left bundle branch block
  2 Structural heart disease
  3 Syncope without prodrome.
- Normal baseline ECG and history of syncope in childhood decreased the likelihood of primary arrhythmia.

Electrophysiologic testing
- The diagnostic yield of electrophysiology studies (EPS) in patients with a structurally normal heart and a normal ECG is low (1% ventricular tachycardia, 10% bradycardia) whereas in patients with organic heart disease, the yield is over 50% (21% ventricular tachycardia, 34% bradycardia). Patients with an abnormal ECG also have a significant diagnostic yield (17% ventricular tachycardia (VT), 19% bradycardia).
- A negative EPS does not necessarily exclude an arrhythmic, cause of syncope and has a poor predictive value in nonischemic cardiomyopathy and long QT syndrome.
- EP testing should be considered in patients with structural heart disease and unexplained syncope.
- It may identify patients with sick sinus syndrome, abnormal AV node conduction (HV of >100 ms, infra-Hisian block), SVT and VT.
- Predictors of abnormal EPS include abnormal left ventricle function, prior MI, bundle branch block, nonsustained VT, male sex and injury during syncope.
- In patients with severe impairment of left ventricular function EPS may have less predictive value. 3 year mortality is 50 % irrespective of EPS findings.

10.2 Neurocardiogenic syncope[1]

- It is the most common cause of syncope. It is reflex mediated.
- Other designations include "vasovagal" or "neurally mediated" syncope.
- Vasovagal syncope is due to a variable combination of reflex bradycardia and hypotension, triggered by prolonged sitting or standing; exposure to pain, blood, or medical procedures; heavy exercise; or getting up and moving abruptly.
- Even in the same patient, the triggers and presentation vary from spell to spell.
- The hypotension may be due to a reduction in peripheral sympathetic neural outflow, leading to venous pooling and vasodepression.
- It typically occurs in upright position but may occur in supine or seated position.
- Neurally mediated syncope (NMS) is characterized by premonitory symptoms of nausea, sweating and pallor (Box 10.1).
- The mortality rate is low.
- An increase in number and upregulation of adenosine A2A receptors and increase in the adenosine plasma levels (APLs), in patients with spontaneous and recurrent episodes of syncope and a positive head-up tilt, has been demonstrated.
- A critical drop in CO, and not a precipitous drop in systemic vascular resistance, is the prime hemodynamic event in patients with neurally mediated hypotension and presyncope.

History and physical examination

- Primary diagnosis of syncope can be made in 45% of patients by clinical history, physical examination, and electrocardiography.
- Vasovagal syncope may be precipitated by the sight of blood, loss of blood, sudden stressful or painful experiences, surgical manipulation, or trauma. History of childhood neurocardiogenic syncope may provide a clue to the cause of vasovagal syncope in adults.
- Prodromal symptoms and signs are usually present.
- Symptoms of epigastric discomfort, nausea, sweating, and a desire to sit down or to leave the room, lightheadedness, fatigue, blurring or fading of vision, palpitations, and tingling of the ears are reported.

Box 10.1 Types of neurally (vagally) mediated syncope

1 Vasovagal faint (common faint)
2 Carotid sinus sensitivity
3 Gastrointestinal stimulation
4 Glossopharyngeal neuralgia
5 Airway stimulation, Cough
6 Micturition syncope
7 Increased intrathoracic pressure, as in wind instrument playing, Valsalva

---

- Signs include facial pallor, sweating, restlessness, yawning, sighing and hyperventilation, and pupillary dilatation. The prodromal phase is often associated with a rapid heart rate. Continuing hypotension and bradycardia results in difficulty in concentrating, lack of awareness of the surroundings, loss of postural tone and then LOC and fall occurs.
- Myoclonic jerks are uncommon in a spontaneous vasovagal syncope.
- The duration of unconsciousness is usually brief, lasting less than 5 min.
- Immediately following the recovery from syncope there is profound fatigue, a persistence of pallor, nausea, weakness, sweating and oliguria. Patient is usually not confused. Syncope may reoccur if the individual is returned to upright position prior to resolution of hypotension and brady-cardia. If the patient sits or lies down promptly, frank syncope may be aborted.

Tilt test[5]
- It is not warranted in the evaluation of a single syncopal episode with clear vasovagal features.
- Tilt table testing is indicated when there is recurrent syncope, or a single episode accompanied by injury or motor vehicle accident, or syncope in a high-risk setting, or recurrent exercise-induced syncope after exclusion of organic heart disease, or syncope due to another established cause whose treatment might be affected by the diagnosis of vasovagal syncope.
- The patient is tilted head-up on a table, with straps and a footplate, at an angle between 60° and 80° for 30–45 minutes.
- Duration of 45 minutes is considered two standard deviations from the mean time to syncope and captures 95% of patients who will faint. Mean time to syncope during tilt test is approximately 25 minutes.
- If the passive stage of the test is negative, the use of provocative agents, such as isoproterenol, epinephrine or nitroglycerin may increase the diagnostic yield by 20 to 25%.
- 80 degree tilt provides 92% specificity which remains unchanged with low dose isoproterenol.
- Tilt test may be reproducible in 60 to 70% of patients.
- The average likelihood of recurrent syncope in the first 2 years after a positive tilt test is about 30% in unselected and untreated patients.
- Factors that predict the likelihood of recurrence of syncope include the frequency and the number of syncopal spells preceding positive tilt tests.
- Age, sex, tilt-test outcome, bradycardia, hypotension during tilt test without syncope and injury during clinical syncope are not useful predictors of the reoccurrence.
- Sensitivity is approximately 50%. Specificity, a measure of how often a head-up tilt-table test does not induce vasovagal syncope in asymptomatic controls is approximately 90%.
- It is not proven to be useful in follow-up evaluation of therapy to prevent recurrence of vasovagal syncope because of the difficulties associated with reproducibility.

Table 10.2 Long-term therapy for vasovagal syncope.

Agents to augment central blood volume	Increase fluids and salt intake, compression hose, mineral corticoids
Agents that increase peripheral vascular resistance	α1-Adrenergic agonist (ephedrine, midodrine)
Parasympatholytic agents	Scopolamine, propantheline, disopyramide
Adenosine blockers	Theophylline, caffeine
Contractility suppressants	β1-Adrenergic blocker, disopyramide
Centrally active agents	Serotonin reuptake inhibitors (fluoxetine proxetine, sertraline), α2-adrenergic agonist (clonidine) central stimulants (phentermine, methylphenidate)
Device therapy	Pacemaker

- Vasovagal responses can be divided into mixed, cardio-inhibitory, and vasodepressor.
- Two additional responses may occur.
- Dysautonomic response in autonomic neuropathy, where the blood pressure gradually falls without significant increase in the heart rate.
- Postural orthostatic tachycardia syndrome, where there is excessive sinus tachycardia in response to orthostatic stress.

Contraindications
- Head-up tilt-table testing is contraindicated in patients with critical obstructive cardiac disease (for example, critical proximal coronary artery stenosis, critical mitral stenosis, or severe left ventricular outflow obstruction) or critical cerebrovascular stenosis.

Treatment[6–8]
- Results of the tilt test (cardioinhibitory or vasodepressor) may influence the choice of the pharmacologic agent in the treatment of neuromuscular syncope. However, it cannot be used to assess the efficacy of the treatment.
- Simple measures such as adequate hydration and salt intake, and avoidance of precipitating stimuli may prevent the reoccurrence of syncope. Medications causing vasodilatation or volume depletion may need to replaced with alternative agents.
- Leg tensing can also abort an imminent faint
- Medical therapy is indicated in a minority of patients, those with recurrent syncope or injury during syncope Table 10.2.
- Beta-blockers may be useful in vasovagal syncope, especially if sinus tachycardia precedes the onset syncope.
- Serotonin reuptake inhibitors, proxetine and fluoxetine have been shown to eliminate or decrease the frequency of syncope.

- Expansion of the intravascular volume with fludrocortisone and use of the α-agonist (vasoconstrictor) midodrine can be helpful for vasodepressor vasovagal syncope and orthostatic hypotension.
- Implantation of dual chamber pacemaker with a "rate drop response" algorithm is indicated in patients with hypersensitive carotid sinus syndrome and cardio-inhibitory type of vasovagal syncope.
- Infrequent episodes of vasovagal syncope that are preceded by prodromal symptoms may only require counseling and observation.
- β-adrenergic blockers are the most widely prescribed first choice therapy for vasovagal syncope.
- Patients did not report any difference between disopyramide and beta-blockers. Beta-blockers may be safer due to lack of proarrhythmias.
- American College of Cardiology and the American Heart Association guidelines suggest a class IIb indication for pacing in patients who experience cardioinhibitory vasovagal syncope unresponsive to drug therapy and reproduced by a head-up tilt with or without isoproterenol or other provocative maneuvers.
- Complete resolution of symptoms is not possible and a satisfactory end point may be reduced frequency or severity of the episodes.
- Patients should be advised to avoid prosyncopal situations such as prolonged static standing, or volume depletion. Drugs that produce volume depletion, peripheral vasodilation, and hypotension should be discontinued.
- Patients with low blood pressure that is aggravated by orthostatic changes may benefit from fludrocortisone, midodrine, and compression hose. Symptomatic resting bradycardia may respond to anticholinergic agents, such as propantheline.
- The duration of pharmacologic therapy should be determined on an individual basis.
- Syncope in the setting of ischemic cardiomyopathy predicts a high risk of sudden death. These patients benefit from implantable cardioverter-defibrillator therapy.
- Prevention of Syncope Trial (POST) metoprolol was not effective in preventing vasovagal syncope in the study population.
- Patients with syncope are encouraged to increase their salt and fluid intake,
- Usual dose of salt tablets is 6–9 g (100–150 mmol) per day.
- Salt supplementation should be avoided in patients with hypertension, renal disease, or cardiac dysfunction.
- Physical counterpressure maneuvers (PCMs). During PCMs, the presyncopal patient does isometric contractions of either the legs (by leg crossing) or the arms and hands (by pulling apart gripped hands) or squats.
- These rely on a prodrome long enough to allow the technique to prevent the progression of presyncope to syncope and usually to prevent syncope during tilt tests.
- PCM works by increasing cardiac output, arterial blood pressure and reducing peripheral resistance.
- Adding leg tension further increased systolic blood pressure and cardiac output peripheral resistance dropped even further.
- Orthostatic training is not helpful and is not recommended.

- Selective serotonin reuptake inhibitors (SSRIs).
- Frequently symptomatic patients might be prescribed serotonin-specific reuptake inhibitors. Debatable effect.

Midodrine

- It is a peripherally active α-agonist, as is its metabolite.
- It counteracts reduction in peripheral sympathetic neural outflow that is responsible for venous pooling and vasodepression that are central to vasovagal syncope.
- It does not cross the blood–brain barrier and has few gastrointestinal side effects.
- Midodrine has demonstrated short- and medium-term therapeutic success while being well tolerated in both adult and pediatric populations.
- Side effects including supine hypertension, nausea, scalp paresthesias, piloerection, and rash. These are dose-related and easily reversible.
- Midodrine, starting at 5 mg three times daily during waking hours. The first dose should be taken when the patient wakes up, with subsequent doses 4 hours apart. Usually the dose level and interval will require modification.
- It should not be used in patients with hypertension or heart failure.
- In the absence of contraindications, frequently symptomatic patients should be prescribed midodrine.
- Vasovagal Pacemaker Study II (VPS II) no significant benefit was seen.
- The Vasovagal Syncope and Pacing trial (SYNPACE). No significant difference was seen between the two groups.
- Blinded trials do not show a benefit with pacing for vasovagal syncope, even when analyzed for patients with marked cardioinhibitory response on tilt table testing.
- In unblinded trials, there seems to be a benefit for pacing, and this might be due to an expectation effect from the patients and the medical staff.
- One unresolved question is whether the subset of patients with vasovagal syncope who have asystolic pauses during syncope might benefit from pacing.
- Pacemakers should not be used routinely to treat vasovagal syncope. Drug-resistant, highly symptomatic patients with documented asystole during syncope might be prescribed dual-chamber pacing with rate-drop sensing.

Carotid sinus hypersensitivity

- Carotid sinus hypersensitivity (CSH) is diagnosed when carotid sinus pressure for five seconds results in a pause of greater than three seconds. It may be produced in 40% of asymptomatic patients.
- Carotid sinus massage has its greatest utility in elderly patients.
- Carotid sinus massage should be avoided in patients with:
  1 Transient ischemic attacks
  2 Strike in last 3 months
  3 Carotid bruits.
- CSH may be the cause of syncope in the elderly.
- Dual chamber pacemaker is recommended for patients with syncope due to CSH.

Syncope and driving privileges

- Patients with syncope should refrain from driving if:
  1 There is potential for reoccurrence.
  2 Presence and duration of warning symptoms.
  3 Posture during syncope.
- Noncommercial drivers should not drive for several months.

Causes of exercise-induced syncope:

- It includes vasovagal syncope, hypertrophic cardiomyopathy, anomalous origin of coronary arteries, right ventricular dysplasia, myocarditis, Wolff–Parkinson–White syndrome, aortic stenosis and long QT syndrome.
- Neurally mediated syncope may occur during or immediately after exercise.
- Neuromuscular syncope during exercise may not be reproduced during exercise test.

References

1 Van Lieshout JJ, Wieling W, Karemaker JM, Secher NH. Syncope, cerebral perfusion, and oxygenation. *J. Appl. Physiol.* 2003;94(3):833–848.
2 Mittal S. Managing orthostatic hypotension: is this inspiration the answer? *Heart Rhythm.* 2007;4(2):136–137.
3 D'Ascenzo F, Biondi-Zoccai G, Reed MJ, et al. Incidence, etiology and predictors of adverse outcomes in 43,315 patients presenting to the Emergency Department with syncope: An international meta-analysis. *International Journal of Cardiology.* 2011. Available at: http://www.ncbi.nlm.nih.gov/pubmed/22192287. Accessed January 21, 2012.
4 Rosanio S, Schwarz ER, Ware DL, Vitarelli A. Syncope in adults: Systematic review and proposal of a diagnostic and therapeutic algorithm. *International Journal of Cardiology.* 2011. Available at: http://www.ncbi.nlm.nih.gov/pubmed/22188993. Accessed January 21, 2012.
5 Guaraldi P, Calandra-Buonaura G, Terlizzi R, et al. Tilt-induced cardioinhibitory syncope: a follow-up study in 16 patients. *Clinical Autonomic Research: Official Journal of the Clinical Autonomic Research Society.* 2011. Available at: http://www.ncbi.nlm.nih.gov/pubmed/22170295. Accessed January 21, 2012.
6 Kuriachan V, Sheldon RS, Platonov M. Evidence-based treatment for vasovagal syncope. *Heart Rhythm.* 2008;5(11):1609–1614.
7 Krediet CTP, Go-Schön IK, van Lieshout JJ, Wieling W. Optimizing squatting as a physical maneuver to prevent vasovagal syncope. *Clin. Auton. Res.* 2008;18(4):179–186.
8 Sheldon R, Connolly S, Rose S, et al. Prevention of Syncope Trial (POST): a randomized, placebo-controlled study of metoprolol in the prevention of vasovagal syncope. *Circulation.* 2006;113(9):1164–1170.

Answers to self-assessment questions

1 B
2 C
3 A
4 D
5 B
6 B

CHAPTER 11

Pharmacologic therapy of arrhythmias

Self-assessment questions

1 Intravenous administration of which of the following agents will result in greatest increase in conduction time?
   A Amiodarone
   B Bretylium
   C Lidocaine
   D Procainamide

2 A 37-year-old African American man was told that he had CYP2D6 deficiency. Which one of the following accurately reflects the pharmacologic effects of this deficiency?
   A If propafenone is administered he is likely to demonstrate excessive beta-blocking effects
   B Analgesic effect of the codeine will be enhanced
   C There will be increased level of 5 hydroxy propafenone
   D Likely to develop lidocaine toxicity when administered with Ca channel blockers and erythromycin

3 Which one of the following characteristics are common between amiodarone and dronedrone?
   A Thyroid dysfunction
   B Pulmonary toxicity
   C Blockade of multiple ionic channels
   D Long elimination half-life

Essential Cardiac Electrophysiology: The Self-Assessment Approach, Second Edition. Zainul Abedin.
© 2013 Blackwell Publishing Ltd. Published 2013 by Blackwell Publishing Ltd.

4 A 50-year-old woman, who has hypertension, and hyperlipidemia, has had two recent episodes of paroxysmal atrial fibrillation, each lasting more than 4 hours. Current medications are lisinopril, 20 mg daily; simvastatin, 40 mg daily; hydrochlorothiazide, 12.5 mg daily; and aspirin, 325 mg daily. Warfarin and amiodarone was added. Two weeks later, the patient reports soreness and weakness in the thigh muscles when she walks up hill.

Which of the following is the most likely cause of the current symptoms?

A Hypothyroidism

B Amiodarone-induced peripheral neuropathy

C Simvastatin-induced myositis

D Intramuscular hemorrhage

11.1 Pharmacologic principles as applied to antiarrhythmic drugs

Antiarrhythmic drugs

- Pharmacokinetics is a study of drug concentration, pharmacodynamics relates to variability in response after administration.
- The term bioavailability describes the amount of drug detected in systemic circulation following oral administration.
- Availability of the drug can be reduced by lack of absorption or rapid metabolism in liver or intestine before reaching circulation.
- Drugs that have poor bioavailability after oral administration require smaller doses when administered intravenously.
- During steady state the amount of drug entering and leaving the plasma or tissues is same.

Elimination half life (EHL)

- In a "first order kinetics" drug elimination is dependent on the plasma concentration. If the drug elimination per unit time is constant irrespective of plasma concentration it is called "zero order kinetics".
- An example of zero order kinetics is ethanol.
- When first order mechanisms are saturated, at high plasma levels of the drug, the mode may switch to zero order kinetics. Thus doubling of the dose may raise plasma concentration by more then twofold.
- Elimination half life is the time required for plasma concentration to fall 50%.
- Drug elimination will be complete in four to five half lives. Fallowing a change in the dose of the drug it takes four to five half lives to reach new steady state. This applies to initiation, termination or dosage change of drug.
- Loading dose may result in early attainment of therapeutic concentration but time to steady state is still dependent on half life. When steady state is achieved the plasma level may not be therapeutic. It means at that dose and plasma level the drug entering and leaving plasma and tissues is same.
- Following a loading dose drug concentration maybe high but by steady state it may become subtherapeutic if the maintenance dose is inadequate.
- Loading dose is desirable for rapid results or when the drugs half life is long.

Clearance

- Clearance is defined as the amount of plasma cleared of drug in a unit time by elimination or metabolism. Its unit is volume/time or ml/min.
- Half life determines time to steady state while clearance and dose of the drug determines actual level of the drug when steady state is achieved. Decrease clearance will result in increase steady state levels of the drug.
- Steady state concentration = dose/clearance.
- Organ specific such as renal or hepatic clearance can be measured.
- A drug can clear the plasma by elimination, metabolism or intracellular uptake (adenosine)

Volume of distribution

- The central volume of distribution is where IV administered drug distributes.
- Steady state volume of distribution is the total volume in to which drug distributes at a steady state.
- In congestive heart failure (CHF) central volume of distribution is reduced.
- Elimination half life varies directly with volume of distribution and inversely with clearance.
- In CHF, lidocaine volume of distribution and clearance is reduced requiring reduced loading and maintenance dose. The elimination half life remains unchanged at two hours and time to steady state at 8 to 10 hours.

Distribution half life

- Time it takes for distribution of the drug from central compartment to peripheral sites. For example lidocaine distribution half life in 8 min and elimination half life is 120 min. This may be responsible for precipitous drop in drug concentration shortly after IV administration.

Protein binding

- Most drugs bind to circulating plasma proteins. Unbound fraction of the drug exerts pharmacologic effect. Change in protein binding can affect amount of free drug available. Drugs bind to plasma albumin.
- Drugs with high affinity for plasma protein (such as warfarin which is 99% bound) may result in large variations in free drug concentration with slight change in protein binding.
- Drugs may bind to acute phase reactants such as alpha1 acid glycoprotein (AAG). Levels of AAG increase with acute illness, such as myocardial infarction (MI). This may result in lower free drug concentration during acute illness.
- In acute MI higher plasma levels of lidocaine may be well tolerated and required to suppress arrhythmias. In these situations level of unbound drug concentration will be more reliable than total drug concentration.
- In general loading dose should be avoided and dose should be reduced if clearance is reduced.
- Clearance can be reduced by
  1 Dysfunction of eliminating organ.
  2 Concomitant drug therapy that inhibits (erythromycin and cisapride) or induces(rifampin and quinidine) metabolic / transport pathway
  3 Defective function of drug eliminating proteins and channels.
- Therapeutic margin is a plasma concentration of the drug above which toxicity occurs and at lower levels effectiveness is lost.
- Drug dosing is determined by elimination rate and lower and upper therapeutic level. Wide therapeutic margin allows infrequent dosing even if the drug is eliminated rapidly. Propranolol administered twice daily even though half life is 4–6 hours.
- With narrow therapeutic margin drug should be administered according to elimination half life.

- To measure steady state level the drug should be administered with frequency of elimination half life. If the frequency of administration is more or less often than the elimination half life than plasma level of the drug may not reflect steady state levels.
- If the drug produces active metabolites then the level of parent drug and metabolite should be measured and expressed individually. Drugs may have multiple pharmacologic effects at different plasma levels.

CYP2D6 (Table 11.1)

- It is an enzyme that belongs to cytochrome P450 (CYP) family and is expressed in liver. It is responsible for metabolism of beta-blockers (timolol, metoprolol), antiarrhythmics (propafenone) and noncardiovascular drugs (phenformin, codeine).
- It is absent in 7% of Caucasians and African Americans. These patients are poor metabolizers.
- In poor metabolizers parent drug will accumulate. In case of propafenone excessive beta blocking effect will be evident. In case of codeine which is metabolized to morphine lack of CYP2D6 will result in ineffective analgesia.
- In ultra rapid metabolizers (increased CYP2D6) there will be accumulation of metabolites.

N acetyltransferase (NAT)

- Procainamide, hydralazine and isoniazide are metabolized by conjugation with acetyl group of NAT. Fifty percent of Caucasians and African Americans are slow acetylators.
- Procainamide is eliminated by kidney and by N acetylation to *N*-acetylprocainamide (NAPA), which is eliminated by kidney.
- Rapid acetylators will be at increased risk of developing NAPA induced torsades de pointes in the presence of renal failure. Slow acetylators are at a higher risk of developing lupus.
- NAT1 is present in everyone however NAT2 is absent in slow acetylators.

CYP3A4

- It is expressed in the liver (Table 11.1).
- Inhibitor of CYP3A4 will allow the substrate level to increase, for example high levels of terfenadine or cisapride when given with erythromycin or ketoconazole or increased risk of rhabdomyolysis with simvastatin and mibefradil or increased levels of cyclosporine with ketoconazole and calcium channel blockers.

P glycoprotein (PG)

- PG acts as a drug efflux pump. Its expression in cancer cells may be responsible for multi drug resistance (MDR).
- PG is also expressed normally at multiple sites important for drug distribution such as intestinal epithelium, hepatocytes, renal tubular cells and capillaries of the blood–brain barrier.
- In intestine PG eliminates drug by efflux back into intestinal lumen.
- In liver and kidney PG eliminates drugs into bile and urine. In blood brain barrier it removes drug from capillary endothelium. PG is integral part of

Table 11.1 Enzymes and drug interactions.

Enzyme	Substrate	Inducer	Inhibitor	Effect
CYP2D6	Codeine Debrisoquine Flecainide Mexiletine Phenformin Propafenone Propranolol Thioridazine Timolol		Flecainide Fluoxetine Mibefradil Propafenone Paroxetine Quinidine	Deficiency results in poor metabolizers
CYP2C19	Mephenytoin Omeprazole		Omeprazole Ticlopidine	
CYP3A4	Astemizole Cisapride Cortisol Cyclosporine HMG-CoA reductase inhibitors HN protease inhibitors Lidocaine Nifedipine Quinidine Terfenadine	Phenytoin Rifampin	Ca channel blockers diltiazem mibefradil Cimetidine Erythromycin & macrolide antibiotics Grapefruit juice Ketoconazole & azole antifungal	Drug toxicity with inhibition
N-acetyltransferase	Hydralazine Isoniazid Procainamide			Increase drug levels in slow acetylators
P-glycoprotein	Cortisol Cyclosporine Digoxin HN protease inhibitors Quinidine Verapamil		Cyclosporine Quinidine Verapamil	Inhibition affects blood brain barrier
Thiopurine methyltransferase	6-mercaptopurine Azathioprine		Sulfasalazine	Marrow aplasia
Pseudocholinesterase	Succinylcholine			Paralysis

blood brain barrier. Inhibition of PG in brain capillaries results in higher levels of the drugs in cerebral tissues.
- Cells that express PG also express CYP3A4.
- Administration of digoxin with quinidine results in doubling of serum digoxin levels. Digoxin is a substrate for PG and quinidine is an inhibitor of PG.

Pharmacodynamics

- The effect of drug represents a net effect of its action on different receptors and channels. For example beta-blocking effects of sotalol occur at a lower dose than the QT prolonging effects. Direct effect of Ca channel blockers may be nullified by vasodilator induced increased sympathetic tone which increases the Ca current.
- Spontaneous and drug induced I_{Kr} blocked results in prolongation of the QT interval and reactivation of inward calcium channel resulting in arrhythmias. Effect of I_{Kr} blockade is variable in different cells of ventricle resulting in dispersion of refractoriness.
- External factors can modulate effect of drug on target channels such as a minor decrease in extra cellular potassium can potentiates the I_{Kr} block and increase in extra cellular potassium reverses this affect.
- Catecholamine stimulation increases I_{Ks} and blunts the effects I_{Ks} blockers.
- Expression of target molecule may be modified in disease.
- Aberrant responses to drug therapy may be due to mutation in target protein. For example patients with drug associated LQT in fact may have mutation in gene expression which becomes manifest after drug challenge. These are aberrant responses to therapeutic drug levels due to mutation in target protein and are not due to high level or toxicity (Table 11.1).

11.2 Antiarrhythmic drugs

- Antiarrhythmic drugs are grouped in to four classes. This grouping is based on their pharmacological action.
- Given antiarrhythmic drug may have multiple pharmacological actions from different groups. For example sotalol has a potassium channel blocking (Class III) action and it also is a beta-blocker (Class II) action (Table 11.8).
- Class I antiarrhythmics are subdivided:

  IA   Prolongs conduction and repolarization

  IB   No effect on conduction shortens repolarization

  IC   Prolongs conduction no effect on repolarization.

Class 1A

Quinidine
- It binds to alpha-1-acid glycoprotein.
- It is metabolized in liver through oxidation by the cytochrome P450 system. Its active metabolite is 3-hydroxy-quinidine.
- Twenty percent is excreted unchanged in the urine.
- It crosses placenta and is excreted in breast milk.
- It blocks sodium and potassium channels thus affecting depolarization and repolarization. It produces greater depression of upstroke velocity in ischemic tissue. It produces use dependent block of Na channel during activated state. This results in suppression of automaticity.
- It also blocks I_{K1} (inward rectifier), I_K (delayed rectifier), steady state sodium current, I_{Ca}, $I_{K,ATP}$, I_{to} and $I_{K,ach}$.

- Quinidine blocks I_{to} and prolongs epicardial action potential duration. It also blocks I_{Kr}.
- Quinidine Blocks α-1 and α-2 adrenergic receptors. Its vagolytic effect is produced by M2 receptor blockade.
- Prolongation of QRS duration is directly related to plasma level of quinidine while QT interval is not. It may produce prominent U waves.
- Alpha blocking effect may cause orthostatic hypotension. It does not cause negative inotropy.
- Vagolytic effect may enhance atrioventricular node (AVN) conduction and may increase ventricular response in atrial flutter (AF).
- Side effects include diarrhea, loss of hearing tinnitus, blurred vision, thrombocytopenia, coombs positive hemolytic anemia, QRS widening and ventricular arrhythmias which may respond to sodium lactate or sodium bicarbonate infusion.
- Proarrhythmias include Torsade de Pointes, which is due prolongation of QT interval. Plasma level does not predict occurrence of arrhythmia. Hypokalemia facilities quinidine induced early after-depolarizations (EAD) and arrhythmias. These arrhythmias are treated by IV infusion of magnesium and pacing.
- It is 50% effective in controlling AF. It blocks conduction in accessory pathway. It is not very effective in controlling ventricular arrhythmias.
- Oral does is 300–600 mg every 6 hours.
- Atrial selective/predominant sodium channel blockers, such as ranolazine are effective in suppressing AF. This atrial selectivity is caused by atrioventricular differences in the action potential characteristics and differences in biophysical properties of atrial and ventricular sodium channels.

Procainamide
- Sixty percent is excreted by kidney, 40% by liver. Protein binding is weak.
- *N*-acetyl procainamide (NAPA) is an active metabolite.
- NAPA has a half life of 6 hours; 90% is excreted by kidney.
- Procainamide therapeutic level is 4–12 µg/ml and for NAPA it is 9– µg/ml. Both are removed by hemodialysis.
- It crosses placenta and is excreted in breast milk.
- Pharmacologic effects are similar to quinidine.
- Neuromuscular side effects may occur when given with amnioglycosides.
- It may cause hypotension when given IV. Other side effects include hemolytic anemia. Antinuclear antibodies may develop in 80% of the patients in first 6 months of therapy. Lupus syndrome occurs in 30%. Antibodies to DNA do not occur commonly.
- Slow acetylators are more likely to develop lupus.
- It may cause Torsades de Pointes.
- It is useful in the treatment of AF in the presence of Wolff–Parkinson–White (WPW) syndrome.
- IV bolus administration should not exceed 50 mg/min and infusion rate of 1–6 mg/min. Oral dose is 3–6 g/day.

Disopyramide

- It is metabolized by N-dealkylation to desisopropyldisopyramide, which is electrophysiologically active.
- It binds to ã 1 acid glycoprotein.
- Fifty percent of the drug is excreted unchanged in urine.
- Plasma half life is 4–8 hours. Dose reduction is warranted in hepatic and renal failure.
- It passes through placenta and is excreted in breast milk.
- It causes use dependent block of I_{Na}. It may also block I_K, I_{K1}, I_{Ca} and I_{to}.
- The time to recovery from the block is 700 ms to 15 s.
- It prolongs QT interval and may cause Torsades de Pointes.
- Its anticholinergic effects are due to block of M2 cardiac, M4 intestinal, and M3 exocrine gland muscarinic receptors.
- It produces significant negative inotropic effect.
- Anticholinergic side effects include dry mouth, constipation and urinary retention.
- Hypoglycemia may occur due to enhanced insulin secretion.
- It may cause cholestatic jaundice and agranulocytosis.
- It is effective in treatment of atrial arrhythmias. It may also suppress digitalis induced arrhythmias.
- It has been effectively used in the treatment of neurocardiogenic syncope and hypertrophic cardiomyopathy.
- Usual dosing is 100–150 mg every 6 hours or 200–300 mg every 12 hours of slow release preparation. Dose should be reduced in the presence of hepatic and renal insufficiency.

Class 1B

Lidocaine

- Lidocaine blocks I_{Na} by shifting voltage for inactivation to more negative. It binds to activated and inactivated state of sodium channel.
- Lidocaine, quinidine, and flecainide exert use-dependent block with fast intermediate and slow kinetics respectively.
- Continuous activation of I_{Na} may cause increase in action potential duration (APD) (long QT syndrome 3 (LQT3)). This current is blocked by lidocaine and mexiletine which may result in correction of long QT interval.
- It is metabolized in liver to glycinexylidide and monoethylglycinxylidide which are less active than the parent compound.
- It binds to αl acid glycoprotein, which is elevated in acute MI and CHF. This protein binding results in decrease level of free unbound drug.
- Its clearance is equal to hepatic blood flow. Decrease in blood flow due to propranolol or CHF will result in decrease clearance.
- The half life of rapid distribution is 8–10 minutes after IV bolus. Elimination half life is 1 to 2 hours.
- In CHF, because of decrease in volume of distribution and clearance, the elimination half life remains unchanged.

- It crosses placenta.
- Its anti arrhythmic effects are the result of sodium channel blocked in its inactivated state.
- Because of rapid binding and unbinding of the drug the conduction slowing occurs during rapid heart rates or in tissue with partially depolarized membrane such as in the presence of ischemia, hyperkalemia and acidosis. In ischemic ventricular muscle cells lidocaine depresses excitability and conduction velocity.
- It suppresses normal and abnormal automaticity in Purkinje fibers. This may result in asystole in the presence of complete AV block.
- EAD and delayed after-depolarizations (DAD) are also suppressed.
- It does not alter hemodynamics.
- Central nervous system (CNS) side effects include perioral numbness, paresthesias, diplopia, slurred speech and seizures. It does not cause proarrhythmias.
- In acute MI lidocaine reduces ventricular tachycardic ventricular fibrillation (VT VF) but does not alter mortality.
- Prophylactic use of lidocaine in post acute MI showed increase in death rate in treated group.
- The bolus dose is 1.5 mg/kg. Continuous IV infusion rate is 1–4 mg/minutes.
- Because of rapid distribution plasma levels falls in 8–10 minutes. Three additional boluses of half of the amount of initial dose can be given every 10 minutes.
- Bolus and infusion dose should be reduced in the presence of CHF and liver disease.
- Renal dysfunction does not affect dosing.

Mexiletine

- It is an oral congener of lidocaine. It is eliminated by liver utilizing P450 system.
- Side effects include tremor, blurred vision, dysarthria, ataxia, confusion, nausea and thrombocytopenia.
- Usual oral dose is 150–200 mg every 8 hours.

Class 1C

Flecainide

- It is a fluorinated analogue of procainamide.
- It is metabolized in the liver to meta-O-dealkylated-flecainide.
- Thirty percent is excreted by the kidneys.
- It is a potent sodium channel blocker. Time constant for recovery from the block is 21 seconds. It causes use dependent block.
- It also blocks I_K and slow inward calcium currents. It prolongs atrial refractor period
- It has negative inotropic effect. Its use is not recommended in CHF. It may be useful in patients with diastolic dysfunction and arrhythmias.
- Its side effects include blurred vision, headache, ataxia and CHF.

- Flecainide-induced proarrhythmias occur in patients with ischemic heart disease, VT and/or left ventricular dysfunction.
- Because of use-dependent block proarrhythmias may occur during exertion. Exercise test is recommended after achieving a steady state.
- Use of beta-blockers and hypertonic sodium bicarbonate has been successful in the treatment of proarrhythmias.
- It is useful in controlling paroxysmal AF.
- The initial dose is 100 mg every 12 hours and it could be increased to 200 mg every 12 hours. A single dose of 300 mg can be used for converting recent onset AF.
- QRS duration should be monitored and it should not be allowed to exceed more than 20% of baseline interval.

Propafenone
- High first pass metabolism results in low bioavailability.
- It is metabolized in the liver to 5-hydroxy propafenone, which is the active metabolite.
- 5-Hydroxylation but not N-dealkylation uses cytochrome P450.
- N-dealkylation produces a weak metabolite N-dealkyl-propafenone.
- Seven percent of Caucasians are poor metabolizers. They have high levels of propafenone and low levels of 5-hydroxy-propafenone.
- Hepatic dysfunction decreases clearance. In renal failure propafenone level remains unchanged however 5-hydroxypropafenone levels double.
- Propafenone and its metabolites are excreted in milk.
- It is an effective Na channel blocker in a use dependent manner. It demonstrates slow binding unbinding.
- 5 hydroxy and N-dealkylpropafenone also block I_{Na}. The 5-hydroxy compound is as potent as parent drug.
- It is a weak I_K and I_{Ca} channel blocker.
- It is a nonselective beta-blocker. This effect is enhanced in slow metabolizers.
- It has negative inotropic effect. Blood pressure may decrease.
- Side effects include nausea, metallic taste, dizziness, blurred vision, exacerbation of asthma, and abnormal liver function test.
- Proarrhythmias occur in 5% of patients. Na lactate can be used to reverse arrhythmogenic effects. It may cause atrial flutter.
- QRS duration monitoring and exercise test is recommended.
- Initial dose is 150–300 mg every 8 hours. Dose adjustment may be necessary in hepatic and renal failure. A single dose of 600 mg can be used in patients with PAF.

11.3 Beta-blockers

Beta-blockers as antiarrhythmic drugs
- Beta-blockers are most effective on tissues under intense stimulation by adrenergic agents.
- β-agonists enhance I_{CaL} and I_f current. This respectively increases inotropy and heart rate. Both these effects are negated by beta-blockers.

- β-blockers decrease the slope of phase 4 depolarization and decrease conduction velocity in the sinoatrial (SA) and AVN.
- Prolongation of AH interval and AVN effective refractory period may cause Wenckebach block.
- Shortening of QTc in post-myocardial infarction (MI) patients and increase in refractoriness in ischemic tissues by counteracting the arrhythmogenic effects of adrenergic agonist has been observed.
- Beta-blockers with ISA may not benefit post-MI patients.
- Most Beta-blockers competitively block β_1 receptors.
- In post-MI patients there may be loss of autonomic receptors and sympathetic denervation which may result in super sensitivity to circulating catecholamines predisposing to heterogeneity of refractoriness and arrhythmias. Beta-blockers may improve survival in post-MI patients.
- Some of the beneficial effects of the beta-blockers may be due to alleviation of ischemia.
- Beta-blockers increase survival in post-MI, LQTS patients. Reduction in mortality in post MI-patients appears to be due to reduction in incidence of VF sudden death. This beneficial effect was observed irrespective of age, sex, race and site of MI. It correlates positively with degree of bradycardia produced. Beta-blockers should be given routinely to post-MI patients.
- Beta-blockers complement the antiarrhythmic effects of amiodarone.
- Patients with congestive heart failure tend to have elevated adrenergic activity. Beta blockers significantly reduce total mortality in patients with heart failure of ischemic and non ischemic etiology.
- Carvedilol, labetalol and bucindolol also have vasodilator activity (Table 11.2).
- Beta-blockers complement device therapy in survivors of cardiac arrest.
- Patients with LQTS who develop arrhythmias due to sympathetic activation respond to beta-blockers. Bradycardia and pause dependent Torsades does not respond to beta-blockers.
- In LQTS the mortality is 25% in the first 3 years after initial syncope and it is reduced to 6% after beta-blockade.
- Implantable cardioverter-defibrillator (ICD) is the treatment of choice after syncope in patients with LQTS.
- PVCs and nonsustained VT in the setting of left ventricular dysfunction increase the incidence of arrhythmic deaths. Suppression of arrhythmias by antiarrhythmic drugs does not improve survival.
- Beta-blockers improve survival by exerting anti ischemic effects, reducing effects of adrenergic stimulation, improve electrical homogeneity and increase heart rate variability.
- Beta-blockers may be effective in controlling catecholamine sensitive ventricular tachycardia but they do not prevent induction of ischemic VT.
- In patients, who survived cardiac arrest and subsequently were found to have an ejection fraction of 45–47%, beta-blockers were as effective as amiodarone in reducing mortality.
- Exercise induced VT and PVCs respond well to beta-blockers.

Table 11.2 Pharmacological properties of beta-blockers.

Name	Plasma half life (h)	Site of clearance	Lipid solubility	ISA	β_1 blocked potency ratio
Non selective					
Propranolol	6	Liver	+++	None	1.0
Nadolol	20	Kidney	None	None	1.0
Sotalol	12	Kidney	None	None	0.3
Timolol	5	Liver & kidney	None	None	6.0
β_1 selective					
Acebutolol	10	Liver & kidney	+	++	0.3
Atenolol	6	Kidney	None	None	1.0
Betaxolol	18	Liver & kidney	None	None	1.0
Bisoprolol	10	Liver & kidney	None	None	10.0
Metoprolol	6	Liver	None	None	1.0
Vasodilator α_1 non selective					
Labetalol	6	Liver	None	++	0.3
Pindolol	4	Liver & kidney	++	+++	6.0
Carvedilol	6	Liver	+	None	10.0
Vasodilator α_1 selective β_1					
Celiprolol	6	Kidney	None	+ β_2	

- Beta-blockers are effective in the treatment of narrow complex supraventricular tachycardia, inappropriate sinus tachycardia, rate control in atrial fibrillation and prevention of post cardiac surgery AF. They should not be used in the presence of pre-excitation.

11.4 Class III antiarrhythmic drugs[1,2]

Balance between conduction velocity and refractoriness of the tissue determines the properties of the reentrant circuit.
- APD influences the refractory period. Short refractory period favors reentrant arrhythmias and long refractory period abolishes re-entry.
- Class III drugs prolong APD and increase refractory period without affecting the conduction velocity. They tend to prolong QT interval and may cause torsades.

- An increase in inward currents (sodium and calcium currents) or reduction in outward currents (potassium or chloride) during plateau phase will increase APD.
- Class III agents prolong APD by inhibiting potassium current.
- Dofetilide and sotalol are selective I_{Kr} blockers. Their actions are more prominent at slow heart rate (reverse use dependence). This limits their efficacy and increases the tendency for induction of proarrhythmias.
- Amiodarone, ambasilide and azimilide are nonselective potassium channel blockers.
- Class III agents delay cardiac repolarization and increase refractoriness. This will manifest as prolongation of QT interval without affecting the PR or QRS duration. Increase refractoriness without slowing conduction makes these agents very effective in terminating reentrant arrhythmias.
- These agents tend to be less effective in terminating AF due to reverse use dependence effect.
- An adverse effect is prolongation of QT interval and Torsades de Pointes. It is a dose related effect likely to occur when drug elimination is impaired. Other factors such as hypokalemia, bradycardia and female gender predispose to drug induced acquired long QTS9 (Box 11.1).
- Agents with I_{Kr} blocking properties mimic mutation of *HERG* that encodes I_{Kr} and causes congenital LQTS.
- Subclinical abnormality in ion channel may be brought to surface by APD prolonging agents.

Amiodarone[1,2]

- Amiodarone is an iodinated benzofuran derivative that has class I, II, III and IV antiarrhythmic properties.

Box 11.1 Factors predisposing to Torsades de Pointes in the presence of Class III agents

Female gender
History of sustained ventricular arrhythmias
LV hypertrophy and heart failure
Use of diuretics
Recent conversion from atrial fibrillation
　↑Sympathetic activity and calcium loading
Hypokalemia
Hypomagnesemia
High drug doses
Factors affecting metabolism and/or excretion e.g. renal failure.
Bradycardia.
Short–long–short coupling interval.
Prolong baseline QTc interval or excessive on-treatment QTc interval prolongation.

- It contains two iodine molecules. It is lipid soluble.
- It demonstrates antiarrhythmic actions of all four classes.
- It blocks I_{Na} in its inactivated state. This results in slowing of conduction and prolongation of the QRS duration in a rate dependent fashion.
- It noncompetitively antagonizes adrenergic effects which may be due to adrenergic receptor blocked, hypothyroidism or Ca channel blocked. This results in blunted heart rate response to adrenergic stimulation
- It prolongs APD by blocking I_{Kr}, I_{Ks} and I_{K1}. It inhibits thyroid hormone binding to the nuclear receptors which results in I_{Ks} block.
- It blocks I_{Ca}, which accounts for its depressant effect on AVN.
- Ca dependent effects of amiodarone appear early and effects on repolarization appear more slowly. This may be due to time dependent accumulation of the metabolite desethylamiodarone (DEA).
- All electrocardiographic intervals are prolonged with chronic administration of the amiodarone. This is a reflection of its electrophysiologic effect across all four classes.
- In the CASCAD trial amiodarone was found to be more effective then conventional antiarrhythmic drugs (Table 11.6).
- In AVID trial ICD was found to be superior to amiodarone.
- Prophylactic administration of amiodarone in patients with CHF did not demonstrate significant reduction in mortality. In post-MI patients, prophylactic administration of amiodarone resulted in reduction of arrhythmic deaths but not in total mortality (Table 11.3).
- In ARREST trial administration of IV amiodarone in VF cardiac arrest patients resulted in increased in successful resuscitation.
- It is 60% effective in maintaining sinus rhythm in patients with AF. Given 7 days prior to surgery it has been shown to be effective in preventing post cardiac surgery AF.
- Amiodarone is the drug of choice in patients with ventricular arrhythmias in whom ICD can not be implanted. It is also effective in the treatment of AF.
- Because of its lipid solubility it accumulates in fatty tissues, consequently its volume of distribution is approximately 5000 liters.
- Its elimination half life is 50 days. It is metabolized in the liver to active metabolite DEA. Dose adjustments are not necessary in renal failure.
- The loading dose is 1 to 1.6 g/day maintenance dose is 200 to 300 mg/day. IV administration should be through the central line to avoid phlebitis. IV infusion rate should not exceed 30 mg/min. Infusion should be prepared in glass containers because of drugs tendency to absorb in to polyvinyl chloride surfaces.
- Twenty to 30% of the patients may discontinue the drug due to side effects.
- It causes bradycardia and hypotension especially with IV infusion. It is less likely to cause TDP (0.3%) in spite of prolonging QT interval.
- Other side effects include interstitial pneumonitis and pulmonary fibrosis.
- Neurologic side effects include anxiety, tremor, headache, myoclonic jerks and neuropathy.
- It may also cause corneal micro deposits, ophthalmic neuritis, and photophobia.

Table 11.3 Adverse reactions to amiodarone.

Reaction	Incidence (%)	Diagnosis	Management
Pulmonary	2	Cough and/or dyspnea, especially with local or diffuse opacities on high-resolution CT scan and decrease in DLCO from baseline	Usually discontinue drug; corticosteroids may be considered in more severe cases; occasionally, can continue drug if levels high and abnormalities resolve; rarely, continue amiodarone with corticosteroid if no other option
Gastrointestinal tract	30	Nausea, anorexia and constipation	Symptoms may decrease with decrease in dose
	15–30	AST or ALT level greater than 2 times normal	If hepatitis considered, exclude other causes
	<3	Hepatitis and cirrhosis	Consider discontinuation, biopsy, or both to determine whether cirrhosis is present
Thyroid	4–22	Hypothyroidism	L-Thyroxine
	2–12	Hyperthyroidism	Corticosteroids, propylthiouracil or methimazole; may need to discontinue drug; may need thyroidectomy
Skin	<10	Blue discoloration	Reassurance; decrease in dose
	25–75	Photosensitivity	Avoidance of prolonged sun exposure; sunblock; decrease in dose
Central nervous system	3–30	Ataxia, paresthesias, peripheral polyneuropathy, sleep disturbance, impaired memory and tremor	Often dose dependent, and may improve or resolve with dose adjustment
Ocular	<5	Halo vision, especially at night	Corneal deposits the norm; if optic neuropathy occurs, discontinue
	≤1	Optic neuropathy	Discontinue drug and consult an ophthalmologist
	>90	Photophobia, visual blurring, and microdeposits	
Heart	5	Bradycardia and AV block	May need permanent cardiac pacing
	<1	Proarrhythmia	May need to discontinue the drug
Genitourinary	<1	Epididymitis and erectile dysfunction	Pain may resolve spontaneously

ALT = alanine aminotransferase; AST = aspartate aminotransferase; DLCO = diffusion capacity of carbon monoxide.

- Nausea abnormal liver function test, photosensitivity and bluish-gray discoloration of the sun exposed parts of the skin.
- Amiodarone may cause hypo or hyperthyroidism. It affects thyroid production, peripheral deiodination to triiodothyronine, entry of the hormone to the tissue and triiodothyronine binding to nuclear receptors.
- Amiodarone may interact with digoxin, quinidine, warfarin, procainamide, and phenytoin.
- Amiodarone is the antiarrhythmic drug of choice, in combination with other appropriate therapies such as beta-blocking agents, in patients who have sustained ventricular tachyarrhythmias associated with structural heart disease, especially if associated with left ventricular dysfunction, who are not candidates for an ICD.
- This recommendation is based on the following observations:
- Efficacy of amiodarone at 2 years to prevent sustained VT/VF or death is approximately 60%.
- It has minimal negative inotropic effects.
- It has low pro-arrhythmic potential.
- Prospective trial data demonstrate long-term neutral effects on survival and safety in patients with post-MI left ventricular dysfunction, and in patients with either ischemic and nonischemic dilated cardiomyopathy;
- Empiric use of amiodarone has been found to be more effective than the use of class I antiarrhythmic drugs even though these drugs had their efficacy guided by serial invasive or noninvasive tests.
- Efficacy of amiodarone is similar to ICD therapy in patients with left ventricular ejection fractions greater than 35%.
- Several prospective trials such as The Antiarrhythmics versus Implantable Defibrillators Study (AVID), Cardiac Arrest Study Hamburg (CASH), Canadian Implantable Defibrillator Study (CIDS) have demonstrated that an ICD is superior to empiric amiodarone in improving survival and preventing sudden cardiac (presumed arrhythmic) death.
- This finding has been demonstrated in patients with a history of sustained VT/VF.
- high risk post-myocardial infarction patients (depressed ejection fraction, nonsustained VT and inducible sustained VT),
- Patients with New York Heart Association (NYHA) II/III heart failure and left ventricular ejection fractions ≤35%.
- Thirty to 70% of ICD patients continue to require concomitant antiarrhythmic drug therapy for suppression of recurrent VT or suppression of or prophylaxis against AF with rapid ventricular rates.
- Majority of patients with ICDs have structural heart disease and left ventricular dysfunction, amiodarone is the drug most often used.
- Because amiodarone may increase the defibrillation threshold as well as slow the slow rate of VT, repeat ICD testing may be helpful to optimally program the ICD.
- The Optimal Pharmacological Therapy in Cardioverter Defibrillator Patients (OPTIC) study demonstrated that amiodarone, in combination with a beta-blocker, can reduce the number of ICD discharges.

- Although amiodarone is not approved for use in the treatment of AF by the FDA, it is the most commonly used antiarrhythmic drug for this purpose.
- One year efficacy rates for maintaining sinus rhythm of greater than 60%, compared to 50% or less for other antiarrhythmic agents.
- The Canadian Trial of Atrial Fibrillation (CTAF) demonstrated that amiodarone was more effective than propafenone or sotalol in preventing AF recurrences; although discontinuation rates due to adverse effects trended to be higher in the patients treated with amiodarone.
- In the Sotalol-Amiodarone Atrial Fibrillation Efficacy Trial (SAFE-T) amiodarone prolonged the median time to AF recurrence compared to sotalol but not in patients with ischemic heart disease.
- Maintenance of sinus rhythm with amiodarone improved quality of life and exercise capacity.
- Amiodarone could be used to treat AF in
  1 Patients post-MI who are not candidates for sotalol or dofetilide;
  2 Patients with CHF and left ventricular dysfunction who are not candidates for dofetilide
  3 Patients with significant left ventricular hypertrophy
  4 Antiarrhythmic drug-refractory, symptomatic patients as a medical alternative to catheter ablation.
- Because of the end-organ toxicity, the drug should be considered after sotalol and/or dofetilide have been tried in the post-MI setting, after dofetilide in patients with left ventricular dysfunction, and only in drug-refractory idiopathic AF.
- Prophylactic Amiodarone for the Prevention of Arrhythmias that Begin Early After Revascularization, Valve Replacement, or Repair (PAPA BEAR), have demonstrated that loading with oral amiodarone prior to aortocoronary bypass surgery can decrease the incidence of postoperative AF, this approach should be considered only in high risk patients (prior history of AF, valve replacement surgery).
- IV amiodarone has a "class IIb" indication in the Advanced Cardiac Life Support (ACLS) guidelines.
- IV amiodarone is now the antiarrhythmic drug of first choice for persistent VF or pulseless VT if standard (non-antiarrhythmic) resuscitative measures are ineffective.
- Amiodarone has also been advocated for treatment of VT VF refractory to lidocaine after acute myocardial infarction and as an adjunct for "electrical storm," defined as multiple episodes of recurrent rapid poorly tolerated VT or VF requiring multiple defibrillation attempts over a short period of time (24 hours or less) in which recurrent VT/VF can be only transiently terminated.
- IV amiodarone, at a dose of 5 mg/kg over 30 minutes followed by 10 mg/kg over 20 hours, was associated with significantly higher conversion rate of AF to sinus rhythm high doses such as this are, however, only rarely used in clinical practice.
- Amiodarone crosses the placental barrier, although fetal serum levels are only 10–25% of maternal levels.

Table 11.4 Recommended laboratory testing in patients receiving amiodarone.

Type of test	Time when test is performed
Liver function tests	Baseline and every 6 months
Thyroid function tests	Baseline and every 6 months
Chest X-ray film	Baseline and then yearly
Ophthalmologic evaluation	At baseline if visual impairment or for symptoms
Pulmonary function tests (including DLCO)	Baseline and for unexplained cough or dyspnea, especially in patients with underlying lung disease, if there are suggestive X-ray film abnormalities, and if there is a clinical suspicion of pulmonary toxicity
High-resolution CT scan	If clinical suspicion of pulmonary toxicity
Electrocardiogram	Baseline and when clinically relevant

DLCO = diffusion capacity of carbon monoxide; ECG = electrocardiogram.

- Fetal thyroid and congenital malformations have been reported. Given the drug's complex pharmacokinetics, effects on thyroid metabolism and significant end-organ toxicity, the drug should not be used in pregnant patients. Currently, it has an FDA class "D" rating.

Follow-up of the patient on amiodarone requires:

- Continued assessment of drug efficacy.
- Titration of drug dose after achieving a steady state.
- Evaluation of adverse and toxic effects (Table 11.3).
- Appropriate management of toxic effects (Table 11.4) and
- Attention to important drug–drug and drug–device interactions (Table 11.5).

Pulmonary toxicity

- Amiodarone-induced pulmonary toxicity is a morbid complication of amiodarone therapy.
- Overall risk of developing pulmonary toxicity is around 2%, and is more common in older patients and with higher doses of therapy.
- Amiodarone pulmonary toxicity can occur with low-dose therapy, and can occur within a week of therapy.
- Patients with pre-existing pulmonary disease may do poorly when they develop pulmonary toxicity. Serial pulmonary function testing has been shown to be a sensitive but nonspecific marker of pulmonary toxicity (likely due to a high incidence of heart failure in the population receiving the drug) and is of unclear clinical benefit.
- Clinical presentation includes acute or sub-acute cough; later manifestations include progressive dyspnea; fever may be present. Pulmonary function testing will show a decreased diffusing capacity (DLCO) and evidence of restriction.
- Chest computed tomography (CT) will reveal diffuse ground glass and reticular abnormalities, evidence of ongoing inflammation, and fibrosis.

Table 11.5 Drug interactions with amiodarone.

Drug	Interaction
Digoxin	Increased concentration and effect with sinus and AV node depression and gastrointestinal tract and neurologic toxicity
Warfarin sodium	Increased concentration and effect
Quinidine, procainamide hydrochloride, or disopyramide	Increased concentration and effect and torsade de pointes ventricular tachycardia
Diltiazem or verapamil	Bradycardia and AV block
Beta blockers	Bradycardia and AV block
Flecainide acetate	Increased concentration and effect
Phenytoin	Increased concentration and effect
Anesthetic drugs	Hypotension and bradycardia
Cyclosporine	Increased concentration and effect
Simvastatin, atorvastatin	Can promote liver function abnormalities

- An increase in lung (as well as liver and spleen) attenuation on CT scan due to parenchymal accumulation of amiodarone may occur but is not predictive of current or future pulmonary toxicity.
- Surgical lung biopsy should be avoided given reports of post-operative acute respiratory distress syndrome (ARDS), but, if performed, reveals a non-specific interstitial pneumonia pattern, with foamy alveolar macrophages filled with amiodarone–phospholipid complexes and focal organizing pneumonia.
- Bronchoscopy has little role in diagnosing pulmonary toxicity, since the findings are non-specific.
- The diagnosis of amiodarone-induced pulmonary toxicity is often one of exclusion. Treatment consists of discontinuing amiodarone and, in more severe cases, starting corticosteroids.
- There are no data to guide dosing and duration of corticosteroid therapy.
- Forty to 60 mg of prednisone (or equivalent) daily has been prescribed; the response is often rapid.
- Because the elimination of amiodarone is slow, prolonged therapy, for months, may be required.
- Dose of steroids can be decreased after the first few months to minimize side effects. Mortality from amiodarone-induced pulmonary toxicity can be lower if the diagnosis is made early.

Effects on thyroid function
- Treatment with amiodarone can lead to both hypo- and hyperthyroidism.
- Acutely, there is an increase in thyroid stimulating hormone (TSH) (although typically it remains <20 mU/L), an increase in both free and total T4, and a decrease in total, and, to a lesser extent, free T3.

Table 11.6 Prophylactic use of class III agents in the prevention of sudden cardiac death Post MI Class III Primary prevention Trials.

Trial	Drug	Inclusion/exclusion	Results
Post MI Class III Primary prevention Trials			
BASIS	Amiodarone vs placebo	Asymptomatic ventricular ectopy	Total mortality: amiodarone 5%; placebo 13%
SWORD	D-sotalol vs placebo	LVEF ≤0.40;	Total mortality: sotalol 5.0%; placebo 3.1%
EMIAT	Amiodarone vs placebo	LVEF ≤0.40	Total mortality: amiodarone 13.9%; placebo 13.7%
CAMIAT	Amiodarone vs placebo	≥10 PVCs/hour or non-sustained VT	Total mortality: amiodarone 6.1%; placebo 8.4%
DIAMOND-MI	Dofetilide vs placebo	LVEF ≤0.35	Total mortality: dofetilide 30.7%; placebo 31.9%
ALIVE	Azimilide vs placebo	15% ≤LVEF ≤35% plus low heart rate variability	Total mortality: azimilide 11.6%; placebo 11.6%
Post CHF Class III Primary prevention Trials			
GESICA	Amiodarone vs control	LVEF ≤0.35; NYHA class II–IV	Total mortality: amiodarone 33.5%; controls 41.4%
CHF-STAT	Amiodarone vs placebo	LVEF ≤0.40; NYHA class I–IV	Total mortality: amiodarone 30.6%; placebo 29.2%
DIAMOND-CHF	Dofetilide vs placebo	LVEF ≤0.35; NYHA class III–IV	Total mortality: dofetilide 41%; placebo 42%
Secondary prevention trials			
CASCADE	Empiric amiodarone	Cardiac arrest or sustained VT	Combined endpoint of cardiac mortality, resuscitated VT or syncopal ICD discharge: amiodarone 47%; other drugs 60%

(Continued)

Table 11.6 (*Continued*)

Trial	Drug	Inclusion/exclusion	Results
CASH	ICD vs empiric drug treatment (propafenone, amiodarone or metoprolol)	Cardiac arrest with documented VT/VF	Total mortality ($p = 0.08$): ICD 36%; amiodarone or metoprolol 44%
AVID	ICD vs amiodarone or EP-guided antiarrhythmic treatment	Cardiac arrest; sustained VT + syncope; sustained VT + LVEF <0.40	Total mortality: ICD 16%; drugs 24%
CIDS	ICD vs amiodarone	Cardiac arrest; sustained VT + LVEF ≤0.35; syncope + sustained VT/inducible VT	Yearly mortality rate: ICD 8.3%; amiodarone 10.2%

ALIVE = Azimilide Post-Infarct Survival Evaluation; AVID = Antiarrhythmics Versus Implantable Defibrillators; BASIS = Basel Antiarrhythmic Study of Infarct Survival; CAMIAT = Canadian Amiodarone Myocardial Infarction Arrhythmia Trial; CASCADE = Cardiac Arrest in Seattle: Conventional versus Amiodarone Drug Evaluation; CASH = Cardiac Arrest Study Hamburg; CHF-STAT = Congestive Heart Failure: Survival Trial of Antiarrhythmic Therapy; CIDS = Canadian Implantable Defibrillator Study; DIAMOND-CHF = Danish Investigators of Arrhythmia and Mortality on Dofetilide in Congestive Heart Failure; DIAMOND-MI = Danish Investigators of Arrhythmia and Mortality on Dofetilide in Myocardial Infarction; EMIAT = European Myocardial Infarct Amiodarone Trial; GESICA = Grupo de Estudio de la Sobrevida en la Insuficiencia Cardiaca en Argentina; SWORD = Survival with Oral D-sotalol.

- After 3 months, a new equilibrium is reached, and TSH normalizes, again becoming the most reliable marker of thyroid status. T4, however, will remain high normal, or even frankly high, while T3 will remain low normal or, rarely, low.
- Due to these acute changes, it is best to avoid checking thyroid function tests during the first 3 months of treatment, if possible.
- In iodine sufficient areas, such as the US, the prevalence of amiodarone-induced hypothyroidism (AIH) is as high as 22%.
- Both female sex and the presence of anti-thyroid antibodies prior to the initiation of therapy increase the risk.
- Typically, AIH occurs within the first 1–24 months of amiodarone treatment.
- The diagnosis should be suspected in the presence of an elevated TSH (generally >20 mU/L) and a low or low-normal free T4.
- Symptoms of hypothyroidism, while nonspecific and often subtle, can also aid in the diagnosis.
- Treatment is accomplished with L-thyroxine, with a goal of normalizing the TSH.

- The majority of patients who do not have underlying Hashimoto's thyroiditis will have resolution of their hypothyroidism after discontinuation of amiodarone.
- Consultation with an endocrinologist may be helpful to decide on whether or not subclinical disease (high TSH but normal T4 in an asymptomatic patient) should be treated.
- Prevalence of amiodarone-induced thyrotoxicosis (AIT) is much lower than that of AIH in iodine sufficient areas.
- AIT can occur quite suddenly and at any time during treatment. The diagnosis is made based on a suppressed TSH with an elevated free T4.
- Given the beta-blocking effects of amiodarone, the classic findings of thyrotoxicosis are often absent. Clinically, the most common findings may be weight loss or a required change in warfarin dose.
- Elevated or high normal T3 indicating thyrotoxicosis.
- The natural history and treatment of AIT should be guided by the underlying etiology. Some patients have pre-existing thyroid disease (e.g., Graves' disease or multi-nodular goiter) aggravated by the iodine load of amiodarone.
- Patients who clearly have underlying thyroid disease should have amiodarone discontinued, and be treated with high doses of antithyroid drugs (propylthiouracil or methimazole).
- Patients who have unequivocal signs of thyroiditis (tender thyroid gland, fever) can be treated with prednisone with continuation of amiodarone.
- The thyroiditis is typically self-limited, and patients often eventually become hypothyroid. Start both antithyroid drugs and prednisone initially. If there is rapid improvement in 1–2 weeks, the disease is prednisone-responsive and discontinuation of the antithyroid drug can be considered.
- The decision to discontinue amiodarone is made based on the cardiac needs of the patient.
- In patients with subclinical disease (low TSH but normal free T4 in an asymptomatic patient), the decision to discontinue amiodarone can be deferred while the response to antithyroid medication is being assessed.
- As the drug effects will last for months, discontinuation will not result in immediate improvement.
- Due to the large iodine load, ablation with radioactive I131 is not possible.
- Potassium perchlorate, an agent effective in AIT, is no longer available in the US. Thyroidectomy is effective in high-risk patients (for example those being treated for VT) who need rapid treatment.
- Iopanoic acid, important for controlling thyrotoxicosis prior to surgery, is no longer available in the US.
- AIT should be evaluated and treated aggressively at the first hint of disease.
- For patients who need to restart the drug after discontinuation for AIT, prophylactic ablative therapy with radioactive I131 is recommended and has proven successful in preventing recurrence.
- Given the significant risk of thyroid side effects, patients should have a TSH, free T4 and total T3 checked prior to initiation of therapy.
- In addition, obtaining anti-thyroid peroxidase antibodies (TPO) can be useful for predicting subsequent hypothyroidism. These tests, excluding TPO, should

be rechecked in 3–6 months to establish a new baseline. Subsequent testing of TSH and free T4 should be conducted every 6 months or sooner based on clinical findings.

Bretylium

- It prolongs APD and refractory period without affecting conduction velocity.
- It causes initial release of norepinephrine followed by inhibition of release and uptake from sympathetic nerve terminal. This may result in initial aggravation of arrhythmia and hypertension fallowed by hypotension.
- It increases VF threshold. It is available for intravenous infusion for refractory ventricular tachyarrhythmias at a dose of 5–10 mg/kg bolus administered slowly.
- It is excreted unchanged in urine. Its half life is 10 hours.
- Adverse effects include hypotension, nausea, vomiting and parotid pain.

Ibutilide

- It is a methanesulfonamide derivative. It is a potent I_{Kr} blocker. It is effective in termination of AF (30% efficacy) and atrial flutter (60% efficacy). It prolongs QT QTc intervals.
- It is administered as 1 mg infusion over a period of 10 min fallowed by 0.5 to 1 mg if necessary. It is eliminated by the liver. Its elimination half life is 6 hours.
- Adverse effects include QT prolongation and polymorphic ventricular tachycardia in 8% of the patients. Patient should be monitored for ventricular arrhythmias 4 to 6 hrs after administration of ibutilide.
- Presence of CHF, female gender, bradycardia and hypokalemia are associated with increased risk of TDP.

Sotalol

- D and L isomers have class III and beta-blocking activity.
- It is a competitive non selective beta-blocker without intrinsic sympathomimetic activity. Its beta-blocking activity resides in the L isomer. Both isomers are I_{Kr} blockers. This action confers class III properties to Sotalol. The D isomer prolongs APD and it is a pure class III compound. At lower dose of 80 mg/day it produces beta-blocking effect with little class III effect. At higher doses of greater then 160 mg/day class III effects become prominent.
- It causes bradycardia, prolongs AH and PR interval and increases atrial ventricular and AV nodal refractory periods. It does not affect QRS duration and HV interval.
- It produces reverse use dependence effects on atrial and ventricular repolarization. This limits its efficacy in terminating AF.
- D Sotalol worsens mortality in post-MI patients with left ventircular dysfunction.
- It is eliminated unchanged in the urine. Dose should be reduced in the presence of renal dysfunction but not if liver disease is present.
- Plasma half life is 15 hours. Dose is from 40 to 460 mg/day. Larger doses are likely to produce Torsades de Pointes.

- Adverse effects include AV block, TDP, LV dysfunction sinus node dysfunction and bronchospasm. Incidence of TDP varies from 3 to 7% depending on the dose and associated factors such as hypokalemia and renal failure.

Dofetilide
- It is a methanesulfonamide compound.
- It selectively blocks I_{Kr} current. It prolongs QT interval. There is close relation between plasma level of dofetilide and QT interval.
- It has no effect on conduction interval or cycle length. It lengthens effective refractory period of the atrium, ventricle, and AP.
- It is eliminated by hepatic and renal clearance. Its elimination half life is 8 hours
- It is metabolized by CYP3A4 thus likely to interact with drugs using the cytochrome P40 such as erythromycin and ketoconazole resulting in higher concentration of dofetilide.
- It is more effective in terminating atrial flutter than AF.
- It is administered orally at a dose of 500 µg twice daily.
- In the Diamond study there was no adverse effect on mortality in patients with CHF and post-MI who received dofetilide.
- Incidence of Torsades de Pointes is 3–5%.
- Therapy should be initiated under monitored conditions. Dose should be reduced or drug should be avoided in the presence of renal insufficiency.

Azimilide
- It blocks both I_{Kr} and I_{Ks} currents.
- It prolongs refractory period, and increases APD and QT interval.
- It does not affect conduction or hemodynamics.
- Its therapeutic effects are rate independent and are maintained during ischemia and hypoxia.
- It is 90% bound to plasma proteins. It can be administered once daily. Dose adjustments may not be required for age, gender, hepatic or renal function.
- It is administered orally as 100 mg /day.
- Alive trial included post-MI patients with low ejection fraction who were at high risk of sudden death.

Dronedarone[3-5]
- Dronedarone is a noniodinated benzofuran approved for the treatment of atrial fibrillation.
- Dronedarone is a modified amiodarone molecule without the iodine and with the addition of a methane-sulfonyl group,
- Iodine is considered the main cause of the thyroid side effect and pulmonary toxicity of amiodarone.
- Dronedarone blocks multiple ion channels including both the rapidly activating and the slowly activating delayed-rectifier potassium currents, the inward rectifier potassium current, the acetylcholine-activated potassium current, the sodium current, and the L-type calcium current, It has an antiadrenergic effect.
- Dronedarone's absorption increases two- to threefold when it is taken with food. Therefore, it is recommended that it is taken with meals.

- Dronedarone undergoes first-pass metabolism that reduces its bioavailability to 15%.
- It is less lipophilic than amiodarone, it does not require loading doses and has a shorter half-life of approximately 24 hours.
- The recommended daily dose of 400 mg twice a day results in steady-state plasma concentrations of 85 to 150 ng/ml in 7 days.
- Elimination is mostly nonrenal. Dronedarone partially inhibits the tubular transportation of creatinine, hence it can increase the serum creatinine level by 10–20%, but does not reduce glomerular filtration.
- Dronedarone is both an inhibitor of and a substrate for CYP3A4.
- It should not be coadministered with potent CYP3A4 inhibitors such as macrolide antibiotics, ketoconazole, and other antifungals or protease inhibitors because the dronedarone exposure may increase by as much as 25-fold.
- If dronedarone is used in combination with verapamil or diltiazem, which are moderate inhibitors of CYP3A4, lower doses of concomitant drugs should be considered to avoid bradycardia or conduction block.
- Through the inhibition of CYP3A4, dronedarone can increase simvastatin levels by two- to fourfold, increasing the risk of statin-induced myopathy.
- Dronedarone also increases digoxin level by 1.7- to 2.5-fold, therefore close monitoring of the digoxin level, and possible dose reduction is suggested.
- No significant difference in total mortality was noted, dronedarone reduced the incidence of stroke by 34% which cannot be attributed to the reduction of AF. A potential explanation is the modest blood pressure reduction observed with dronedarone therapy, because even small reductions in blood pressure have been reported to significantly reduce stroke.
- Dronedarone is not recommended for patients with acute or recently worsening heart failure Caution should also be exercised when using dronedarone in patients with chronic heart failure.
- Dronedarone did not exhibit pulmonary or thyroid toxicity.
- Bradycardia, QT prolongation, diarrhea, nausea, and rash occurred significantly more frequently among patients taking dronedarone.
- Only one case of torsade de pointes ventricular tachycardia was noted out of 3282 patients treated with dronedarone.
- Amiodarone is more effective than dronedarone in the treatment of AF.

Vernakalant[6]

- It blocks the atrially selective potassium channel and ultrarapid potassium current (I_{Kur}) (as well as the acetylcholine activated potassium current), These currents are not expressed in the ventricular myocardium.
- Vernakalant is the atrially selective antiarrhythmic agent.
- Vernakalant is also bioavailable by oral administration.
- Vernakalant mainly blocks the ultrarapid potassium channel but also blocks other ion currents such as the transient outward current and the inward sodium current.
- Intravenous vernakalant hydrochloride, 4 mg/kg over 10 min followed by 1 mg/kg/h for 35 min, prolonged atrial effective refractory period by a mean of 25 ms without significantly prolonging the ventricular effective refractory period.

- There was a small but significant prolongation of atrioventricular nodal refractoriness, and the sinus node recovery time also increased.
- Vernakalant was most effective for atrial fibrillation of less than 3 days' duration (conversion efficacy of 70–80%), while only converting 8% of patients with atrial fibrillation of longer than a week.
- It was also relatively ineffective in patients with atrial flutter, with a conversion rate of less than 10%.
- Vernakalant was well tolerated, the most common side effects being dysgeusia and nausea.
- Less ventricular arrhythmia occurred than in the placebo group (9.0% vs 17.4%), with no torsade de pointes ventricular tachycardia reported.

Celivarone
- Celivarone is a noniodinated benzofuran derivative similar to dronedarone, with multiple channel-blocking properties.
- It showed a borderline efficacy of preventing recurrence of atrial fibrillation
- celivarone 300 mg a day reduces appropriate ICD therapy by 46% compared with placebo celivarone is being investigated in the prevention of ICD therapies for ventricular arrhythmias.

Ranolazine[7–10]
- Ranolazine, like amiodarone, was developed as an antianginal agent, but later it was found to have blocking effects on multiple ion channels including the late sodium current, both the rapidly activating and the slowly activating delayed-rectifier potassium currents, and the L-type calcium current.
- The use-dependent blockade of sodium channels by ranolazine is atrially selective which would make it useful in the treatment of atrial fibrillation.
- The Metabolic Efficiency with Ranolazine for Less Ischemia in Non ST-Elevation Acute Coronary Syndrome Thrombolysis in Myocardial Infarction 36 (MERLIN-TIMI36) large randomized trial showed a significant decrease in the incidence of new-onset atrial fibrillation, supraventricular tachycardia, and ventricular tachycardia in patients with acute coronary syndrome.
- The effect of ranolazine on arrhythmias and microvolt T-wave alternans is currently being investigated in patients with significant left ventricular dysfunction.

11.5 Calcium channel blockers

Calcium channel blockers
- Six classes of calcium channels have been identified; only L and T types are found in the heart.
- Dihydropyridines do not affect AVN conduction. Their depressant effects are over ridden by reflex action from vasodilatation.
- In spite of anti-ischemic anti hypertensive properties there is no effect on mortality in post MI patients.

- Calcium channel blockers increase refractory period and slow AVN conduction velocity by slowing phase 4-depolarization in SA and AV nodes. This property may be useful in controlling the heart rate during AF.
- Bepridil blocks fast sodium channel and prolongs repolarization.
- Ca channel blockers may be beneficial for coronary spasm inducted ventricular arrhythmias and may also be effective in exercise induced idiopathic LV VT.
- There is no effect on ischemic VT.
- There is marked prolongation of QTc interval in hypothyroidism, chronic amiodarone therapy and hypocalcemia yet Torsade is rare perhaps due to depressed I_{Ca} activity.
- Calcium channel blockers are effective in treatment of SVT where one of the limbs of the reentrant circuit is AVN. Verapamil at a dose of 7.5 mg IV was effective in terminating 90 % of the AV node dependent SVT. Reinitiation is less likely with verapamil.
- The use of calcium channel blockers should be avoided in the presence of pre-excitation.

11.6 Adenosine

Adenosine
- Adenosine is produced in the heart by two different pathways.
  1 Adenosine monophosphate (AMP) can undergo dephosphorylation by enzyme 5-nucleotidase to adenosine. Reverse reaction is mediated by adenosine kinase.
  2 Reversible conversion of S-adenosylhomocysteine to adenosine by enzyme S-adenosylhomocysteine hydrolase.
- Metabolism of the adenosine occurs by deamination to inosine.
- Myocardial ischemia or hypoxia increases the production of adenosine using both pathways.
- Adenosine receptors have been classified in to A1, A2A, A2B and A3.
- A_1 receptors are responsible for electrophysiologic and inotropic effects on heart.
- Adenosine acts on A_1 receptor via guanine nucleotide binding protein complex.
- Direct effect of A_1 stimulation is enhancement of IK-Ado outward potassium current.
- $I_{K\text{-}Ado}$ is present in atrium, SA and AV node but not in ventricular myocytes.
- Activation of $I_{K\text{-}Ado}$ results in shortening of atrial APD, hyperpolarization of membrane and prolongation of APD in AV node.
- Other direct effects include inhibition of I_f in SA and AV node and inhibition of I_{Ca}.
- The indirect effect of adenosine is produced by decrease in intracellular cAMP due to inhibition of adenylyl cyclase. Additional indirect effects include inhibition of catecholamine stimulated I_{Ca}.
- Adenosine suppresses catecholamine stimulated DAD and EAD.

- Adenosine and Acetylcholine produce similar G protein mediated effect on heart but through different receptors. Acetylcholine effects are mediated by the M2 receptor.
- Methylxanthines block A_1 receptor and nullifies the effects of adenosine. Increase activity of adenosine deaminase will also decrease the effectiveness of adenosine.
- Dipyridamole enhances the effects of adenosine by blocking its reuptake.
- AV block in inferior MI maybe adenosine mediated and could be reversed by aminophylline.
- Adenosine prolongs AH interval. It has no effect on HV interval. It slows or blocks antegrade conduction over slow and fast pathway.
- Adenosine has minor effects on junctional and ventricular escape pacemaker.
- In atrium it shortens ERP may induce AF.
- It does not affect conduction over accessory pathway. Preexcitation becomes prominent due to delay in AV conduction.
- Slowly conducting accessory pathways may respond to adenosine.
- Continuous infusion causes sinus tachycardia and lowers diastolic pressure.
- Sinus tachycardia is mediated by adrenergic reflex by activation of aortic arch chemo receptors. Pulmonary and systemic vascular resistance decreases.

Pharmacology
- Once injected it is rapidly cleared by cellular uptake and enzyme metabolism. Its half life is 0.5 to 5 seconds.
- Site and speed of injection and circulation time determines the response to bolus injection.
- It is effective in termination of SVT by inducing block at the AV node. If ATP is used it degrades to adenosine before being effective.
- Adenosine produces atrial and ventricular extra systole.
- Its effect occurs within 15–30 seconds after injection.
- Adenosine does not accumulate between injections. 12 mg dose is effective in terminating 90% of the AV node dependent SVT. Fallowing a bolus injection frequent PACs, PVCs, AF, and reinitiation of tachycardia may occur.
- It is also effective in pediatric age group at a dose of 37.5 to 300 µg/kg.
- Verapamil could be used when adenosine is contraindicated in patients with bronchial asthma.
- Adenosine is preferable in patients with left ventricular dysfunction, who recently received beta-blockers, in neonates and in patients where electrocardiographic diagnosis is uncertain.
- Adverse effects from adenosine infusion include flushing, dyspnea, and chest pain.
- Chest pain is not prevented by acetylcholine or beta-blockers. It is aggravated by dipyridamole. It is relieved by theophylline. These observations suggest that the chest pain is due to direct effect of adenosine on adenosine receptors.
- Adenosine increases respiratory drive by chemoreceptor activation.
- Flushing is due to vasodilatation mediated by increase in sympathetic activity.

Proarrhythmias

- Frequent PAC, PVC, sinus bradycardia, sinus arrest, AF, or AV block may occur.
- Bradycardia dependent polymorphic VT may occur specially in LQTS.
- It may cause AF by shortening atrial refractory period. In patients with WPW syndrome this could be potentially dangerous.
- Acceleration of tachycardia may occur due to increase in adrenergic tone.
- It may facilitate induction of AVNRT.
- Adenosine has no direct effect on ventricular myocardium.
- Exercise induced ventricular tachycardias in structurally normal hearts with RB and inferior axis QRS morphology which are induced by isoproterenol and terminated by verapamil and vagal maneuver are mediated by catecholamine-induced cAMP dependent triggered activity. These arrhythmias can be terminated by adenosine.
- Adenosine inhibits catecholamine stimulated calcium current. It inhibits isoproterenol induced EAD and DAD.
- It does not inhibit quinidine induced EAD or ouabain-induced DAD.
- Adenosine is useful in differential diagnosis of wide complex tachycardia
- Infusion may help in the diagnosis of sick sinus syndrome and during tilt test.

11.7 Digoxin

- It is a combination of aglycon, related to sterols, and sugar molecules attached to lactone ring. Pharmacologic actions are mediated by aglycon.
- At high blood levels digoxin increases intracellular calcium and causes DAD.
- Digoxin inhibits NA/K ATPases. It increases intracellular calcium concentration by inhibiting sodium / calcium exchange. These actions contribute to positive inotropic effect.

Pharmacologic effects

- The pharmacologic effects of digoxin result from increase vagal tone. It slows AVN conduction and increases refractory period.
- In atrium it shortens refractory period and increases conduction velocity due to increase vagal tone.
- At the toxic level automaticity is increased.
- Digoxin shortens refractory period of accessory pathways therefore its use in preexcitation is not advisable.
- It may cause ST and T changes.

Pharmacokinetics

- After an oral dose 60–80% is absorbed.
- Eubacterium lentum in the intestine metabolizes digoxin to inactive dihydrodigoxin. Use of antibiotic may change the bacterial flora and make more digoxin available.
- Cholestyramine, colestipol, antacids, kaolin and sucralfate decrease digoxin absorption.

- It takes 6–12 hours after an oral dose to achieve adequate serum concentration.
- It is excreted by kidneys. Its half life is 30 hours. Its desired therapeutic level is between 0.8 to 2 mg/ml.
- Quinidine displaces digoxin from binding site and reduces renal excretion.
- Amiodarone, propafenone and verapamil decrease renal and non renal clearance
- Cyclosporine and benzodiazepines raise serum digoxin level.

Clinical uses
- Digoxin is used for rate control during atrial arrhythmias; however, increased sympathetic tone nullifies this effect.
- Digoxin alone maybe effective in controlling the rate in sedentary patients.
- Calcium channel blockers and beta-blockers provide more efficient rate control.
- There could be marked fluctuations in heart rate in 24 hour period. Pauses of 2.8 s during the day and 4 s during sleep could be considered normal.
- Digoxin could be added if left ventricular dysfunction is present.
- Magnesium deficiency reduces effectiveness of digoxin.

Toxicity
- In the presence of sick sinus syndrome, digoxin causes bradycardia and exit blocks.
- Electrolyte abnormality, renal failure, thyroid disease and hypoxia increase the risk of digoxin toxicity.
- Digoxin toxicity is manifested by anorexia, headaches, hyperkalemia and visual changes.
- Cardiac toxicity of digoxin includes bradycardia, DAD due to calcium overload, AV block and bidirectional VT.
- Digoxin may inhibit sodium/potassium exchange resulting in hyperkalemia.
- Treatment of digoxin toxicity includes discontinuation of digoxin correction of hypokalemia and hypomagnesemia.
- Lidocaine and phenytoin have been used in controlling digoxin induced ventricular arrhythmias.
- Cardioversion during high digoxin level may result in VF.
- In the presence of hyperkalemia avoid calcium administration. It may potentiate calcium overload and arrhythmia
- Digoxin-specific Fab antibodies should be used to reverse severe digoxin toxicity.
- They bind to digoxin and are excreted in the urine. In the presence of renal failure this complex may not be excreted.
- Dose of Fab antibodies can be calculated by:

$$\frac{\text{digoxin level} \times \text{body weight in kg}}{100}$$

Table 11.7 summarizes the electrophysiologic properties of antiarrhythmic drugs.

Table 11.7 Summary electrophysiologic properties of antiarrhythmic drugs.

Drug	APD	ERP	VFT	Contractility	Autonomic effects
Quinidine	↑	↑	↑	0	Vagolytic; alpha-blocker
Procainamide	↑	↑	↑	0	Vagolytic
Disopyramide	↑	↑	↑	↓	Central: vagolytic, sympatholytic.
Lidocaine	↓	↓	↑	0	0
Mexiletine	↓	↓	↑	↓	0
Phenytoin	↓	↓			0
Flecainide	0 ↑	↑		↓	0
Propafenone	0 ↑	↑	↑	↓	Sympatholytic
Moricizine	↓	↓	0		0
Propranolol	0 ↓	↓		↓	Beta-blocker
Amiodarone	↑	↑	↑	0 ↑	Sympatholytic
Bretylium	↑	↑	0 ↑	↓	Sympatholytic
Sotalol	↑	↑	0	↓	Beta-blocker
Ibutilide	↑	↑		0	0
Dofetilide	↑	↑		0	0
Azimilide	↑	↑		0	0
Verapamil	↓	0	0	↓	0
Adenosine	↑	↑	0	0	Vagomimetic.

APD = action potential duration, ERP = effective refractory period, VFT = ventricular fibrillation threshold.

Antiarrhythmic drugs and pregnancy

- Maternal and fetal arrhythmias occurring during pregnancy may jeopardize the life of the mother and the fetus.
- Well tolerated minimally symptomatic arrhythmias should be treated conservatively by observation, rest or vagal maneuvers.
- Arrhythmias causing debilitating symptoms or hemodynamic compromise can be treated with antiarrhythmic drugs.
- Although no antiarrhythmic drug is completely safe during pregnancy, most are well tolerated and can be given with relatively low risk (using FDA labeling guidelines) (Table 11.8).
- Drug therapy should be avoided, if possible, during the first trimester of pregnancy, and drugs with the longest strongest safety record should be used first (Table 11.9).

Table 11.8 Definitions of US Food and Drug Administration (FDA) classifications (use in pregnancy ratings).

Category A: No risk to pregnant women or fetus
Category B: No evidence of risk in humans. Animal studies show risk, but human studies do not; **or**, if no adequate human studies have been done, animal findings are negative
Category C: Risk cannot be ruled out. Human studies are lacking, and animal studies are either positive for fetal risk, or are lacking as well.
Category D: Positive evidence of risk. Investigational or post-marketing data show risk to the fetus.
Category X: Contraindicated in pregnancy.

- Quinidine has the longest record of safety during pregnancy, and is generally well tolerated. Procainamide is also well tolerated, and can be used for acute treatment of undiagnosed wide complex tachycardia.
- All IA agents should be administered in the hospital under cardiac monitoring due to the potential risk of ventricular arrhythmias (Torsades de Pointes).
- Lidocaine is well tolerated as an antiarrhythmic agent.
- Phenytoin should be avoided.
- Flecainide has been shown to be very effective in treating fetal supraventricular tachycardia complicated by hydrops.
- Beta-blockers are well tolerated and can be used. They may cause intrauterine growth retardation if administered during the first trimester.
- Amiodarone should be avoided during the first trimester and used only to treat life-threatening arrhythmias.
- Adenosine is the drug of choice for acute termination of maternal supraventricular tachycardia.
- Digoxin can be safely used during pregnancy.
- Direct current cardioversion to terminate maternal arrhythmias is well tolerated and effective, and should not be delayed if indicated.
- The use of an ICD should be considered for women of childbearing potential with life-threatening ventricular arrhythmias.

Herbal medicine and cardiac arrhythmias
- *Ma huang*, or Chinese ephedra (*Ephedra distachya* and *Ephedra vulgaris*) is also known as ephedra.
- Its principal alkaloid constituents are ephedrine and pseudoephedrine, both of which are nonselective α- and β-receptor agonists.
- Ephedra is taken orally for weight loss and to enhance athletic performance.
- Ephedra is associated with life-threatening cardiac adverse effects, including cardiomyopathy, hypersensitivity myocarditis, chest tightness, myocardial infarction, cardiac arrest, cardiac arrhythmias, and sudden cardiac death.
- Prolonged QT interval and premature atrial contractions can occur after ingestion of ephedra.
- The FDA banned the sale and marketing of ephedra-containing products in the United States in 2004.

Table 11.9 FDA class and pharmacodynamics of antiarrhythmic drugs.

Drug	FDA class	Placental transfer	Excretion through breast milk	Adverse effects	Teratogenic	Injury to the fetus
Quinidine	C	Yes	Yes	Thrombocytopenia, rarely oxytocic	No	Minor
Procainamide	C	Yes	Yes	Fetal AV block, Lupus	No	Minor
Disopyramide	C	Yes	Yes	Uterine contraction	No	Minor
Lidocaine	B	Yes	Yes	Bradycardia, CNS adverse effects	No	Minor
Mexiletine	C	Yes	Yes	Bradycardia; low birth weight, low APGAR, low blood sugar	No	Minor
Phenytoin	D	Yes	Yes	Mental and growth retardation, fetal hydantoin syndrome	Yes	Significant
Flecainide	C	Yes	Yes	Rare	None	Minor
Propafenone	C	Yes	Unknown	Rare	No	Minor
Propranolol	C	Yes	Yes	Growth retardation, bradycardia, apnea hypoglycemia	No	Minor
Atenolol	C	Yes	Yes	Low birthweight	No	Minor
Sotalol	B	Yes	Yes	Beta-blocker effects, Torsades de Pointes	No	Minor
Amiodarone	D	Yes	Yes	Hypothyroidism, growth retardation, premature birth, large fontanels	Yes	Significant
Bretylium	C	Unknown	Unknown	Hypotension	Unknown	Unknown
Ibutilide	C	Unknown	Unknown	Torsades de Pointes	Unknown	Unknown
Verapamil	C	Yes	Yes	Bradycardia, AV block, hypotension	No	Unknown
Digoxin	C	Yes	Yes	Low birthweight	No	Minor
Adenosine	C	No	Unknown	None	No	Minor
Diltiazem	C	No	Yes	Bradycardia hypotension	Unknown	Moderate

Weight loss supplements and cardiac arrhythmias[10].

- *Bitter orange* (*Citrus aurantium*), is also known as green orange, aurantium, synephrine HCl, and synephrine.
- Bitter orange fruit and peel, which are taken orally for weight loss, contain the adrenergic agonists synephrine and octopamine.
- Structurally, synephrine is similar to epinephrine, and octopamine is similar to norepinephrine.
- Cardiac side effects include tachycardia, tachyarrhythmias, QT prolongation, variant angina, myocardial infarction, cardiac arrest, VF, syncope, and death. Most of these side effects occurred when bitter orange was taken with caffeine or ephedrine.
- Because bitter orange can inhibit the metabolism of drugs by cytochrome P450 3A4 (CYP3A4), taking bitter orange with CYP3A4-metabolized drugs can increase blood levels of those drugs and thus increase the risk of adverse effects.
- *Ginseng* is also known as Panax ginseng and Korean ginseng.
- Orally, ginseng is used as an adaptogen for increasing resistance to Zenvironmental stress. It may improve abstract thinking, mental arithmetic skills, and reaction times in healthy middle-aged people.
- There are no reports on its efficacy for weight loss.
- Ginseng has several constituents, including ginsenosides, various flavonoids, B vitamins, and pectin.
- Using ginseng concomitantly with bitter orange may prolong the QT interval, because these two substances have synergistic sympathomimetic effects.
- Similarly, ginseng has been reported to have an additive effect with ephedra, increasing the risk of life-threatening ventricular arrhythmias.
- Ginseng can increase the QT interval in healthy adults on the first day of use.
- Ginseng's effects have not been studied in individuals with cardiovascular disease. Ginseng can diminish the effects of warfarin.
- *Licorice* (*Glycyrrhiza glabra*), is also known as Gan Cao, glycyrrhizinic acid, and isoflavone.
- The applicable part of licorice is the root.
- There is conflicting information about the effectiveness of licorice for weight loss. Licorice has antispasmodic, anti-inflammatory, laxative, and soothing properties.
- The mineralocorticoid effects of licorice can induce fluid retention and worsen congestive heart failure.
- Licorice can also cause severe hypokalemia, increasing the risk of arrhythmias.
- Patients with heart disease should avoid licorice.
- Licorice can reduce the effects of antihypertensive drugs, and it may have adverse interactions with other drugs, including warfarin, digoxin, and furosemide.
- *Caffeine anhydrous*, scientifically known as 1,3,7-trimethylxanthine, is commonly called caffeine.
- Its uses include weight loss and treating type 2 diabetes.
- Caffeine is a methylxanthine compound and is structurally related to theophylline, theobromine, and uric acid.
- It is 100% bioavailable after oral administration.

- Its possible mechanisms of action include adenosine receptor blockade and phosphodiesterase inhibition.
- Caffeine is thought to act on adenosine receptors to increase the release of dopamine and other neurotransmitters.
- In large doses, caffeine can stimulate massive catecholamine release, causing sinus tachycardia, metabolic acidosis, hyperglycemia, and ketosis.
- In rare cases, caffeine overdose can result in death from ventricular fibrillation.
- Using caffeine in combination with bitter orange or caffeine-containing herbs, such as green tea, black tea, oolong tea, guarana, mate, kola nut, and ephedra, increases the risk of serious life-threatening or debilitating adverse effects such as hypertension, myocardial infarction, stroke, seizure, and death.
- Caffeine's deleterious effects occur almost exclusively when caffeine is combined with other stimulants or taken in massive doses.
- *Guarana* (*Paullinia cupana*) is also known as and Brazilian cocoa.
- Taken orally, guarana is used for weight loss and enhancing athletic performance.
- Oral guarana may promote weight loss when used in combination with mate and damiana.
- Guarana contains 3.6–5.8% caffeine (compared with 1–2% in coffee), which is responsible for guarana's pharmacologic effects.
- When taken in combination with other caffeine-containing herbs or with bitter orange, guarana can increase blood pressure and heart rate in otherwise healthy, normotensive adults, potentially increasing their risk of serious cardiovascular adverse effects.
- Use of a product containing both ephedra and guarana may cause jitteriness, hypertension, seizures, temporary loss of consciousness, and hospitalization requiring life support.
- *Buckwheat* is also known as buchweizen, grano turco, and sarrasin.
- The active constituents of buckwheat include tocopherols, phenolic acids, and flavonoids.
- Buckwheat is taken orally to treat diabetes, improve vascular tone, and prevent hardening of the arteries.
- In both adults and children, allergic reactions to ingested buckwheat can include skin sensitization, allergic rhinitis, asthma, and anaphylaxis.
- *nyan-mien*, or Korean buckwheat noodles may cause sudden death.
- The greatest use was among women aged 18–34 years (16.7%), and 73.8% of the supplements used by these women contained one or more stimulants, including ephedra, caffeine, and bitter orange.
- Serious adverse events reported with supplemental drugs are predominantly cerebrovascular (ischemic or hemorrhagic stoke) or cardiovascular (arrhythmias, myocardial infarction, sudden death).
- Three out of the four FDA-approved drugs for weight loss work by activating the sympathetic nervous system.
- *Orlistat* (Alli™; GlaxoSmith Kline and Xenical™; Roche), acts in the intestinal mucosa with minimal absorption.
- *Sibutramine* (Meridia™; Abbott), one of the currently approved diet control pills, acts by inhibiting the reuptake of norepinephrine, serotonin, and dopamine.

- It can increase heart rate and blood pressure and has been reported to be associated with serious adverse effects.
- Ephedrine and other sympathomimetic agents such as synephrine and octopamine, the active ingredients in *Citrus aurantium* (bitter orange), another weight-loss supplement, work by the direct stimulation of adrenergic receptors and/or the indirect release of norepinephrine from presynaptic nerve terminals.
- Hyperstimulation of the sympathetic nervous system, particularly in the setting of cardiovascular disease, increases the risk of ventricular tachyarrhythmias.
- Sympathetic stimulation is mediated through activation of myocardial β-adrenergic receptors coupled to stimulatory guanosine triphosphate regulatory protein (Gs).
- The subsequent triggering of the second messenger pathway activates the L-type calcium channel, promoting calcium entry into the myocardial cells.
- This triggers further release of calcium from the sarcoplasmic reticulum via the ryanodine R2 channel.
- Alterations in calcium homeostasis have been implicated in sympathetically mediated ventricular tachyarrhythmias.
- The increase in cytosolic calcium can trigger delayed after-depolarization, explaining the mechanism of adrenergically mediated ventricular tachyarrhythmias.

References

1 Goldschlager N, Epstein AE, Naccarelli GV, et al. A practical guide for clinicians who treat patients with amiodarone: 2007. *Heart Rhythm.* 2007;4(9):1250–1259.
2 Latini R, Tognoni G, Kates RE. Clinical pharmacokinetics of amiodarone. *Clin Pharmacokinet.* 1984;9(2):136–156.
3 Singh BN, Connolly SJ, Crijns HJGM, et al. Dronedarone for maintenance of sinus rhythm in atrial fibrillation or flutter. *N. Engl. J. Med.* 2007;357(10):987–999.
4 Hohnloser SH, Crijns HJGM, van Eickels M, et al. Effect of dronedarone on cardiovascular events in atrial fibrillation. *N. Engl. J. Med.* 2009;360(7):668–678.
5 Køber L, Torp-Pedersen C, McMurray JJV, et al. Increased mortality after dronedarone therapy for severe heart failure. *N. Engl. J. Med.* 2008;358(25):2678–2687.
6 Kowey PR, Dorian P, Mitchell LB, et al. Vernakalant hydrochloride for the rapid conversion of atrial fibrillation after cardiac surgery: a randomized, double-blind, placebo-controlled trial. *Circ Arrhythm Electrophysiol.* 2009;2(6):652–659.
7 Antzelevitch C, Belardinelli L, Zygmunt AC, et al. Electrophysiological effects of ranolazine, a novel antianginal agent with antiarrhythmic properties. *Circulation.* 2004;110(8):904–910.
8 Antzelevitch C, Burashnikov A, Sicouri S, Belardinelli L. Electrophysiologic basis for the antiarrhythmic actions of ranolazine. *Heart Rhythm.* 2011;8(8):1281–1290.
9 Burashnikov A, Di Diego JM, Zygmunt AC, Belardinelli L, Antzelevitch C. Atrium-selective sodium channel block as a strategy for suppression of atrial fibrillation: differences in sodium channel inactivation between atria and ventricles and the role of ranolazine. *Circulation.* 2007;116(13):1449–1457.
10 Nazeri A, Massumi A, Wilson JM, et al. Arrhythmogenicity of weight-loss supplements marketed on the Internet. *Heart Rhythm.* 2009;6(5):658–662.

Answers to self-assessment questions

1 D
2 A
3 C
4 C

CHAPTER 12

Electrical therapy for cardiac arrhythmias

Self-assessment questions

1 What is the likely cause of the absence of ventricular pacing at longer AV interval?

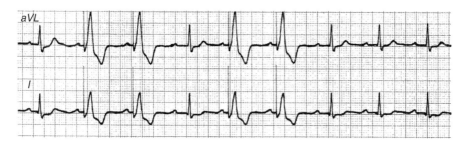

   A Lack of ventricular sensing
   B Inappropriate AVI programming
   C Lack of atrial sensing
   D Loss of pacemaker output

2 What is the correct interpretation of the following ECG tracing?

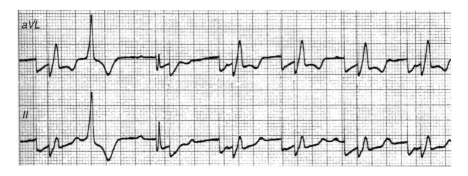

Essential Cardiac Electrophysiology: The Self-Assessment Approach, Second Edition. Zainul Abedin.
© 2013 Blackwell Publishing Ltd. Published 2013 by Blackwell Publishing Ltd.

A Pacemaker is functioning in asynchronous mode
B Pacemaker is functioning normally in DDD mode
C Pacemaker is functioning normally in VDD mode
D Pacemaker is functioning normally in DVI mode

3 An ICD was implanted in a 57-year-old male 4 years ago for ischemic cardiomyopathy. He was recently seen in the clinic because he had received two ICD shocks in the last 24 hours. Intracardiac electrograms from that episode are shown.

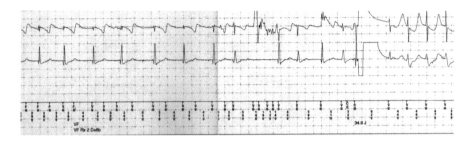

What will be your recommendations?
A Reprogram sensitivity to avoid T wave sensing
B Replace high voltage lead
C Replace pace sense lead
D Initiate amiodarone

4 A 54-year-old man is brought to the hospital after he lost consciousness while walking near his home. Cardiac catheterization reveals normal coronary arteries and left ventricular ejection fraction of 30%. Fifteen beat nonsustained ventricular tachycardia associated with palpitations was noted on telemetry monitor. A dual chamber ICD was implanted. One day later following recording was obtained.

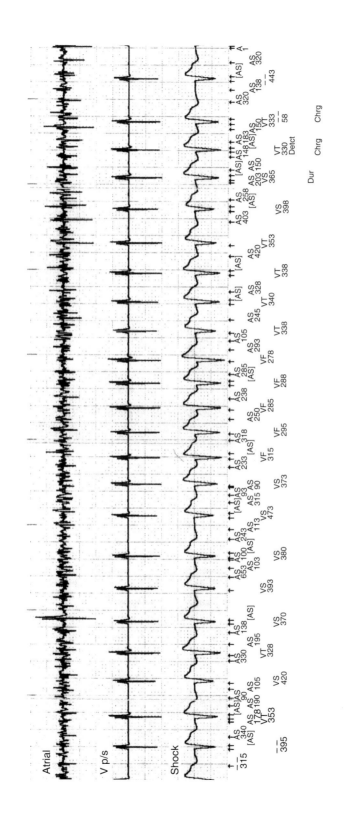

Which of the following is the most appropriate therapeutic maneuver?

A Replace atrial lead

B Reprogram the ICD to perform antitachycardia pacing prior to delivering a shock

C Begin treatment with flecainide

D Begin treatment with sotalol

5 A 62-year-old man, who has a history of myocardial infarction and a left ventricular ejection fraction of 29%, receives an implantable cardioverter-defibrillator for primary prevention of sudden cardiac death.

Which of the following is the most appropriate recommendation regarding the patient's operation of a motor vehicle?

A He may resume driving immediately if he feels well

B He may resume driving one week after implantation if there are no complications

C He may resume driving three months after implantation in the absence of syncope or ICD shock

D He may resume driving 6 months after implantation in the absence of syncope or ICD shock

6 A 58-year-old man had two episodes of syncope without any prodromal symptoms. First episode occurred when he was sitting at the breakfast table. Second episode occurred while he was working in his yard. He sustained bruises over his face and shorter. There is no history of cardiac disease, he takes no medications and there is no family history of sudden cardiac death or syncope.

Physical examination is normal.

Chest x-ray, Laboratory data, echocardiogram are normal.

Electrocardiogram shows a PR interval of 220 ms, right bundle branch block and left anterior fascicular block. Carotid sinus pressure results in the 3 second pause.

During treadmill exercise test heart rate of 160 bpm is achieved and no arrhythmias are recorded.

What will be your recommendation?

A Thirty day loop event recorder.

B Electrophysiologic study programmed ventricular stimulation.

C Permanent dual chamber pacemaker insertion.

D Coronary angiography.

12.1 Cardioversion, defibrillation[1,2]

- The success of defibrillation depends on waveform and electrode characteristics.
- The waveform characteristics include – shape, duration, tilt, number of phases.
- The electrode characteristics include – number, location, size, material.

Waveform

Shape of the waveform
- Damped sinusoidal (used for external defibrillators requires a large inductor).
- Straight capacitor discharge.
- Truncated capacitor discharge (used for internal defibrillators).

Waveform duration
- Rheobase is defined as the minimal amount of electrical energy that is required to produce a physiologic response; any stimulus of lower strength will not produce response even if it is maintained for long duration.
- Chronaxie is defined as smallest amount of time that is required to produce stimulation (pulse width) when the electrical energy is maintained as twice the threshold.
- Monophasic waveform requires larger current at shorter duration. In biphasic waveform the duration of the second phase could be same as the first phase or longer.

Waveform tilt
- It is defined as percentage difference in the leading edge and trailing edge voltage of the waveform.
- A square waveform occurs with large capacitors, high resistance or short duration of the pulse and tends to have small tilt.
- In a defibrillation system with a fixed tilt the duration of the waveform changes with impedance.
- In a system with a fixed duration of the waveform the tilt is determined by impedance.
- Commonly 50–65% tilt is used.

Waveform polarity
- Defibrillation thresholds are lower when right ventricular electrode is an anode for mono phasic waveform of greater then two milliseconds in duration and for biphasic waveform when the second phase is longer then the first phase.

Number of phases
- A biphasic waveform requires less energy to defibrillate. Which of the two phases results in defibrillation is unknown. The possibilities include that the first phase results in defibrillation and second phase removes the residual current from the cell membrane. This phenomenon is called burping of cell membrane.

- The second possibility is that the first phase preconditions the cell membrane by activating Na channels and the second phase depolarizes the cell membrane.
- The amplitude of the second phase is more important than the duration of this phase.
- A defibrillating electric shock produces electrical potential gradient throughout the heart. It tends to be greatest near the defibrillating electrode.
- For a successful defibrillation minimal potential gradient has to be achieved throughout the heart.
- Subthreshold shocks produce multiple areas of activation and results in unsuccessful defibrillation.
- Stronger shocks produce more effective defibrillation.
- A biphasic waveform is superior to monophasic waveform because it eliminates the conditions necessary for reentry.

Action potential
- When shock is delivered to a cell that has recovered from previous depolarization it generates a new response. If the cell is refractory, when the shock is delivered, no response is elicited.
- A strong electric shock may depolarize partially refractory cells and produce extension of refractoriness.
- Cathodal stimuli depolarize tissue whereas anodal stimulus hyperpolarizes the tissue.
- Myocardial discontinuities and anisotropic conduction may affect the depolarization of the tissue from the shock.

Detrimental effects of the shock
- High potential gradients created by shock may cause bradycardia, atrioventricular (AV) block, and ventricular fibrillation.
- Potential gradient exceeding 100 V/cm can cause tissue necrosis.
- At transmembrane potential of grater than 200 mV, pores form in the cell membrane this is called electroporation and results in ion leak and arrhythmias.

Defibrillation cardioversion
- The unit of energy for cardioversion defibrillation is Joules (J) or watts/second (W/s).
- The amount of energy selection depends on type of arrhythmia being treated.
- The synchronized shock of 50 J may be sufficient for atrial flutter, 100 to 150 J for atrial fibrillation (AF) and ventricular tachycardia (VT). For ventricular fibrillation (VF) 200 to 300 J of unsynchronized energy is delivered. For the pediatric age group the dose is 1 J per pound (0.45 J per kg).
- The success of cardioversion and maintenance of sinus rhythm depends on duration of arrhythmia and left atrium size.
- Prior to cardioversion for AF or atrial flutter patient should be anticoagulated for 3 to 4 weeks maintaining the INR between 2–3 or a negative transesophageal electrocardiogram.

- The flow of transthoracic current depends on electrode position. Anteroposterior or apex to right infrascapular position provides satisfactory results.
- Only 4% of the current flows through the myocardium.
- The size of electrodes determines the transthoracic impedance and current flow. For adults the size of the electrodes should be between 8 to 12 cm in diameter. Contact area should be at least 50 cm²/electrode or 150 cm² for both electrodes.
- Two electrodes must remain apart without any water or gel between them to avoid short circuiting of the current.
- Current flow is influenced by amount of energy and transthoracic impedance.
- Impedance depends on inter electrode distance (chest size), electrode size, electrode chest wall contact, couplant and respiratory phase.
- Impedance decreases after repeat shock perhaps due to tissue hyperemia.
- The average transthoracic impedance in an adult is 75 Ω.
- The minimum current necessary to defibrillate is constant but amount of energy required to achieve that current varies with impedance.
- Transthoracic impedance can be determined prior shock by passing low level of current between the electrodes. If impedance is determined to be high then higher energy level or a longer pulse width should be used.
- Current based defibrillation is independent of transthoracic impedance.
- Current and shock success relationship is parabolic. Highest success occurs with 30–40 A for defibrillation and 15–25 A for cardioversion. Lower current strengths were ineffective and higher currents produced toxicity.
- The biphasic wave from is superior and requires less energy for cardioversion defibrillation.
- Early defibrillation using external automated defibrillators in public places may improve survival after cardiac arrest.
- Successful defibrillation can be associated with immediate cessation of all activity (type A defibrillation) There are no vulnerable periods Type A successful defibrillation is usually associated with a higher shock strength.
- If defibrillation is followed by a brief period of rapid repetitive activity before eventual successful defibrillation (type B).
- Electrical shock that falls into a vulnerable period might induce repetitive responses, which may result in unsuccessful defibrillation or type B successful defibrillation depending on whether or not repetitive responses degenerated into VF.

12.2 Pacemakers

Permanent pacemakers[3]

NBG Code (developed by North American and British electrophysiology groups) for Pacemaker function designation is shown in Table 12.1.

- Pacemaker syndrome may occur with any pacing mode if AV dissociation occurs.
- Symptoms include dyspnea, dizziness, fatigue, cough, pulsation in neck and apprehension.
- If the AV conduction remains intact up to the heart rate of 120–140 bpm then the incidence of AV block is less than 2%.

Table 12.1 NBG pacemaker function designation.

Chamber Paced	Chamber Sensed	Effect of sensing	Rate modulation	Multisite pacing
0=None	0=None	0=None	0=None	0=none
A=Atrium	A=Atrium	T=Triggered	R=Rate modulation	A=Atrium
V=Ventricle	V=Ventricle	I=Inhibited		V=Ventricle
D=Dual	D=Dual	D=Dual		D=Any combination

ACC/AHA/HRS Guidelines for device based therapy
Class I = generally indicated.
Class II A = possibly indicated but limited published data.
Class II B = possibly indicated disagreement exists.
Class III = not indicated

Recommendations for permanent pacing in sinus node dysfunction (SND)

Class I
- Permanent pacemaker implantation is indicated for SND with documented symptomatic bradycardia, including frequent sinus pauses that produce symptoms.
- Permanent pacemaker implantation is indicated for symptomatic chronotropic incompetence.
- Permanent pacemaker implantation is indicated for symptomatic sinus bradycardia that results from required drug therapy for medical conditions.

Class IIa
- Permanent pacemaker implantation is reasonable for SND with heart rate less than 40 bpm when a clear association between significant symptoms consistent with bradycardia and the actual presence of bradycardia has not been documented.
- Permanent pacemaker implantation is reasonable for syncope of unexplained origin when clinically significant abnormalities of sinus node function are discovered or provoked in electrophysiological studies.

Class IIb
- Permanent pacemaker implantation may be considered in minimally symptomatic patients with chronic heart rate less than 40 bpm while awake.

Class III
- Permanent pacemaker implantation is not indicated for SND in asymptomatic patients
- Permanent pacemaker implantation is not indicated for SND in patients for whom the symptoms suggestive of bradycardia have been clearly documented to occur in the absence of bradycardia
- Permanent pacemaker implantation is not indicated for SND with symptomatic bradycardia due to nonessential drug therapy.

Recommendations for permanent pacing in AV blocks

Class I
- Permanent pacemaker implantation is indicated for third-degree and advanced second-degree AV block at any anatomic level associated
    1 With bradycardia with symptoms (including heart failure) or ventricular arrhythmias presumed to be due to AV block.
    2 Medical conditions that require drug therapy that results in symptomatic bradycardia.
    3 Awake, symptom-free patients in sinus rhythm, with documented periods of asystole greater than or equal to 3.0 seconds or any escape rate less than 40 bpm, or with an escape rhythm that is below the AV node.
    4 Awake, symptom-free patients with AF and bradycardia with 1 or more pauses of at least 5 seconds or longer.
    5 After catheter ablation of the AV junction.
    6 Postoperative AV block that is not expected to resolve after cardiac surgery.
    7 Neuromuscular diseases with AV block, such as myotonic muscular dystrophy, Kearns–Sayre syndrome, Erb dystrophy (limb-girdle muscular dystrophy), and peroneal muscular atrophy, with or without symptoms.
    8 Second-degree AV block with associated symptomatic bradycardia regardless of type or site of block.
    9 Average awake ventricular rates of 40 bpm or slower if cardiomegaly or left ventricular dysfunction is present or if the site of block is below the AV node.
    10 Second- or third-degree AV block during exercise in the absence of myocardial ischemia.

Class IIa
- Permanent pacemaker implantation is reasonable
    1 For persistent third-degree AV block with an escape rate greater than 40 bpm in asymptomatic adult patients without cardiomegaly.
    2 For asymptomatic second-degree AV block at intra- or infra-His levels found at electrophysiological study.
    3 For first- or second-degree AV block with symptoms similar to those of pacemaker syndrome or hemodynamic compromise.

4 For asymptomatic type II second-degree AV block with a narrow QRS. When type II second-degree AV block occurs with a wide QRS, including isolated right bundle-branch block, pacing becomes a Class I recommendation.

Class IIb
- Permanent pacemaker implantation may be considered
  1 For neuromuscular diseases such as myotonic muscular dystrophy, Erb dystrophy (limb-girdle muscular dystrophy), and peroneal muscular atrophy with any degree of AV block (including first-degree AV block), with or without symptoms, because there may be unpredictable progression of AV conduction disease.
  2 Permanent pacemaker implantation may be considered for AV block in the setting of drug use and/or drug toxicity when the block is expected to recur even after the drug is withdrawn.

Class III
- Permanent pacemaker implantation is not indicated
  1 For asymptomatic first-degree AV block.
  2 For asymptomatic type I second-degree AV block at the supra-His (AV node) level or that which is not known to be intra- or infra-Hisian.
  3 For AV block that is expected to resolve and is unlikely to recur (e.g., drug toxicity, Lyme disease, or transient increases in vagal tone or during hypoxia in sleep apnea syndrome in the absence of symptoms.

Recommendations for permanent pacing in chronic bifascicular block

Class I
- Permanent pacemaker implantation is indicated for
  1 Advanced second-degree AV block or intermittent third-degree AV block.
  2 Type II second-degree AV block.
  3 Alternating bundle-branch block.

Class IIa
- Permanent pacemaker implantation is reasonable for
  1 Syncope suspected to be due to AV block when other likely causes have been excluded, specifically ventricular tachycardia (VT).
  2 An incidental finding, at electrophysiological study, of a markedly prolonged HV interval (greater than or equal to 100 milliseconds) in asymptomatic patients.
  3 An incidental finding at electrophysiological study of pacing-induced infra-His block that is not physiological.

Class IIb
- Permanent pacemaker implantation may be considered in the setting of neuromuscular diseases such as myotonic muscular dystrophy, Erb dystrophy

(limb-girdle muscular dystrophy), and peroneal muscular atrophy with bifascicular block or any fascicular block, with or without symptoms.

Class III
Permanent pacemaker implantation is not indicated for
1 Fascicular block without AV block or symptoms.
2 Fascicular block with first-degree AV block without symptoms.

Recommendations for permanent pacing after the acute phase of myocardial infarction (MI)

Class I
• Permanent ventricular pacing is indicated for
1 Persistent second-degree AV block in the His Purkinje system with alternating bundle-branch block or third-degree AV block within or below the His Purkinje system after ST-segment elevation MI.
2 Transient advanced second- or third-degree infranodal AV block and associated bundle-branch block. If the site of block is uncertain, an electrophysiological study may be necessary.
3 Persistent and symptomatic second- or third-degree AV block.

Class IIb
1 Permanent ventricular pacing may be considered for persistent second- or third-degree AV block at the AV node level, even in the absence of symptoms.

Class III
• Permanent ventricular pacing is not indicated for
1 Transient AV block in the absence of intraventricular conduction defects.
2 Transient AV block in the presence of isolated left anterior fascicular block.
3 New bundle-branch block or fascicular block in the absence of AV block.
4 Persistent asymptomatic first-degree AV block in the presence of bundle-branch or fascicular block.

Recommendations for permanent pacing in hypersensitive carotid sinus syndrome and neurocardiogenic syncope

Class I
1 Permanent pacing is indicated for recurrent syncope caused by spontaneously occurring carotid sinus stimulation and carotid sinus pressure that induces ventricular asystole of more than 3 seconds.

Class IIa
1 Permanent pacing is reasonable for syncope without clear, provocative events and with a hypersensitive cardioinhibitory response of 3 seconds or longer.

Class IIb

1 Permanent pacing may be considered for significantly symptomatic neurocardiogenic syncope associated with bradycardia documented spontaneously or at the time of tilt-table testing.

Class III

1 Permanent pacing is not indicated for a hypersensitive cardioinhibitory response to carotid sinus stimulation without symptoms or with vague symptoms.
2 Permanent pacing is not indicated for situational vasovagal syncope in which avoidance behavior is effective and preferred.

Recommendations for cardiac resynchronization therapy (CRT) in patients with severe systolic heart failure

Class I

1 For patients who have left ventricular ejection fraction (LVEF) less than or equal to 35%, a QRS duration greater than or equal to 0.15 seconds, and sinus rhythm, CRT with an ICD is indicated for the treatment of NYHA functional Class III or ambulatory Class IV heart failure symptoms with optimal recommended medical therapy.

Class IIa

• For patients who have LVEF less than or equal to 35%, with NYHA functional Class III or ambulatory Class IV symptoms who are receiving optimal recommended medical therapy CRT with an ICD is reasonable for:
  1 QRS duration greater than or equal to 0.12 seconds, and AF,
  2 Patients who have frequent dependence on ventricular pacing, CRT is reasonable.

Class IIb

1 For patients with LVEF less than or equal to 35% with NYHA functional Class I or II symptoms who are receiving optimal recommended medical therapy and who are undergoing implantation of a permanent pacemaker and/or ICD with anticipated frequent ventricular pacing, CRT may be considered.

Class III

1 CRT is not indicated for asymptomatic patients with reduced LVEF in the absence of other indications for pacing.
2 CRT is not indicated for patients whose functional status and life expectancy are limited predominantly by chronic noncardiac conditions.

Pacemaker timing cycle (Figure 12.1)

• If the timing circuit is not reset it will result in release of stimulus at its completion.
• Output is inhibited by sensed ventricular/atrial event.

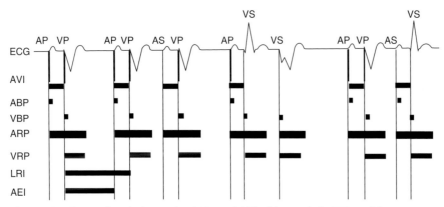

Figure 12.1 Pacemaker timing cycle. ABP=atrial blanking period. AEI=atrial escape interval. AVI=AV interval. ARP=atrial refractory period (includes AVI and PVARP). LRI=lower rate interval. VBP=ventricular blanking period. VRP=ventricular refractory period.

- The refractory period is initiated after a sensed or paced atrial (ARP)/ventricular (VRP) event.
- Any event occurring during refractory period is not sensed and does not reset the timing cycle.
- A blanking period is initiated during and immediately after the pacemaker stimulus is released and during which the opposite channel of the dual chamber pacemaker is blinded.
- With ventricular-based timing the atrial escape interval (AEI) is fixed. Ventricular-sensed events occurring during AEI reset this timer.
- In an atrial-based timing system AA interval is fixed. A ventricular-sensed event during AEI will reset AA interval as apposed to AEI in V-based timing system.
- The timing cycle in DDD consists of a lower rate (LR) limit, an atrioventricular interval (AVI), a post-ventricular atrial refractory period (PVARP), and an upper rate limit. The AVI and PVARP together comprise the total atrial refractory period (TARP). If intrinsic atrial and ventricular activity occurs before the LR times out, both channels are inhibited and no pacing occurs. If no intrinsic atrial or ventricular activity occurs, there is atrioventricular (AV) sequential pacing (complex 1, 2). If no atrial activity is sensed before the ventriculoatrial (VA) interval is completed, an atrial pacing artifact is delivered, which initiates the AVI. If intrinsic ventricular activity occurs before the termination of the AVI, the ventricular output from the pacemaker is inhibited, that is, atrial pacing (complex 4). If a P wave is sensed before the VA interval is completed, output from the atrial channel is inhibited. The AVI is initiated, and if no ventricular activity is sensed before the AVI terminates, a ventricular pacing artifact is delivered, that is, P-synchronous pacing (complex 3) (Figure 12.1).
- In rate-adaptive pacing AAIR/VVIR mode paced rate may vary and may reach programmed upper limit for the sensor (see Table 12.1).

Table 12.2 Pacing modes and indications.

Mode of pacing	Indications	Pitfalls
VVI/VVIR	Chronic AF slow rate.	Pacemaker syndrome if SR
AAI/AAIR	SSS bradycardia normal AV conduction.	Ineffective if AV block develops. Does not recognize/respond to ventricular events. Far field sensing from ventricle may inhibit A pacing.
DDI	A and V sensing No competitive A pacing. Inhibited, no P wave tracking. V pace rate will not exceed programmed base pacing rate. Useful for mode switches.	Acts as VVI during high atrial rates.
DVI	SSS bradycardia. Like atrial based pacemaker that response to ventricular events.	Competitive atrial pacing whenever V pacing is required.
VDD	P tracking (triggered), responds to ventricular events (inhibition). Normal SA node and AVN disease. Single lead pacing system.	Unable to pace in atrium if SAN dysfunction occurs. Acts as VVI in the absence of sensed atrial activity. May track atrial signal in SVT.
DDD	Normal sinus function and AV block.	May track atrial signal during SVT.

SR = sinus rhythm. SSS = sick sinus syndrome. SVT = supraventricular tachycardia.

- Tracking rate refers to when the pacemaker is tracking the intrinsic atrial activity. MSR refers to maximum rate allowed under sensor control.
  1 The V-A interval is calculated by the following equation:

$$V - A \text{ interval} = \text{lower rate limit interval} - \text{paced AV delay}$$

- In patient with sinus node dysfunction, but normal AV conduction, as demonstrated by 1:1 AV node conduction to rates of 120 to 140 beats/min, occurrence of clinically significant AV node disease is <2% per year.
- Non P wave synchronous AV sequential pacing with dual chamber sensing (DDI) is like DDD pacing without atrial tracking. The DDI pacing mode could be considered for patients with intermittent atrial tachyarrhythmias.
- In the VDD mode a sensed atrial signal initiates AVI (AV interval). If intrinsic QRS occurs before the end of the AVI the ventricular output is inhibited and lower rate timer (LRT) is reset. If paced beat occurs at the end of AVI it will also reset LRT. In the absence of atrial signal-paced ventricular complex (VVI) occurs. VDD pacing may be appropriate for the patient with normal sinus node function and conduction disease of the AV node or if the intent is to pace in the atrium and have the backup ventricular pacing should AV conduction fail (Table 12.2).

Table 12.3 Rate adaptive pacing sensors and mechanism of action.

Type of sensor	Mechanism
Piezoelectric crystal	Senses vibration from up and down motion
Accelerometer	Also senses anterior posterior motion
Minute ventilation	Transthoracic impedance, which varies with respiration is used to calculate minute volume
Closed loop system (CLS)	Responds to ↑ sympathetic activity, contractility

- In the DDD mode during lower rate pacing the timing cycle is divided in to AVI and VA interval. AV interval is initiated by spontaneous or paced atrial event and terminates with spontaneous or paced ventricular event. Maximum tracking rate is limited by total atrial refractory period which includes AVI and PVARP.
- In rate responsive DDD pacemakers increase in heart rate may be atrial or sensor driven.
- Rate responsive pacemakers use sensors to detect vibrations, motion, respiration or other parameters of physical activity (Table 12.3).
- Some pacemakers combine more than one sensor to smooth the effect of different type of physical activities.
- Complications may occur during pacemaker implant and include cardiac perforation, infection and pneumothorax.

Factors influencing pacing mode selection
- Underlying rhythm.
- Exercise capacity.
- Chronotropic response.
- Associated medical problems.

Pacemaker follow-up

Output programming:
- The output must be high enough to allow an adequate safety margin for pacing; this will maximize pacemaker longevity.
- A strength–duration curve plots voltage and pulse width thresholds and allows determination of appropriate values to ensure an adequate safety margin.
- Output programming options include doubling the voltage amplitude at threshold, tripling the pulse width at threshold, or programming output parameters to achieve triple the threshold, determined in microjoules.

AV interval

- In dual-chamber pacemakers it is the interval between paced or sensed atrial event and paced ventricular event. This corresponds to intrinsic PR interval. It must be programmed to optimize hemodynamic benefit from the pacemaker. It is desirable to maintain intrinsic ventricular activation by programming a longer AVI, thus avoiding the potential adverse effects of right ventricular apical pacing.

Potential adverse effects of programmed long AV delay

1 A long programmed AV delay may promote pacemaker-mediated tachycardia, as delayed ventricular pacing can result in retrograde conduction through a no longer refractory AV node.
2 Programmed long AV delays may interfere with mode switch functions. As the atrial blanking period is prolonged, atrial events may go undetected.

Lead impedance

- Lead impedances should be measured to assess the integrity of the pacing system.

Mode switch

- Mode switching is the ability of the dual chamber pacemaker to automatically switch from one mode to another in response to paroxysmal supraventricular tachyarrhythmias. In the DDD or DDDR pacing modes, supraventricular tachyarrhythmias may result in rapid ventricular pacing.
- Pacing modes such as DDI, DDIR, DVI, or DVIR eliminate tracking of atrial activity.
- Mode switching allows DDD or DDDR mode, during sinus rhythm to switch to a non-tracking mode, such as DDIR, during atrial tachyarrhythmias and than back to DDD/R mode on termination of the arrhythmia.

Analysis of pacemaker ECG

- The following pacemaker functions should be evaluated.
  1 Which chamber(s) is/are paced?
  2 Which chamber(s) is/are sensed?
- If pacemaker spikes are present, which event follows the stimulus? Is it QRS complex, P wave, both or neither?
- Is QRS induced by pacemaker stimulus or is pacemaker stimulus is occurring coincidentally with spontaneous QRS.
- Is sensing of the P and QRS is appropriate? Loss of sensing results in asynchronous pacing.
- Atrial or ventricular events that occur during refractory or blanking period are not sensed.
- Analysis of the pacemaker ECG is facilitated by the assessment of the timing cycles, such as escape interval, lower rate interval.
- In dual chamber pacemaker sensed P wave terminates the atrial escape interval and initiates AV interval. This will allow AV sequential pacing up to upper rate limit, referred to as maximum tracking rate (MTR).

- MTR is defined by TARP. It is the sum of AV interval and PVARP. When the atrial rate exceeds this limit every other P wave will fall in the refractory period and will not be sensed, resulting in 2:1 pacemaker AV block.
- Other upper rate responses include pacemaker AV Wenckebach, fall back and rate smoothing.
- Tachycardia with a ventricular paced rhythm of sudden onset the possibilities include ventricular tracking of a native atrial tachycardia and a pacemaker-mediated tachycardia.
- Endless-loop, pacemaker-mediated tachycardia (PMT) will terminate by magnet application.

Cardiac pacing and cardiac memory
- T-wave inversions (TWI) caused by right ventricular pacing may be difficult to distinguish from the diffuse TWI due to anterior wall ischemia.
- Following electrocardiographic criteria may help differentiate between the two.
- Combination of:
  1 Positive T wave in aVL,
  2 Positive or isoelectric T wave in lead I, and
  3 Maximal precordial TWI > TWI in lead III
- This provides 92% sensitive and 100% specific for CM, discriminating it from ischemic precordial TWI regardless of the coronary artery involved, especially if cardiac enzymes and other parameters of ischemia are negative.
- Altered ventricular activation during ventricular pacing initiates cardiac memory via induction of altered contractile patterns and altered stretch.
- Cardiac memory is a change in T-wave morphology induced by ventricular pacing or arrhythmias that persists after resumption of atrial pacing or sinus rhythm. Cardiac memory may be of short (lasting minutes to hours) or long (lasting weeks to months) duration,
- Long-lasting atypical ventricular activation such as permanent right ventricular pacing produces a new ventricular gradient (a significant inverse relationship between the activation time and the action potential duration (APD)) to the new activation sequence.
- "cardiac memory" reaches a steady-state in the human heart within one week of the onset of the right ventricular endocardial pacing at physiological rates.
- Right ventricular apical (RVA) pacing induces electrophysiological, contractile, and structural remodeling of the ventricles.
- If normal conduction resumes, ECG signs of cardiac memory appear, such that the T vector tracks the vector of the previously altered QRS complex.
  Sensing abnormalities could include (Table 12.4):
  1 Undersensing – failure to recognize normal cardiac activity.
  2 Oversensing – unexpected sensing of intrinsic or extrinsic signal. Normally functioning pacemaker may fail to sense premature beats.
  3 Functional under sensing occurs when intrinsic cardiac event is not sensed because it falls in refractory period such as atrial event falling in PVARP will not be sensed.

Table 12.4 Causes of abnormal pacemaker ECG.

Absence of pacer spikes	Lack of capture	Altered pacing rate
1 Battery depletion	1 Asynchronous mode/magnet	1 Altered recording speed
2 Circuit failure	application	2 Circuit failure
3 Conductor coil fracture	2 Battery depletion	3 Cross talk
4 EMI	3 Functional noncapture	4 Hysteresis
5 Lack of anodal contact	(stimulus on refractory period)	5 Magnet rate
6 Loose set screw	4 High threshold, spontaneous	6 Over sensing
7 Over sensing	or drug and metabolic induced	7 Sensor rate
noncardiac signal	5 Inadequate output	
8 Over sensing P & T	6 Insulation defect	
wave	7 Lead dislodgment	
	8 Perforation	
	9 Poor connection	
	10 Under sensing PVC, PAC	

- Programming the pacemaker temporarily to triggered mode may reveal the source of abnormal sensing.
- When a cardiac event has morphology between intrinsic and paced beat it is called a fusion beat.
- Pseudo fusion occurs when the pacer spike falls on an intrinsic event but does not contribute to or alter that event. This is due to insufficient cardiac voltage to inhibit sensing circuit. Pseudo fusion may occur when there is intraventricular conduction delay.
- Class IC drugs may increase pacing thresholds may also cause sensing abnormalities.
- Electrolyte and metabolic abnormalities like hyperkalemia, acidosis, hypoxia hyperglycemia, and myxedema may affect pacing and sensing thresholds.
- Ventricular pacing may result in pacemaker syndrome manifested by shortness of breath, dizziness, fatigue, pulsations in the neck or abdomen, cough, and apprehension.
- When the device detects the programmer telemetry wand, it ceases all automatic testing algorithms.
- Evoked response is used to test for ventricular capture when programmed "on."
- In the DAVID Trial the primary study outcome measure – death or hospitalization for new or worsened heart failure – was lower in the ventricular-paced group compared with the dual-chamber paced group.
- Patients with left ventricular dysfunction who were more frequently paced in the ventricle were more likely to experience an adverse outcome.
- The Mode Selection Trial (MOST) substudy reported adverse effects of frequent ventricular pacing on the development of heart failure and AF.
- Ventricular pacing >40% of the time in the DDDR group was associated with increased risk of developing congestive heart failure (CHF).
- Patients who were more frequently paced in the ventricle were also more likely to develop AF.

- The risk of developing AF increased by 0.7% to 1% for each 1% increase in ventricular pacing in the DDDR and VVIR groups, respectively.
- Although chronotropic incompetence is common in the pacemaker population, not all patients require rate adaptation.
- The rate response setting may promote ventricular pacing if rate adaptive AV delays are programmed.
- Increased incidence of nonsustained ventricular tachycardia and worsening of some measures of quality of life may be associated with rate response.
- Exercise tolerance as assessed by a 6-minute walk test does not differ between DDD and DDR groups.
- The Advanced Elements of Pacing Trial (ADEPT) compared DDD or DDDR pacing No differences was noted in some of the clinical endpoints.
  1 The DDDR group were more likely to experience hospitalization for heart failure. Clinical superiority of a "more physiologic" pacing mode has not been established.
  2 "Physiologic pacing" modes may aggravate AF and heart failure.
- Programming rate response resulted in more frequent ventricular pacing, thus increasing the risk of heart failure. Clinical benefit of rate response has been questioned.
- Persistent right ventricular apical pacing may cause ventricular dysfunction over time in individuals with normal systolic function at the time of pacemaker implant.
- Patients with sinus node disease who are treated with atrial pacing alone (AAI) have higher survival and lower cardiovascular death compared with those treated with ventricular pacing (VVI).
- Patients treated with atrial pacing were less likely to develop AF, thromboembolism, or symptomatic heart failure.
- AAIR mode when compared to the DDDR mode with either a short (150 ms) or long AV delay (300 ms) with sinus node disease results in higher incidence of AF in the DDDR group.
- There is detrimental effect of ventricular pacing even in an AV synchronous mode with a prolonged AV delay that minimized but did not completely eliminate ventricular pacing.
- In Canadian Trial of Physiologic Pacing (CTOPP) a higher incidence of paroxysmal and persistent AF was observed in the ventricular pacing group, and this effect persisted over 6 years of follow-up.
- In MOST significantly higher incidence of AF and hospitalization for heart failure was observed among the ventricular pacing group.
- United Kingdom Pacing and Cardiovascular Events (UKPACE) Trial, patients with high-grade AV block were treated with dual-chamber or ventricular pacing. No significant difference was observed between the two groups.
- Atrial or dual-chamber pacing should be considered only for patients with sinus node disease and intrinsic AV conduction.
- Dual-Chamber and VVI Implantable Defibrillator (DAVID) Trial death or hospitalization for new or worsened heart failure was lower in the ventricular-paced group compared with the dual-chamber paced group.

- Patients with left ventricular dysfunction who were more frequently paced in the ventricle were more likely to experience an adverse outcome.
- Atrial Pacing Periablation for Paroxysmal Atrial Fibrillation (PA3) Study subgroup, proarrhythmic effect of ventricular pacing occurs in patients with AF.
- Right ventricular pacing appears to be harmful for the following reasons
  1 Right ventricular apical pacing may cause ventricular dysfunction by creating ventricular dyssynchrony due to an abnormal ventricular activation sequence.
  2 Changes in the timing sequence of the mitral valve apparatus induced by right ventricle pacing may cause mitral regurgitation due to left ventricle papillary muscle dysfunction.
  3 This may lead to left atrial stretch/enlargement and electrophysiologic changes that leads to AF.
  4 Right ventricular pacing may induce abnormalities of myocardial blood flow.
- These detrimental effects appear to be greatest in patients with significant left ventricular systolic dysfunction and in those with an underlying intraventricular conduction delay.
- The degree of ventricular dysfunction is directly linked to the duration of ventricular pacing.
- Right ventricular apical pacing precipitating ventricular dysfunction and/or AF in patients with sinus node dysfunction and in patients with left ventricle ysfunction puts patients at risk for sudden cardiac death.
- To avoid right ventricle pacing:
  1 Programme long AV delays
  2 Avoid rate adaptation programming.
- The majority of patients with SND have intrinsic AV conduction in the absence of major intraventricular conduction delays, and up to 20% of these patients are candidates for AAIR pacing.
- Even those patients with AV node conduction abnormalities have intrinsic AV conduction most of the time.

Programming to minimize right ventricle pacing

- In patients with SND and normal AV conduction, the AAIR mode should be considered.
- The risk of progression to AV block requiring ventricular pacing over time is <1% per year if patients are carefully selected.
- Programming long AV delays (e.g., >300 ms) may reduce the amount of ventricular pacing.
- Doing initial implant position the atrial lead in a location to minimize intra-atrial conduction delay otherwise, prolonged atrial conduction may result in a significant amount of ventricular pacing.
- Adaptive AV interval hysteresis algorithms have been developed to promote intrinsic AV conduction. This may reduce ventricular pacing by 90% in DDDR mode.
- Algorithms that enable mode switching from the AAIR mode to the DDDR mode have reduced the proportion of ventricular pacing in patients with dual-chamber

ICDs from 74% when programmed to the DDDR mode with traditional AV delays to 4% when programmed to the managed ventricular pacing mode.

- In patients with SND managed ventricular pacing mode reduced the cumulative percent ventricular pacing compared with the DDDR mode. This may also be useful in patient with AV block.
- In the DAVID II Trial the effect of atrial pacing on event-free survival and quality of life was not substantially worse than, and was likely equivalent to, backup-only ventricular pacing.

Alternate RV sites for lead placement
- Parahisian pacing
- RV outflow tract
- High RV septum.

Left ventricular or biventricular pacing
- Left ventricular or biventricular pacing may be superior to right ventricular apical pacing, particularly in patients with systolic dysfunction.
- Patients with initially normal ventricular function who were right ventricle apical paced and followed long term (up to 7 years) after AV junction ablation for rate control of AF. Ventricular remodeling with increases in left ventricle dimensions and left atrial diameter, as well as increased mitral regurgitation and decreased LVEF, has been reported.
- Biventricular pacing has been reported to provide a significant improvement in the 6-minute hallway walk test and ejection fraction compared with right ventricular pacing in patients with impaired systolic function or with symptomatic heart failure.

Pacing recommendations
- In patients without systolic dysfunction, pacing the right ventricle apex may not be harmful.
- In patients paced for congenital complete AV block, the probability of developing left ventricle dysfunction was low (6%) during an average follow-up of 10 years.
- Right ventricle pacing should be minimized.
- AAIR mode should be considered for patients with SND, a normal PR interval, and an intraventricular conduction delay <120 ms. In these patients, the risk of progression to heart block is 0.6% per year (range 0–4.5%).
- In patients without evidence of chronotropic incompetence, backup VVI pacing (e.g., 40–50 bpm) could be considered, as most of the patients require pacing <1% of the time. Algorithms that automatically adapt the AV delay to promote intrinsic conduction or that mode switch from AAI to DDD pacing could be used.
- In patients with heart block, the choice of pacing system should be based on whether heart block is intermittent or permanent and whether systolic function is normal or abnormal.
- For intermittent AV block, dual-chamber pacemakers with algorithms to minimize right ventricular pacing should be chosen.

- Rate adaptation should not be programmed unless there is evidence of symptomatic chronotropic incompetence.
- For patients with complete heart block and normal systolic function, alternative right ventricle pacing sites could be considered, but more clinical studies are required to validate this approach. Support for biventricular pacing in this subgroup is weak.
- In patients with symptomatic left ventricular dysfunction and an AV block indication for pacing, cardiac resynchronization therapy should be considered. Whether this option is chosen in a bradycardia device or ICD depends on a number of clinical factors.
- Rate response should not be programmed on unless there is evidence of chronotropic incompetence.
- Leaving a device set at the nominal parameters at the time of implant is unacceptable. Pacemaker programming must be tailored to the individual patient.
- Every effort should be made to preserve spontaneous atrial activity and to promote intrinsic conduction.
- Pacing algorithms to minimize right ventricular pacing should be considered. MVP and AAISafeR modes are examples of these algorithms for reducing ventricular pacing.

Pacemaker-related complications

- Subclavian puncture may be associated with traumatic pneumothorax and hemopneumothorax, inadvertent arterial puncture, air embolism, arteriovenous fistula, thoracic duct injury, subcutaneous emphysema, and brachial plexus injury.
- Hematoma at the pulse generator site may occur with spontaneous or therapeutically induced coagulation abnormality. Aspiration is not advised.
- Cardiac perforation and tamponade may occur.
- Venous thrombosis of the subclavian vein may occur.
- Lead related complications include lead dislodgment, loose connector pin, conductor coil (lead) fracture, and insulation break.
- Pocket erosion and infection may occur. Impending erosion should be dealt with as an emergency. Once any portion of the pacemaker has eroded through the skin, pacemaker system should be removed and implanted at different site.
- Infection may be present even without purulent material. Culture should be obtained and proven negative before pocket revision. Adherence of the pacemaker to the skin suggests an infection, and salvage of the site may not be possible.
- The incidence of infection after pacemaker implantation should be less than 2%. Prophylactic use of antibiotics before implantation and in the immediate postoperative period remains controversial. There appears to be no significant difference in the rate of infection between patients who received prophylactic antibiotics and those who did not.
- Irrigation of the pacemaker pocket with an antibiotic solution at the time of pacemaker implantation may help prevent infection.

- Septicemia is uncommon.
- Early infections are caused by *Staphylococcus aureus*. Late infections are caused by *Staphylococcus epidermidis*.
- Superior vena cava (SVC) obstruction in association with implantation of pacemaker or defibrillator leads is estimated at 0.2 to 3.3% of all device implants.

Electromagnetic interference (EMI)[4]

- EMI may be caused by intrinsic or extrinsic signals of such frequency that is detected by sensing circuit.
- Biological signals are T waves, myopotentials, after potentials, P wave, and extrasystole.
- Nonbiological signals include electrocautery, cardioversion, magnetic resonance imaging (MRI), lithotripsy radiofrequency ablation, diathermy, electroshock, and radio frequency signals (cell phones).
- Welding equipment, degaussing equipment, cell phone, and antitheft devices are potential sources of EMI.
- Patient should avoid having an "activated" cell phone directly over the pacemaker or ICD, either from random motion of the phone or by carrying the activated phone in a breast pocket over the device.
- Patients should avoid leaning on or lingering near electronic equipment for surveillance of articles. Passing through these equipments is unlikely to adversely affect the pacemakers/ICDs.
- mp3 players placed within 2 inches (5 cm) of implanted pacemakers monitored via the telemetry wand can cause interference with pacemakers.
- Cosmic radiation is a well-known cause of single-event upsets (SEU) on disruption to electrical circuits in electronic devices. It occurs in devices such as laptop computers, cell phones, and personal digital assistants.
- Cosmic radiation originates from the Sun, other stars, and cataclysms in outer space, some having occurred millions of years ago, and is made up of protons, electrons, and neutrons. At sea level, cosmic radiation contributes 13% of the natural background radiation.
- There are four predominant factors contributing to cosmic radiation.
  1 Altitude: the earth's atmosphere shields cosmic radiation. At higher altitude the shield decreases, therefore the density of cosmic radiation increases. At flying altitude, cosmic radiation is 100 times greater than at sea level.
  2 Latitude: the earth's magnetic field deflects cosmic radiation. Shielding cosmic rays is greatest at the equator and decreases at the outer poles. Cosmic radiation at either the North or the South Pole is twice as great as at the equator.
  3 Solar activity: the sun's activity cycles every 11 years, with periods of high and low activity. During a quiet solar year, large amounts of cosmic radiation shower down through the atmosphere.
  4 Solar proton events: these are large, explosive ejections of charged particles. This increased ejection of solar energy can cause a sudden surge in cosmic radiation.

- Patients may be reassured that although these interactions may not be completely preventable, in general they result only in temporary "soft" resets that do not affect the lifesaving features of their ICD.

12.3 Implantable defibrillators

Implantable cardioverter defibrillators (ICD) design

- An ICD is housed in stainless steel or titanium case that also serves as an active electrode. ICD is implanted subcutaneously in the prepectoral region.
- Pace sense leads are connected to generator header using IS-1 connector and defibrillation leads are connected using DF-1 connector. The header is made of clear polymethylmethacrylate.
- Other components of ICD include battery, capacitor, telemetry coil and microprocessor.
- The battery is made of lithium silver vanadium oxide. It stores 18 kJ of energy. It generates 3.2 V; a battery voltage of less than 2.2 V indicates elective replacement parameter has been reached.
- Aluminum electrolyte capacitors are used to store 30–40 J using DC/DC converter. Capacitor is capable of charging and delivering 750 V to the heart in 10–15 ms. Capacitor charging begins after tachycardia detection criteria are met. Capacitor charge time should be less than 15 s.
- A long charge time would result in a longer period of circulatory arrest. In addition to battery voltage longer charge time is also an indication for ICD replacement.
- A single ventricular lead incorporates pace sense and defibrillation electrode.
- A defibrillation electrode consists of two coils, made of platinum-iridium alloy or carbon and is capable of delivering high voltages. The distal coil is located in the right ventricle and the proximal coil is located in the SVC.
- The pace sense component consists of bipolar electrodes. Some systems use intergraded bipolar electrodes that records between the tip and distal coil. Other systems use true bipolar electrodes that record between the tip and the ring electrode.
- A dual chamber ICD uses standard bipolar atrial lead. In addition to atrial pacing, atrial lead provides intracardiac electrograms which are helpful in differentiating VT from SVT.
- Virtually all ICD systems are implanted transvenously and include antitachycardia pacing (ATP) and ventricular bradycardia pacing, dual-chamber pacing with rate-adaptive options. In addition, atrial defibrillation and CRT features, are available.
- Defibrillating current is directly proportional to the voltage and inversely proportional to lead impedance. Polarization at lead tissue interface may occur.

Sensing

- Ventricular heart rate is the cornerstone of tachyarrhythmia detection by the ICD.
- Each and every electrogram must be detected and interval analyzed for proper sensing and detection of the tachycardia.

- Detection of the electrogram depends on the quality of signal received from the ventricular myocardium.
- Assessment of far field signal detection by ventricular lead should be performed at the time of implant. If far field signals are detected in spite of sensitivity reprogramming the lead should be repositioned.
- A band pass filter is utilized to filter out very low and very high frequency signals that are out of range of ventricular signal.
- Ventricular repolarization, atrial events, post pacing and post depolarization polarization, myopotentials and external environmental signals may be detected by the ventricular lead resulting in false detection of tachyarrhythmia and spurious shock or inhibition of the pacemaker.
- In addition to the amplitude of the signal the frequency contents of the signal (Slew rate V/Sec) are important for better detection of the signal.
- Large signal improves specificity of detection. Small signal (4–6 mV), but with good frequency contents, as represented by slew rate of >1 V/s, is better than larger signal with poor frequency content and slew rate of <0.1 V/s.
- The device must quickly and accurately identify the amplitude variation that occurs between normal beat of 10 mV, pacing spike of >500 mV, VF with amplitudes of 0.2 to 10 mV and asystole, where the amplitude of the electrogram may be 0 to 0.15 mV.
- This limitations have been overcome by using the autogain or autosensing threshold function. Autogain technique uses fixed amplitude voltage threshold and amplifies it for better detection. In the autothreshold technique amplification is fixed and a continuously varying amplitude voltage is detected.
- Adequate signal during sinus rhythm may be inadequate during VF therefore assessment of adequacy of signal detection should be performed by inducing VF at the time of implant.
- Failure to detect <10% of the VF signals during detection period would still result in proper detection and treatment of VF.
- Ventricular electrogram amplitude of 5 mV during sinus rhythm predicts reliable detection of VF.
- The Medtronic Sprint Fidelis ICD lead has a higher than expected incidence of conductor fractures.
- Its identification is important to the prevention of inappropriate shocks.
- The sensing integrity counter, which stores the cumulative number of nonphysiologically short ventricular intervals ≤130 ms, is a diagnostic feature designed to enhance early identification of lead failures.
- Failure of the ICD lead pace-sense conductor results in oversensing of high-frequency signals ("noise") on stored electrograms, abnormal lead impedance (often transient), and sensing of nonphysiologic short intervals near the ventricular blanking period with frequent, ICD-detected rapid nonsustained tachycardias.
- Even if no evidence of inappropriate sensing is found with one device, the change of device manufacturer itself may result in clinically significant sensing

problems. Inappropriate ventricular sensing related to differences in signal processing between manufacturers may result in oversensing of T waves.
- The St Jude Riata lead has demonstrated externalization of conductor coil resulting in lead malfunction and inappropriate shocks.

Detection
- After the detection of the electrogram the algorithm to detect and classify the intervals between electrogram is activated.
- This algorithm differentiates between bradycardia that may require pacing, VT that may require antitachycardia pacing and VF requiring shock.
- The primary features for the detection of the ventricular arrhythmias are heart rate and the duration of the arrhythmia.
- For faster rhythm shorter detection intervals should be programmed. Rate detection alone does not describe the hemodynamic status of the patient. An algorithm, where X number of intervals out of the total number of intervals Y, that meet the detection criteria, may improve the sensitivity of detection.
- SVT with overlapping rate with ventricular detection may result in inappropriate therapy.
- Additional criteria such as suddenness of onset (to differentiate from sinus tachycardia), beat to beat variation in cycle length (to differentiate from AF) and use of the atrial electrogram and its relationship to ventricular electrogram have been used.
- The presence of AV dissociation will confirm the diagnosis of VT. If there is 1:1 relationship between ventricular and atrial electrogram then it could be due to VT with 1:1 retrograde conduction or SVT.
- Ratio of the AV to VA interval may help in differentiating these arrhythmias. These additional features may delay the detection and decrease the sensitivity of detection.
- Algorithms should be programmed to deliver shock immediately for rapid arrhythmias irrespective of their origin. Sensitivity should not be sacrificed at the expanse of specificity. Lower rate cutoff may result in inappropriate shocks.
- A reconfirmation feature reconfirms the presence of arrhythmia during charging period. This may avoid unnecessary shocks in the presence of nonsustained arrhythmias which might terminate spontaneously during charging period.
- A redetection feature detects the occurrence of arrhythmia few beats after its successful termination. Reducing the number of intervals required for redetection can shorten redetection time.

Neodymium-iron-boron magnets
- Neodynium is a naturally occurring, powerful, concentrated magnetic substance found in the earth's crust.
- Magnets interfere with the implanted devices up to a distance of 3 cm.
- Persistent magnetic interference of a pacemaker can deplete the battery and cause undesirable hemodynamic effects because of rapid pacing at the magnet rate.

- Induction of life-threatening ventricular tachyarrhythmia may occur by pacing during the ventricular vulnerable period as the result of magnet-induced asynchronous pacing.
- Similarly, induction of AF or atrial flutter or other supraventricular tachyarrhythmia can happen as the result of asynchronous atrial pacing.
- Persistent magnet application may disable the tachyarrhythmia detection and therapy of ICD.
- The "beep on magnet" function can be turned on to warn the patients about ongoing magnet interference, but a patient with impaired hearing (very common in the elderly) may not hear the beeping.
- These magnets can be contained in brooches, necklaces, bracelets, name tags, apparel, reading glasses, or other products that could potentially be placed at a short distance from an implanted pacemaker or ICD.
- Headphones with a measured magnetic field strength ≥10 gauss at 2 cm were much more likely to cause magnetic interference than were those with lower magnetic field strength. Magnetic interference was not observed when headphones were placed ≥3 cm from the skin surface.
- Headphone magnets are used to vibrate the speaker (and thus the air in front of the speaker) to create sound waves that can be heard. Portable headphones typically contain the magnetic substance neodymium,
- Magnets or RF signals from cellular telephones, antitheft devices, and airport security wands may interfere with pacemaker and ICD functions.

Energy, load and tilt
- Manufacturers report ICD capacity as stored energies or as delivered energy under a typical 40-Ω clinical load and nominal 65% tilt waveform.

Indications for ICD implant
- EF of <35% irrespective of etiology (ischemic or nonischemic).
- Cardiac arrest due to VF or VT not due to a transient or reversible cause.
- Spontaneous sustained VT associated with structural heart disease.
- Syncope, associated with structural heart disease, and clinically relevant, hemodynamically significant sustained VT or VF induced at electrophysiologic study.
- Nonsustained VT in patients with coronary disease, prior MI, EF 40–45%, and inducible VF or sustained VT at electrophysiologic study.
- Familial or inherited conditions with a high risk for life-threatening ventricular tachyarrhythmias such as long-QT syndrome or hypertrophic cardiomyopathy

Class I indications
- In patients who are survivors of cardiac arrest due to VF or hemodynamically unstable sustained VT after evaluation to define the cause of the event and to exclude any completely reversible causes.
- In patients with structural heart disease and spontaneous sustained VT, whether hemodynamically stable or unstable.
- In patients with syncope of undetermined origin with clinically relevant, hemodynamically significant sustained VT or VF induced at electrophysiological study.

- In patients with LVEF less than 35% due to prior MI who are at least 40 days post-MI and are in NYHA functional Class II or III.
- In patients with nonischemic DCM who have an LVEF less than or equal to 35% and who are in NYHA functional Class II or III.
- In patients with LV dysfunction due to prior MI who are at least 40 days post-MI, have an LVEF less than 30%, and are in NYHA functional Class I.
- In patients with nonsustained VT due to prior MI, LVEF less than 40%, and inducible VF or sustained VT at electrophysiological study.

Class IIa indications
- In patients with unexplained syncope, significant left ventricular dysfunction, and nonischemic dilated cardiomyopathy.
- In patients with sustained VT and normal or near-normal ventricular function.
- In patients with hypertrophic cardiomyopathy who have 1 or more major risk factors for sudden cardiac death (SCD).
- For the prevention of SCD in patients with ARVD/C who have 1 or more risk factors for SCD.
- To reduce SCD in patients with long-QT syndrome who are experiencing syncope and/or VT while receiving beta-blockers.
- For nonhospitalized patients awaiting transplantation.
- For patients with Brugada syndrome who have had syncope.
- For patients with Brugada syndrome who have documented VT that has not resulted in cardiac arrest.
- For patients with catecholaminergic polymorphic VT who have syncope and/ or documented sustained VT while receiving beta-blockers.
- For patients with cardiac sarcoidosis, giant cell myocarditis, or Chagas' disease.

Class IIb indications
- In patients with nonischemic heart disease who have an LVEF of less than or equal to 35% and who are in NYHA functional Class I.
- For patients with long QT syndrome and risk factors for SCD.
- In patients with syncope and advanced structural heart disease in whom thorough invasive and noninvasive investigations have failed to define a cause.
- In patients with a familial cardiomyopathy associated with sudden death.
- In patients with left ventricular noncompaction.

Class III nonindications
- ICD therapy is not indicated for patients who do not have a reasonable expectation of survival with an acceptable functional status for at least 1 year, even if they meet ICD implantation criteria specified in the Class I, IIa, and IIb recommendations above.
- ICD therapy is not indicated for patients with incessant VT or VF.
- ICD therapy is not indicated in patients with significant psychiatric illnesses that may be aggravated by device implantation or that may preclude systematic follow-up.

- ICD therapy is not indicated for NYHA Class IV patients with drug-refractory congestive heart failure who are not candidates for cardiac transplantation or CRT-D.
- ICD therapy is not indicated for syncope of undetermined cause in a patient without inducible ventricular tachyarrhythmias and without structural heart disease.
- ICD therapy is not indicated when VF or VT is amenable to surgical or catheter ablation (e.g., atrial arrhythmias associated with the Wolff–Parkinson–White syndrome, right ventricular or left ventricular outflow tract VT, idiopathic VT, or fascicular VT in the absence of structural heart disease).
- ICD therapy is not indicated for patients with ventricular tachyarrhythmias due to a completely reversible disorder in the absence of structural heart disease (e.g., electrolyte imbalance, drugs, or trauma).

Exclusion criteria
- Terminal illnesses with projected life expectancy < 6 months.
- Coronary revascularization in last 3 months.
- NYHA Class IV drug-refractory congestive heart failure in patients who are not candidates for cardiac transplantation.

Subcutaneous ICD
- Subcutaneous ICD systems do not use transvenous leads and may be considered in the pediatric population because of concerns about venous patency and lead failure with patient growth and potentially greater difficulty with lead extraction.
- Subcutaneous coil is placed in the parasternal area. Device provides satisfactory detection and treatment of ventricular arrhythmias by delivering shock.
- Pacing therapies are not available.

Prognosis after ICD implant
- With the ICD, survival may be extended by a mean of 4 months over a 6-year follow-up period (Table 12.5).
- There seems to be an association between appropriate ICD discharges and death from progressive heart failure.
- In CAT (Cardiomyopathy Arrhythmia Trial), only 50% of patients with appropriate ICD discharges survived, in contrast to 85% of patients without appropriate ICD discharges after 5 years.
- Beneficial effects of ICD therapy become apparent a year or more after implantation of the device. Cost per life-year saved starts to look reasonable 5 years or more after device implantation.
- ICDs seem to be more effective in older patients and those with more advanced cardiac disease.
- Rapid heart rate is a recognized independent predictor of adverse cardiovascular outcomes in:
  1 In general population
  2 Following acute MI
  3 In chronic heart failure (HF)
  4 Isolated bradycardia identifies patients at lower risk for HF and mortality.

Table 12.5 Prevention trials.

Study	Inclusion criteria	Endpoint(s)	Treatment arms	Key results
Secondary prevention trials				
AVID	Survivor of cardiac arrest VT with syncope Symptomatic sustained VT with LVEF ≤ 0.40.	Total mortality Mode of death Quality of life Cost benefit	Amiodarone or sotalol or ICD	Significant improvement in overall survival with ICD
CASH	Survivor of cardiac arrest	Total mortality Recurrences of arrhythmias requiring CPR Recurrence of unstable VT	ICD Amiodarone, propafenone, or metoprolol.	Significant improvement in overall survival with ICD
CIDS	Survivor of cardiac arrest Syncope with sustained or inducible VT. EF ≤ 35	Total mortality	Amiodarone or ICD	No significant improvement in survival with ICD
Primary prevention trials				
MADIT	Q wave MI ≥ 3 weeks Asymptomatic NSVT LVEF ≤ 35% Inducible VT during EPS and nonsuppressible with procainamide NYHA Classes I–III	Overall mortality	ICD Conventional therapy	ICDs reduced overall mortality by 54%
CABG- PATCH	Scheduled for elective CABG surgery LVEF < 36% Abnormal SAECG	Overall mortality	ICD v/s Standard treatment	Survival not improved by prophylactic implantation of ICD at time of elective CABG
MUSTT	CAD EF ≤ 40% NSVT Inducible VT or VF	Sudden arrhythmic death or spontaneous sustained VT	ICD in nonsuppressible group	> 70% risk reduction in arrhythmic death or cardiac arrest and > 50% reduction in total mortality
BEST-ICD	Acute MI EF ≤ 0.40 SDRR < 70 ms or ≥ 109 PVCs/h or abnormal SAECG	All-cause mortality	EPS: if inducible, ICD and BB; if noninducible, BB	No significant survival improvement with ICD too few patients enrolled

Table 12.5 (*Continued*)

Study	Inclusion criteria	Endpoint(s)	Treatment arms	Key results
MADIT-II	Prior MI EF ≤0.30	All-cause mortality	Conventional therapy or ICD	With ICD, 31% reduction in mortality
SCD-HeFT	Ischemic or nonischemic cardiomyopathy EF ≤35% NYHA Class II or III No history of sustained VT/VF	All-cause mortality	Placebo, Amiodarone or ICD	significant survival improvement with ICD

AVID = Antiarrhythmics Versus Implantable Defibrillators. BB = beta blocker. BEST-ICD = Beta-Blocker Strategy Plus Implantable Cardioverter-Defibrillator. CABG = coronary artery bypass graft. CABG-PATCH = Coronary Artery Bypass Graft Patch Trial. CASH = Cardiac Arrest Study Hamburg. CIDS = Canadian Implantable Defibrillator Study. MADIT = Multicenter Automatic Defibrillator Implantation Trial. MI = myocardial infarction. MUSTT = Multicenter Unsustained Tachycardia Trial. SCD-HeFT = Sudden Cardiac Death in Heart Failure Trial.

Therapy

- The ICD functions by continuously monitoring the patient's cardiac rate and delivering therapy when the rate exceeds the programmed rate "cutoff".
- ICD provide separate bradycardia and post-shock pacing. In dual chamber ICD routine bradycardia pacing could be programmed to AAI if AVN conduction is adequate. This will obviate the need for ventricular pacing with its possible detrimental effects on LV function.
- ATP consists of delivering a specified number of ventricular pacing impulses at a faster interval than the programmed ventricular detection interval.
- Number of sequences of ATP could be programmed. If the interval between pulses is constant the technique is called burst pacing if the interval progressively decreases then it is termed ramp. If the pacing interval decreases from one sequence to the next, although it remains constant within that sequence, the technique is called scan. Combination of scan and ramp will result in more aggressive ATP protocol.
- ATP may be effective in terminating VT in 90% of the episodes.
- ATP may accelerate the tachycardia.
- Electrical shock is delivered by the device through the coils in to myocardium.
- Placement of the distal coil along the interventricular septum improves the efficacy of defibrillation. Speed with which total output is delivered depends on impedance of the electrodes and duration and tilt of the pulse width.
- The device may contain two capacitors each capable of 250 to 300 μF capacitance maximum voltage of 350 to 375 V. Capacitors are charged simultaneously in parallel however the shock is delivered in series so the total voltage is doubled 700 to750 V. This configuration reduces the capacitance by

one-half to 120 to 150 µF. High voltage lead impedance is between 30 to 60 Ω. This combination of low capacitance and low impedance allows 60 to 90% of the stored energy delivered in <20 ms.

Defibrillation threshold (DFT) and safety margin

- VF is induced and progressively lower amount of energy is delivered. Lowest amount of energy that successfully defibrillates is called the DFT. This may necessitate repeated induction of VF. Alternatively, two consecutive successful defibrillations using energy with 10 J margin has been shown to provide success rate of 98% during follow-up.
- Using biphasic shock a margin of twice the DFT provides 95% probability of successful defibrillation.
- The upper limit of vulnerability (ULV) can be used to assess DFT. A test shock is delivered on the T wave. Normally low energy shock delivered on T wave will induce VF. If the test shock fails to induce VF it is believed to be above the DFT. The shock of lowest energy that fails to induce VF is considered the DFT.
- One of the advantage of ULV include that the DFT can be determined without inducing VF. The disadvantage includes inability to determine the sensing from electrodes during VF.
- Both methods can be combined to achieve high success rate without inducing VF repeatedly. First the VF is induced and 15 J of energy is delivered if successful then ULV is determined by delivering 5 J on T wave. If VF is not induced then DFT is greater than 5 J.
- Amiodarone may increase DFT, the effect is very small. Therefore, DFT reassessment after the institution of antiarrhythmic drug therapy with amiodarone or sotalol is not routinely required.

ULV

- Shock strength above which a defibrillation shock given during the vulnerable period of the cardiac cycle cannot induce ventricular fibrillation (VF), and that this ULV corresponds to the DFT.
- A weak shock cannot induce reentry in the heart. However, a stronger shock can, if timed during the vulnerable period, causing an arrhythmia that often decays into ventricular fibrillation.
- An even stronger shock does not induce reentry.
- The strongest shock that causes re-entry is the ULV.
- ULV is often similar to the defibrillation threshold.
- Successful defibrillation shock must not only halt pre-existing fibrillation, but also must not re-induce fibrillation by the same mechanism responsible for the ULV.

Biphasic wave front

- The capacitor discharge is divided in to two phases with opposite polarity. After the first phase the polarity is reversed. First phase is longer than second phase. Switching capacitor from series to parallel configuration in second phase could double the second phase voltage.
- The magnitude of the wave form is characterized by its amplitude (peak voltage or current) and tilt. Percent change in amplitude of the wave form

from its initial value to its terminal value is described as tilt. If the amplitude is reduced by ½ then the tilt for that wave form is 50%.

- Current is delivered from cathode (negative) electrode located in the RV to a can and SVC coil configured as anode (positive electrode). Sometime this configuration does not provide satisfactory DFT and reversal of polarity using the right ventricle as an anode is required.
- ICD provides defibrillation cardioversion and antitachycardia pacing for termination of sustain ventricular arrhythmias.
- Shocks are synchronized during VT (cardioversion) or are asynchronous during VF (defibrillation).
- The device can be programmed in to three zones depending on the rate cutoff. Slower rates are labeled as VT zone and faster rates are labeled as VF zone. Fast VT may fall in to VF zone and will be treated according to the programmed criteria for VF zone.
- The DFT remains stable over years; antiarrhythmic drugs do not significantly affect biphasic DFT.
- Low energy cardioversion defibrillation has advantage of short charge time rapid conversion, with less battery consumption.
- Acceleration of VT may occur fallowing a low energy cardioversion or ATP in 3 to 5% of patients. ATP has a success rate of 90% in terminating VT.
- Faster VT in patient with low EF is likely to accelerate if short coupling intervals are used.
- ATP can be programmed empirically in patients who did not have spontaneous or sustained VT.
- Follow up ICD testing should be limited to patients in whom device malfunction is suspected or antiarrhythmic drugs have been added that might alter defibrillation threshold.

Device selection
- Patients who have bradycardia may benefit from dual chamber ICD programmed in a AAI mode to prevent ventricular pacing.
- As suggested by the Dual-chamber and VVIT Implantable Defibrillator (DAVID) trial, ventricular pacing may increase mortality and incidence of CHF.
- Devices that combine CRT and ICD therapy can be considered for patients who meet CRT criteria.
- The survival benefit of ICD was noted in patients with ejection fraction of <35%.
- The systematic shortening of the AV delay during exercise is not recommended because, in a high proportion of patients, the optimal AV delay tends to be longer during exercise than at rest.

DFT
- DFT can be defined as the minimal energy that terminates VF.
- An acceptable DFT is a value that ensures an adequate safety margin for defibrillation, usually being at least 10 J less than the maximum output of the ICD, which ranges from 30 to 41 J of stored energy

- Generally, the preference is to implant the ICD in the left pectoral region because of a more favorable vector for delivery of the shock.
- QRS duration ≥200 ms can be used to identify patients at high risk of elevated DFTs.
- Women experience fewer episodes of spontaneous VT or VF during follow up.

Management of high DFTs

Use of a high-output device
- In patients who are expected to have an elevated DFT (e.g., patients receiving chronic amiodarone therapy or with hypertrophic cardiomyopathy) may benefit from high output devices.

Right ventricular lead location
- Proximal location of the distal coil, towards tricuspid annulus, is likely to result in high DFTs. Distal coil should be placed as distally as possible towards the apex of the right ventricle.
- Repositioning the RV lead to the anterior high interventricular septum in the right ventricular outflow tract (RVOT) is an alternative strategy.

Addition of a subcutaneous array
- Subcutaneous (SQ) array can be added to lower DFTs. After placing the RV lead and confirming a high DFT, a curved tunneling rod introducer is advanced through the standard infraclavicular incision into the SQ tissue until the tip rests inferior to the scapula and just lateral to the spine. Then the SQ array is advanced to this position through the introducer.

Repositioning of the proximal electrode
- Placement of the proximal coil in the left subclavian vein may improve DFTs.

Removal of the SVC coil
- Standard ICD configuration consists of an active can and dual coil, single lead with electrodes in the right ventricle apex and SVC–right atrium junction. Sometime removing the proximal coil and changing the configuration from distal coil to the can may improve DFTs.

Addition of a coronary sinus lead
- Placement of a coil in a posterior or lateral branch of the coronary sinus (CS) can result in substantial (up to 45%) reductions in mean DFTs.

Changing polarity
- In standard setting distal coil is used as a cathode; using the distal coil as the anode is the reverse configuration. Reverse polarity may lower DFTs by 15 to 20%.

Waveform
- Adjustment to the tilt of the biphasic waveform is an option for managing high DFTs. Based on lead impedance and device capacitance observed ratio of

the tilt between first and second phase can be calculated from the published tables. This may result in significant reductions in DFTs.

Pneumothorax
- Pneumothorax is a complication of subclavian vein access. It may result in high DFTs during device implantation. A high DFT with high impedance could be the result of pneumothorax. Inspection of the thorax with fluoroscopy during the procedure may assist in early detection of this complication.

Medications
- Chronic amiodarone use has been demonstrated to increase DFTs. Dofetilide and sotalol appears to lower the DFT.
- Prolonged procedure time and repeated unsuccessful DFT testing.
- Recurrent unsuccessful shocks can cause transient ventricular dysfunction. In addition, anesthetic agents, myocardial ischemia, hypoxia, acidosis and increased circulating catecholamines may lead to increase in DFTs.
- In this situation previously effective defibrillation becomes ineffective. When this occurs, repeat DFT testing at a later time should be considered.

Magnets and ICDs[5]
- Magnets interact with pacemakers and ICDs by closing the reed switch. The reed switch consists of two flat, ferromagnetic reeds, separated by a small gap, enclosed in a glass capsule filled with an inert gas. The magnetic switch is designed to close when it is exposed to an approximately 10-Gauss magnetic field.
- Closure of the magnetic reed switch disables sensing, resulting in temporary asynchronous pacing in a pacemaker or suspending therapies in an ICD.
- The switch is reactivated when the magnetic field is removed.
- The ability to close the magnetic switch by applying a magnet over pacemakers or ICDs is necessary in certain circumstances when the telemetric programmer or the expertise to use it are not readily available.
- Magnet application can also be used to trigger specific features in some devices, such as electrogram storing capability or event markers.
- Static magnetic fields in the normal environment or even in most industrial environments are unlikely to be strong enough to close the magnetic switch because the magnetic field strength dissipates quickly as distance from the source increases.
- Cardiac devices can be affected if patients are close enough to objects that can generate strong magnetic fields, such as stereo speakers or bingo wands.
- Inadvertent application of a magnet over pacemakers or ICDs is not uncommon because of the increasing number of objects that contain or are made of magnets.
- Even a small magnet can affect pacemakers or ICDs if it is strong enough and placed close enough to the device.
- Commercially available neodymium magnets are much smaller in size than conventional magnets but have a much higher magnetic field strength.

- Neodymium magnets are commonly used in jewelry, decoration, and the apparel industry, objects that contain magnets can be inadvertently placed over an implanted device and may cause interaction the maximum distance between the magnet and the device at which interference was noted was 3 cm.
- Similar to stereo speakers, headphones use magnets to produce sound waves. Although the magnet inside the headphone is very small, the magnetic field it generates is quite strong.
- A neodymium iron-boron magnet fixed to the frame of the headphone is used to create a static magnetic field while a dynamic driver made of a coil attached to a diaphragm is used to create sound. When a current is passed through the coil, it creates a temporary magnetic field, which reacts to the fixed magnetic field, resulting in motion of the coil and the diaphragm.
- Magnetic field strengths of both clip-on and in-ear headphones tend to be highest right at the surface of the headphones and markedly decreased with distance.
- A magnetic field strength ≥10 gauss, which is strong enough to close the magnetic switch, seen in clip-on headphones at a 2-cm distance and in none of the headphones at 3 cm.
- It may result in asynchronous pacing in pacemakers or suspension of tachycardia detection and therapy in ICDs.
- Magnet interference was not observed when headphones were placed at least 3 cm away from the device pocket.

Complications associated with ICD implant

- These include infection, pneumothorax, cardiac tamponade, and dislodgement of the leads.
- Inappropriate shock may occur in 10% of the patients in first year and up to 30% of the patients may receive inappropriate therapy by 4 years after implant.
- AF is the most common cause of inappropriate therapy. Stability and onset criteria may help prevent inappropriate shocks due to AF.
- In patients with advanced heart failure bradycardia and pulseless cardiac electrical activity are the commonest cause of death.
- At 5 years, the cumulative incidence of lead malfunctions was 2.5%. Lead malfunction may lead to inappropriate ICD shocks.
- Those who receive shocks for any arrhythmia have a substantially higher risk of death than similar patients who do not receive such shocks.
- There is 4.9% prevalence of pocket hematoma, which required reoperation in 1.0% of these complications Pocket bleeding emerged more often in generator or lead revisions than in first device implantation or replacement.
- Vitamin K antagonists maintenance in high-risk patients, for example, with a mitral valve prosthesis, is safe,

Magnetic fields MRI[6]

Force and torque

- Ferromagnetic devices in a magnetic field are subject to static and gradient magnetic field-induced force and torque.

- The potential for movement of an implanted device in the MRI environment depends on:
  o Magnetic field strength
  o Ferromagnetic properties of the device
  o Implant distance from the magnet bore
  o Stability of the implant.
- A 1.5-T MRI scanner exerts less than 100 g maximal force acting upon devices.
- This amount of force is unlikely to dislodge a chronic device that is anchored to the surrounding tissue. This observation has led to recommendation of a 6-week waiting period prior to MRI after device implantation.

Current induction
- The radiofrequency and pulsed gradient magnetic fields in the MRI environment may induce electrical currents in leads within the field.
- Lead length (vs radiofrequency wavelength) and conformations such as loops favor improved transition of energy to the implanted device.
- Under conventional implant conditions (without additional lead loops), the magnitude of induced current likely to be less than 0.5 mA. In the presence of multiple lead loops, current induction at greater than 30 mA is possible and may result in myocardial capture.

Heating
- The extent of radiofrequency energy deposition in tissues is described by the specific absorption rate (SAR).
- Metallic devices and leads can act as an antenna, thus amplifying local radiofrequency energy deposition, which may lead to heating and tissue damage at the device–tissue interface.
- Fractured leads or lead loop configurations may increase the potential for heating. Epicardial leads that are not cooled by blood flow may also be prone to increased heating.
- There is poor correlation of heating at different SAR of sequences across different scanners, even within the same manufacture.

Steps to be taken before MRI
- Device selection – choose MRI compatible devices.
- Programme device to minimize inappropriate activation or inhibition of brady/tachyarrhythmia therapies. Pacing mode can be changed to an asynchronous mode for pacemaker-dependent patients and to demand mode for other patients.
- Limit system-estimated whole-body average SAR to 2.0 W/kg.
- Blood pressure, ECG, oximetry, and symptoms should be monitored.
- Do not perform MRI on pacemaker-dependent ICD patients.
- Retained leads are prone to previously described risks of movement, heating, and current induction.
- Depending on their length and configuration, retained segments may be prone to significant temperature rises than leads that are attached to pulse generators.

- Exclude patients with retained lead fragments and unused capped leads from MRI.
- Avoid MRI in patients with less than 6 weeks' time since device implant or patients with no fixation (superior vena cava coil) leads.
- Patients with mature active and passive fixation endocardial (and coronary sinus) leads of any diameter can safely undergo MRI.
- Avoiding MRI when device leads that are prone to heating, such as nontransvenous epicardial and abandoned (capped) leads, are present.
- To reduce the risk of inappropriate inhibition of pacing due to detection of radiofrequency pulses, device should be programmed to an asynchronous, dedicated pacing mode in pacemaker-dependent patients.
- To avoid inappropriate activation of pacing due to tracking of radiofrequency pulses, device should be programmed, in patients without pacemaker dependence, to a nontracking ventricular or dual-chamber inhibited pacing mode.
- Rate response, premature ventricular contraction response, ventricular sense response, and conducted atrial fibrillation response should be deactivated to ensure that sensing of vibrations or radiofrequency pulses does not lead to unwarranted pacing.
- To minimize asynchronous pacing in patients without pacemaker dependence magnet mode should be deactivated when possible.
- Tachyarrhythmia monitoring should be deactivate to avoid battery drainage that results from recording of multiple radiofrequency pulse sequences as arrhythmic episodes.
- Reed switch activation in ICD systems disables tachyarrhythmia therapies. However, reed switch function in the periphery versus the bore of the magnet is unpredictable; therefore, therapies should be disabled to avoid unwarranted antitachycardia pacing or shocks.
- Limit the estimated whole-body averaged SAR of MRI sequences (<2.0 W/kg when possible) to reduce the risk of thermal injury and changes in lead threshold and impedance.
- Blood pressure, ECG, pulse oximetry, and symptoms should be monitored for the duration of the examination.
- Radiologist and cardiac electrophysiologist, or an individual trained in advanced cardiac life support familiar with device programming and troubleshooting should be present during scans.
- At the end of the examination, all device parameters should be checked, and programming should be restored to pre-MRI settings.

Lead extraction
- Abandoning a nonfunctioning lead appears to be safe and does not pose a clinically significant additional risk of future complications.
- When a malfunctioning lead requires replacement, options include capping or extracting the old lead.
- Arguments in favor of lead extraction include (Table 12.6).
- Elimination of the potential for noise when the abandoned lead contacts the new lead.

Table 12.6 Indication for lead removal.

Strength of recommendation	Indication
Class I	• Sepsis (including endocarditis) as a result of documented infection of any intravascular part of the pacing system, or as a result of a pacemaker pocket infection when the intravascular portion of the lead system cannot be separated • Life-threatening arrhythmias secondary to a retained lead fragment • A retained lead, lead fragment, or extraction hardware that poses an immediate or imminent physical threat to the patient • Clinically significant thromboembolic events caused by a retained lead or lead fragment • Obliteration or occlusion of all useable veins, with the need to implant a new transvenous pacing system • A lead that interferes with the operation of another implanted device
Class II	• Localized pocket infection, erosion, or chronic draining sinus that does not involve the transvenous portion of the lead system, when the lead can be cut through a clean incision that is completely separate from the infected area • An occult infection for which no source can be found, and for which the pacing system is suspected • Non-functional lead in a young patient • Leads preventing access to the venous circulation for newly required implantable devices • Chronic pain at the pocket or lead insertion site that causes significant discomfort for the patient that is not manageable by medical or surgical technique without lead removal • A lead that poses a threat to the patient, though not immediate or imminent if left in place • A lead that interferes with the treatment of malignancy
Class III	• The risk of removal of the lead is significantly higher than the benefit of removing the lead • A single non-functioning lead that may be reused at the time of pulse generator replacement, provided the lead has a reliable performance history • A single non-functional lead in an older patient

- Potential for high DFT values caused by shunting of energy along the abandoned lead.
- Risk of venous obstruction due to the presence of multiple leads and the fact that increased implant duration influences the success and complication rates of percutaneous lead extraction.

- Risk of failed extraction doubles for every 3 years of implant duration, most likely because scar tissue formation appears to increase over time.
- Risks include tamponade, hemothorax, pulmonary embolism, lead migration, and death as a result of either central venous tear or myocardial perforation.
- Patient-specific risk factors include fibrous attachment to intravascular and cardiac structures.
- Common binding areas are at the site of entry of the lead into the subclavian/ axillary vein, especially under the clavicle, at the superior vena cava-right atrial junction, and at the distal electrode–cardiac interface.
- Lead-lead binding in patients with multiple leads and along each of the shocking coils/electrodes of ICD leads.
- The difficulty of lead removal and possibility of complication depends on number of risk factors:
  a. Duration of lead implant.
     - The longer a lead has been implanted, the more difficult it is to remove.
     - Risk of a major complication increased progressively with implant duration.
     - Leads in place for less than one year can be removed with manual traction.
  b. Physician inexperience
  c. Younger patient age
  d. Female sex
  e. Presence of calcification involving the leads noted on chest radiograph
  f. Presence of multiple leads (due to lead-lead binding)
  g. ICD leads appear riskier to remove due to increased size and complexity. The coils seem to stimulate more fibrosis at the interface with the vasculature and myocardium.
- Single coil ICD lead is preferred
- New ICD coil coatings (e.g., ePTFE) and silicone back-filling have the potential to significantly reduce the tissue ingrowth that has hampered ICD lead extractions in the past.
- Several factors favor successful lead extraction as well.
  1 Leads that are severely infected often can be removed with less resistance than those being extracted for other reasons and therefore have a better chance of removal with manual countertraction alone
  2 History of prior cardiac surgery may reduce the risk of tamponade due to scarring of the pericardium and mediastinum. A history of prior surgery, however, has the potential to complicate emergent surgical exploration should this be necessary.
  3 Because passive tined leads rely on entanglement within trabeculae and eventual fibrosis for stability at the distal electrode–cardiac muscle interface, active fixation leads with an extendable-retractable helix tend to be easier to remove than passive fixation leads.

Infection

- Incidence of device infection of 1.9 per 1000 device-years with the cumulative probability higher in patients with defibrillators compared to those with pacemakers.

- In addition, subsequent generator changes are associated with a significant rate of device infections with a rate reported of 3.4% in a recent study.
- Staphylococcal species are the most common causative organism.
- Pocket infection without blood stream infection is the most common clinical presentation followed by pocket infection with bloodstream infection and device-related endocarditis.
- Lead extraction is the recommended treatment for patients with pacemaker system infection, especially associated with bacteremia or sepsis and evidence of intravascular lead involvement or coexistent pocket infection.
- Concern of embolization of vegetations adherent to leads with transvenous removal.
- Management of the infected pacemaker-dependent patient who requires removal of the pacing system.
- Superficial or low-grade infections involving the suture line may be treated conservatively, but must be observed carefully. If the infection fails to improve or recurs, complete removal of the system should be considered.

Lead malfunction and abandoned leads
- Lead malfunction can result in pacing system failure or inappropriate ICD therapy.
- Alternative to lead extraction is to abandon the lead with placement of a new lead on the ipsilateral side or placement of an entirely new system on the contralateral side.
- If possible remove any abandoned or redundant leads.

Device upgrades
- New indications for ICDs and the development of biventricular pacing for the treatment of heart failure has led to the need to "upgrade" patients with existing devices.
- This may include upgrading a pacemaker to an ICD or a pacemaker or ICD to a biventricular pacing device.
- Venous occlusion is relatively common at the time of device replacement or upgrade occurring in 9–12% of patients.
- If leads prevent access to venous circulation for newly indicated implantable devices, lead extraction to regain vascular access can be considered.

Other indications
- Lead extraction can be considered for relief of SVC syndrome, late lead perforation, and thromboembolism caused by a lead or lead fragment.
- Device and lead extraction could be considered for chronic pain at the pocket or lead insertion site that is unresponsive to other management. If generator and leads interfere with treatment of malignancy it may have to be repositioned.

ICD and athletes
- The Bethesda guidelines state that patients with an ICD can participate only in "Class IA" activities, such as bowling or golf, restricting competition in sports such as track, basketball, lacrosse, and field hockey, as well as sports with a likelihood of severe impact to the ICD, such as football and hockey.

- Exercise substantially increases the risk of SCD.
- Exercise is known to exacerbate ventricular arrhythmias in HCM, arrhythmogenic right ventricular dysplasia, and the long QT syndrome.
- High-catecholamine states may render arrhythmias more difficult to terminate
- In the Physician's Health Study, although SCD increased during exercise, habitual vigorous exercise, reduced the risk of SCD during exercise.
- "Weekend athlete" phenomenon of intermittent high-intensity exercise should be discouraged, and patients wishing to exercise vigorously should do so regularly.
- Gradual increases in impedance above the alert threshold do not indicate lead failure; they are likely caused by changes at the electrode–myocardial interface.
- Abrupt changes in impedance without oversensing may be caused by intermittent contact of the lead's ring electrode with the header's connector.
- Spot radiographs of the pocket may diagnose this situation preoperatively.
- Follow-up without surgical revision may be appropriate if pacing and sensing are reliable and no oversensing occurs with provocative maneuvers.

Management of the patient with a pacemaker or ICD during an operative procedure

- Prior to surgery device should be interrogated and detection and therapy should be deactivated. After the procedure, the device should be reinterrogated and ICD therapy reinitiated. During the time ICD therapy is "off," the patient must be monitored.
- For pacemaker-dependent patients, the pacemaker could be programmed to an asynchronous pacing mode, VOO or DOO, or same effect can be achieved by placing a magnet over the pacemaker throughout the procedure.
- The potential effects of electrocautery on the device include, reprogramming; permanent damage to the pulse generator; pacemaker inhibition; reversion to a fall-back mode, noise reversion mode, or electrical reset; and myocardial thermal damage.
- If cardioversion and defibrillation is required in a patient with a pacemaker or ICD, place paddles in the anteroposterior position, keep the paddles at least 4 inches (10 cm) from the pulse generator, have the appropriate pacemaker programmer available, and interrogate the pacemaker after the procedure.

Effect of antiarrhythmic drugs and metabolic abnormalities on pacemaker/ICD

- Flecainide and propafenone have the potential to increase pacing/sensing thresholds and DFT.
- These agents may alter the detection of ventricular tachycardia and produce proarrhythmic effects. Drug-induced slowing of ventricular tachycardia rate can result in inadequate detection of the arrhythmia. Amiodarone can cause increase in DFT.
- Electrolyte and metabolic abnormalities can also affect pacing and sensing thresholds. Hyperkalemia, severe acidosis or alkalosis, hypercapnia, severe hyperglycemia, hypoxemia, and hypothyroidism can alter thresholds.

Causes of multiple ICD shocks
- Frequent VT or VF (electrical storm).
- Unsuccessful ICD therapy due to inappropriately low-output shock or elevation of defibrillation threshold.
- Lead fracture.
- Lead dislodgment.
- Detection of supraventricular rhythms.
- Oversensing separate pacing system, electromagnetic interference or other intracardiac signals such as P or T waves.
- Detached Header: detached header can lead to sudden and unpredictable disruption of the feed-through wire.
- If increased impedance and stimulation threshold are observed the following steps could be taken:
  ○ Perform sensing and capture threshold test
  ○ Evaluate real-time and stored electrograms for noise, artifacts, and other abnormalities
  ○ Perform X-ray and fluoroscopic studies to verify lead and ICD header integrity.
- Noise on the intracardiac EGM may affect sensing and result in inappropriate therapy in implanted cardiac rhythm management devices.
- Commonly encountered sources of noise include:
  ○ Electromagnetic interference,
  ○ Extracardiac muscle signals,
  ○ Lead conductor fractures,
  ○ Llead insulation breach,
  ○ Improper lead-to-pulse generator connection.
- These noise sources typically result in low-amplitude, high-frequency signals on the intracardiac EGM.
- Lead conductor fractures, insulation breaches, and improper lead-to-pulse generator connections are also associated with abnormal lead impedance or threshold values.

Device follow-up
- Follow-up can be accomplished through office based assessment; transtelephonic follow-up, or Internet-based device follow-up.
- Once a year, appropriateness of rate-adaptive pacing mode should be assessed.
- The appropriateness of delivered therapy or other changes in the patient's medical status or drug regimen that could affect ICD therapy should be analyzed.
- The aspects of follow-up include history with specific emphasis on awareness of delivered therapy and any tachyarrhythmic events, device interrogation to assess battery status; charge time, lead impedances, pacing thresholds and retrieval and assessment of stored diagnostic data.
- Periodic radiographic assessment of the leads should be performed.
- Arrhythmia induction in the electrophysiology laboratory to assess DFTs and detection should be considered specially if there is change in patient's clinical or therapeutic status.

- Age, left ventricular ejection fraction, NYHA functional class, Charlson comorbidity index, and use of antiarrhythmic drug predicted ICD shock probability.
- Antiarrhythmic drug use may contribute to increased mortality.
- Beta-blocker and angiotensin-converting enzyme inhibitor use may improve survival.
- A persistent arrhythmic risk even after prolonged shock-free intervals indicates the need for continued ICD therapy in all patients with appropriate ICD indications.
- The analysis of the first postpacing interval (FPPI) can be used to differentiate induced VT and SVT.

Recommendations on driving for individuals with ICDs placed for primary prevention

- Patients receiving ICDs for primary prevention should be restricted from driving a private automobile for at least 1 week. Thereafter, driving privileges should not be restricted in the absence of symptoms potentially related to an arrhythmia.
- Patients who have received an ICD for primary prevention who subsequently receive an appropriate therapy for ventricular tachycardia or ventricular fibrillation, especially with symptoms of cerebral hypoperfusion, should then be subject to the driving guidelines for patients who received an ICD for secondary prevention.
- Patients who received ICDs for primary prevention must be instructed that impairment of consciousness is a possible future event.
- These recommendations do not apply to the licensing of commercial drivers.
- In-hospital complications and mortality rate is much higher in end-stage renal artery disease patients.

EMI from radiofrequency identification devices (RFIDs)

- Composed of two parts: a tag attached to the item of interest and a reader that collects information from the tag.
- Active systems contain a battery that is the source of energy for the tag's antenna and circuitry.
- In a passive system, the tag contains no battery, but an antenna coil in the tag is energized by radio waves emitted by a transmitter located in the reader. These radio waves are a potential source of EMI.
- RFIDs were capable of interfering with infusion pumps and temporary external pacemakers.
- EMI with pacemakers and implanted defibrillators has been demonstrated by portable media players, mobile phones, and induction cooktops.
- Low-frequency RFIDs causes the greatest degree of interaction, high-frequency RFID causes less interaction, no reactions to the ultra-high-frequency RFIDs.
- The probability of an interaction is inversely proportional to the distance from the RFID device.
- All clinically significant reactions occurred within 40 cm of the reader.

- For medical applications in reference to implantable pacemakers and defibrillators, ultra-high- and high-frequency RFIDs should be preferentially used.
- Ultra-high frequency cannot be used in patient applications as human tissue absorbs radiofrequency in this range.
- Maintaining distance from the reader is critical to avoiding clinically significant reactions.

Cardiac resynchronization therapy (CRT)[7]

- CRT is an effective treatment for advanced drug-refractory heart failure in selected patients.
- It improves symptoms and functional capacity, reduces admissions for heart failure, and prolongs survival.
- Approximately 20% of patients do not respond clinically. The lack of response may be due to:
  - Nondelivery of left ventricular pacing (because of high pacing thresholds or atrial arrhythmias with uncontrolled ventricular rate).
  - Inappropriate lead positioning.
  - Suboptimal device programming.
  - Inappropriate patient selection.

Left bundle branch resynch

- Right ventricular pacing creates an iatrogenic "left bundle branch block-like" pattern that is known to impair cardiac function and leads to adverse clinical outcomes.
- Dual-chamber device may result in high rates of right ventricular pacing compared with ventricular backup pacing only, resulting in higher rates of hospitalizations for heart failure. These outcomes correlate with the percent of right ventricular pacing and paced QRS duration.
- In VALIANT (Valsartan in Acute Myocardial Infarction Trial) left bundle branch block was found to be an independent risk factor for cardiovascular and total mortality, myocardial infarction, and the composite endpoint of death, heart failure, or myocardial infarction
- Heart failure patients with chronic atrial fibrillation and left bundle branch block or dependent on right ventricular pacing should be considered for BiV pacing.

CRT trials

- Clinical and electrocardiographic parameters appear to be superior to echocardiographic parameters in selecting patients for CRT.
- Myocardial scar location is more important than scar burden in determining outcome in CRT patients. posterolateral scar location is associated with a low symptomatic response rate, failed reverse left ventricular remodeling, and a high mortality and morbidity after CRT.
- In patients with renal failure, CRT is associated with a poor survival despite good medical treatment.
- Plasma creatinine appears to be a strong independent predictor of cardiovascular mortality in patients with heart failure undergoing CRT.

- In the Multicenter Automatic Defibrillator Implantation Trial II (MADIT-II each 10-unit reduction in glomerular filtration rate, the risk of mortality increased by 16%, whereas no ICD benefit was observed in patients with end-stage renal disease.
- Patients with the largest left ventricular end-systolic volumes appear to be nonresponders to CRT.
- Right bundle branch block and ICD result in less clinical improvement or worsened survival after CRT.
- Reverse remodeling with CRT is likely to occur in those patients who are paced more than 80% of the time.
- CRT has been demonstrated to be clinically effective in 60% to 70% of patients.
- The PROSPECT trial has shown that none of the echocardiographic measures provides a consistent basis for clinical decisions regarding CRT implants.
- The ECG QRS duration (QRSd) is deemed to be the most clinically relevant measure for CRT.
- CRT has been shown to benefit symptomatic patients with wide QRSd >150 ms.
- RethinQ trial showed that CRT is not beneficial for patients with narrow QRSd.
- Long-term follow-up of the Comparison of Medical Therapy, Pacing and Defibrillation in Heart Failure (COMPANION) and CArdiac REsynchronization-Heart Failure (CARE-HF) studies showed that mortality is reduced with CRT as well.
- Benefit of CRT has been shown among patients with mild HF.
- REsynchronization reVErses Remodeling in Systolic left vEntricular dysfunction (REVERSE) and Multicenter Automatic Defibrillator Implantation Trial with Cardiac Resynchronization Therapy (MADIT-CRT) demonstrated clinical benefit with reductions in hospitalizations as well as reverse remodeling among patients with New York Heart Association (NYHA) class I-II HF, LV systolic dysfunction, and QRS prolongation.

Stages versus symptom classes of heart failure

- The four stages of heart failure progression linked to goals of therapy have been defined largely in terms of heart failure with reduced ejection fraction.
- Progression in stages occurs in only one direction, regardless of possible improvement in symptoms.
- Stage A is the presence of risk factors such as hypertension, diabetes, or previous chemotherapy, without detectable cardiovascular disease.
- Stage B is objective evidence of abnormal cardiac structure/function, most often a previous myocardial infarction or decreased LVEF, without apparent heart failure symptoms. In this stage, the focus of therapy is on prevention of disease progression by interrupting molecular and structural changes that lead to further ventricular dilation and dysfunction, and the prevention of unexpected fatal tachyarrhythmias in patients who have substantial risk of sudden death despite absence of symptoms.

- Stage C includes most patients who have been diagnosed with heart failure. There is no returning back to stage B once a patient has ever had clinical symptoms of heart failure, which can encompass NYHA class I to IV symptom severity at any given time. For stage C patients who responded to therapy and currently have few symptoms, the focus is on stabilization and prevention of disease progression and sudden death, as for stage B. For stage C patients who have more advanced heart failure symptoms that limit daily life (class III or IV), a major focus is on relieving symptoms and increasing daily activity.
- Stage D defines patients with refractory or frequently recurrent class IV symptoms despite repeated attempts to adjust recommended therapies. Even within this group there are varying degrees of severity. "Ambulatory" patients with recurrent but not persistent symptoms may benefit from interventions that not only relieve symptoms but can still impact on disease progression.
- Prognosis is likely to be poor regardless of choice of therapy for patients who:
  1 Continue to have symptoms at rest.
  2 Demonstrate deteriorating renal function
  3 Havre symptomatic hypotension
  4 Are no longer able to tolerate neurohormonal antagonist therapy
  5 Require frequent intravenous therapy for hemodynamic support
- Right ventricular dysfunction, which worsens with disease progression, predicts worse prognosis overall and has been associated with a decreased chance of clinical benefit with cardiac resynchronization therapy (CRT).
- QRS duration remains the primary descriptor of patients considered for CRT.
- Length of the QRS increases with disease severity and predicts higher mortality, more commonly from pump failure than sudden death.
- QRS duration does not correlate reliably with echocardiographic measures of dyssynchrony, and QRS shortening does not correlate reliably with clinical improvement after CRT.
- Clinical benefit has been highest in groups with the highest baseline QRS duration and has not been shown for groups of patients with QRS <150 ms.
- Patients undergoing implantation of defibrillator/pacing devices who are likely to require chronic ventricular pacing may be considered for CRT in the absence of prolonged native QRS. This may be particularly important for patients undergoing AV nodal ablation for rate control of AF.
- Etiology of left ventricular dysfunction can influence the decision for CRT. The largest improvements in ejection fraction continue to be seen in patients without coronary artery disease, whether spontaneously, while taking on beta blockers, or with CRT.
- Cardiomyopathies with smaller ventricular size may be accompanied by a component of fibrosis that restricts improvement.
- Patients with cardiomyopathy related to chemotherapy with doxorubicin (Adriamycin), trastuzumab (Herceptin), and newer small-molecule inhibitors

have ventricular size and QRS duration less distorted than in other low ejection fraction cardiomyopathies.

- CRT should be considered an elective procedure to improve the level of chronic compensation, not a rescue therapy from acute decompensation.
- In patients with heart failure 1-year survival even if all sudden deaths could be prevented appears to be 50% after three heart failure hospitalizations, or after two heart failure hospitalizations and estimated glomerular filtration rate less than 60 cm³/min.

Definition of cardiac dyssynchrony
- Heart failure may be associated with mechanical dyssynchrony at various levels.
- Atrioventricular dyssynchrony may be present due to long PR intervals.
- Delayed relaxation of the left ventricle associated with heart failure, resulting in fusion of the E and A waves of mitral inflow, which in turn limits left ventricle filling time.
- Interatrial conduction delay, which results in delayed contraction of the left atrium and premature closure of the mitral valve by ventricular contraction before the end of atrial systole.
- Interventricular dyssynchrony may result from delayed ejection of one of the ventricles, usually the left ventricle in the setting of left bundle branch block.
- Intraventricular dyssynchrony refers to delay in contraction of segments within the left ventricle, usually of the basal lateral wall.

Conventional Doppler echocardiography
- Pre-ejection intervals from QRS onset to the beginning of ventricular ejection is measured at the pulmonary and aortic valve levels using pulsed-wave Doppler.
- Normally there is <40 ms delay.
- In the presence of interventricular dyssynchrony, difference between pulmonary and aortic preejection period is prolonged (>40 ms).
- Patients with interventricular mechanical delay of >40 ms show greater improvement in response to biventricular pacing.
- Patients with an aortic preejection interval >160 ms show greater improvement in clinical outcomes, such as quality-of-life scores, 6-minute walking distance, and peak VO_2, compared with those having an interval ≤160 ms.

Tissue Doppler imaging
- Data can be acquired using either pulsed-wave tissue Doppler imaging samples or color tissue Doppler imaging velocity curves.
- Tissue Doppler imaging measurements should not be performed on akinetic segments. The low-velocity signals recorded are difficult to interpret and most likely reflect passive motion rather than true contraction.
- Interventricular dyssynchrony is assessed by difference in onset of contraction between the lateral wall of the right ventricle and interventricular septum, lateral wall of the left ventricle, or most delayed segment of the left ventricle. Delay in right ventricular activation by approximately 30 ms is considered abnormal.

- Intraventricular dyssynchrony of the left ventricle is defined as the difference in the onset of contraction between the septal and lateral walls, or as the standard deviation of delays in the 12-segment model.
- In normal subjects, there is no significant difference in activation between the different segments of the left ventricle as assessed using color tissue Doppler imaging to peak systolic motion or pulsed-wave tissue Doppler imaging to systolic motion onset. Continuing contraction of the segments of the left ventricle after closure of the aortic valve (a parameter otherwise known as delayed longitudinal contraction) is suggestive of intraventricular dyssynchrony.
- It is inappropriate to deny CRT to patients who fulfill currently accepted criteria (i.e., drug-refractory NYHA functional class III or IV, LV ejection fraction ≤0.35, and QRS width >150 ms simply because dyssynchrony may not be demonstrable by echocardiography.

Sleep disordered breathing (SDB)
- Prevalence of SDB is high among patients with heart failure and MI. SDB is associated with increased morbidity and mortality secondary to multiple contributing factors.
- Proarrhythmic effect of repetitive nocturnal episodes of hypoxia, coupled with myocardial ischemia, augmentation of sympathetic nerve activity, and increased serum catecholamine concentrations.

References

1 Cakulev I, Efimov IR, Waldo AL. Cardioversion: past, present, and future. *Circulation.* 2009;120(16):1623–1632.
2 Deakin CD. Advances in defibrillation. *Curr Opin Crit Care.* 2011;17(3):231–235.
3 Epstein AE, DiMarco JP, Ellenbogen KA, et al. ACC/AHA/HRS 2008 Guidelines for Device-Based Therapy of Cardiac Rhythm Abnormalities. *Heart Rhythm.* 2008;5(6):e1–e62.
4 Wolber T, Ryf S, Binggeli C, et al. Potential interference of small neodymium magnets with cardiac pacemakers and implantable cardioverter-defibrillators. *Heart Rhythm.* 2007;4(1):1–4.
5 Jongnarangsin K, Thaker JP, Thakur RK. Pacemakers and magnets: An arranged marriage. *Heart Rhythm.* 2009;6(10):1437–1438.
6 Nazarian S, Halperin HR. How to perform magnetic resonance imaging on patients with implantable cardiac arrhythmia devices. *Heart Rhythm.* 2009;6(1):138–143.
7 Kass DA. Pathobiology of cardiac dyssynchrony and resynchronization. *Heart Rhythm.* 2009;6(11):1660–1665.

Answers of self-assessment questions

1 C
2 D
3 C
4 D
5 B
6 C

Index

Page numbers in *italics* refer to figures; those in **bold** to tables or boxes. Abbreviations are listed in full at the beginning of the book

Essential Cardiac Electrophysiology: The Self-Assessment Approach, Second Edition. Zainul Abedin.
© 2013 Blackwell Publishing Ltd. Published 2013 by Blackwell Publishing Ltd.